Routledge Revivals

International Studies
Volume 3

First published in 1931, this book is the third of a three volume set which focuses on medical work, and in particular, public administration in relation to the prevention of disease. This volume provides the most in depth account of the countries it surveys: England and Wales, Scotland, and Ireland.

International Studies
Volume 3

Prevention and Treatment of Disease

Sir Arthur Newsholme

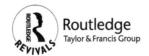

Routledge
Taylor & Francis Group

First published in 1931
by George Allen & Unwin

This edition first published in 2015 by Routledge
2 Park Square, Milton Park, Abingdon, Oxon, OX14 4RN
and by Routledge
711 Third Avenue, New York, NY 10017

Routledge is an imprint of the Taylor & Francis Group, an informa business

© 1931 Arthur Newsholme

Publisher's Note
The publisher has gone to great lengths to ensure the quality of this reprint but
points out that some imperfections in the original copies may be apparent.

Disclaimer
The publisher has made every effort to trace copyright holders and welcomes
correspondence from those they have been unable to contact.

A Library of Congress record exists under LC control number: 32001245

ISBN 13: 978-1-138-91277-9 (hbk)
ISBN 13: 978-1-315-69176-3 (ebk)
ISBN 13: 978-1-138-91282-3 (pbk)

INTERNATIONAL STUDIES

ON THE RELATION BETWEEN THE

PRIVATE *&* OFFICIAL PRACTICE *of* MEDICINE

WITH SPECIAL REFERENCE TO

THE PREVENTION OF DISEASE

conducted for

THE MILBANK MEMORIAL FUND

by

SIR ARTHUR NEWSHOLME, K.C.B., M.D., F.R.C.P.

Volume Three

ENGLAND AND WALES

SCOTLAND, IRELAND

LONDON: GEORGE ALLEN *&* UNWIN LTD

BALTIMORE: WILLIAMS *&* WILKINS CO

FIRST PUBLISHED IN 1931

FOREWORD[1]

ON BEHALF OF THE MILBANK MEMORIAL FUND

ONE of the major problems in present-day public health administration is that of ascertaining the proper sphere of the private physician in the field of public health. Upon a number of occasions during the past few years this matter has been earnestly discussed by private physicians and public health administrators in joint assemblies arranged for the purpose, and some progress has been made in indicating what should be the relationship between private medicine and public health to ensure co-operative service in conserving the health of the public.

During the past seven years the Trustees of the Milbank Memorial Fund have had occasion to consider this problem very seriously, in connection with the opposition of some sections of local members of the medical profession to public health work, which the Milbank Memorial Fund helped to inaugurate by means of participation in certain of the New York State Health Demonstrations. This opposition led the Fund to re-examine the initial tenets upon which its participation in the health demonstrations was based, in order to make sure that its philanthropic service in the field of public health was not such as would in any way embarrass or impede fulfilment of the legitimate professional aspirations of the private medical practitioner. Finding in the history of public health development in the United States few precedents to guide them, the Trustees decided to arrange for an international investigation to be made objectively and without bias, the purpose of the study being to throw light on the relationship in different countries between the fields of activity of private practising physicians and of physicians and laymen engaged

[1] These introductory remarks, which also preface the other volumes in the present series, are reprinted here since they treat of public health matters which are common to all countries, whatever differences there may be as regards methods, special local problems, and results achieved.

in public health work. It was felt that studies of what was being done elsewhere in public health might be valuable in indicating not only solutions of problems, particularly affecting the relation between private physicians and physicians engaged in public health work, but also in showing how the co-operative services of private physicians may be utilised to the highest advantage by public authorities.

These problems have arisen whenever preventive medicine has become in part clinical in character. In various countries medical treatment of the poorer members of the community is provided apart from private medical practice:

1. By the Poor Law authorities for the destitute;
2. By voluntary organisations, in hospitals, dispensaries, and similar institutions, for those who are destitute in the sense of not being able to pay for specially skilled help;
3. Under public insurance schemes, which may be limited to medical aid or may also give financial assistance, and in which the State and the employer are, or may be, partially responsible, as well as the beneficiary;
4. By public health authorities, given as in medical assistance to the destitute at the expense of the taxpayer, as, for instance, in fever and smallpox hospitals, and in sanatoria for tuberculosis, in venereal disease clinics, and to a smaller extent in maternity and infant consultation centres; and
5. By school or public health authorities in school clinics, at which eye defects, skin complaints, adenoids and tonsils, dental caries and other defects are treated either gratuitously or at a small cost proportionate to the resources of the patient.

In different countries the activities under these and allied headings vary enormously. The public increasingly realise that each member of the community must have prompt and adequate medical care. By this means protraction of illness can be avoided, which in itself is a great public health gain; subsequent crops of such diseases as tuberculosis and the venereal diseases can be prevented; and the general standard of health and efficiency of the community can be raised.

As public health becomes more advanced and personal

hygiene forms an increasing part of it, the stimulus to provide medical services either through voluntary or official organisations increases, and the delicacy of the relation between private medical practitioners and voluntary and official organisations becomes accentuated.

Hitherto, most countries have evolved measures for reaching their hygienic objective only as each pressing need has emerged. There has been irregular and unbalanced progress, or stagnation has continued when opposition has been severe. The different countries have not learned adequately from each other; and at the present time, except as regards insurance schemes in England and Germany, but little international information of an accurate and authentic character is available for the medical profession and for social workers.

For the reasons incompletely set forth above, the Trustees of the Milbank Memorial Fund, in the summer of 1928, secured the services of Sir Arthur Newsholme, M.D., K.C.B., former chief medical officer of the Local Government Board of England and Wales, and lecturer on public health administration, School of Hygiene and Public Health, the Johns Hopkins University, to make on their behalf: (1) an objective study of what is being done for the treatment of disease as related to its prevention in the chief European countries, including Great Britain and Ireland; and (2) an impartial study of the philosophy of the subject, with the hope that from the study and deductions made from it there will emerge further possibilities of action which will be for the public good, and will at the same time not be inimical to the real interests of the medical profession. The Trustees of the Milbank Memorial Fund are confident that the two interests are essentially identical; but they believe it important to base any conclusions and recommendations that may be reached on the foundation of a wide and international investigation, which has been objective in character. In securing the services of Sir Arthur Newsholme to make the inquiries included in this series, the Milbank Trustees had confidence that his long experience with the problems discussed in the studies and his familiarity with conditions both in England and in America qualified him to present an accurate account in perspective of the pitfalls and triumphs of preventive medicine and public health administration in the different countries concerned. It is understood, of course, that the Trustees of the Milbank Memorial Fund in submitting herewith the findings of Sir Arthur Newsholme's international investigation do not commit the Fund to endorse his views in any respect or to approve the methods of public health work described. It is to be remembered that the essence of the investigation is to throw light on the relationship in different countries between practising physicians on the one hand, and physicians in public health work and their authorities on the other hand; and this consideration explains the choice of subjects discussed in each chapter, which are selected as best illustrating this main problem.

As Volume III of these studies goes to press, it is gratifying to note the high commendation with which the preceding volumes in this series have been received.

JOHN A. KINGSBURY
Secretary

AUTHOR'S PREFACE TO
VOLUME THREE

THE present volume contains the most detailed of the international studies included in my investigation. The explanatory notes given in Volumes I and II need not be repeated here, though they are relevant to the contents of this volume.

The greater detail arises in part from my having been engaged during more than forty years with most of the medical problems which are outlined in the following pages. I can thus claim a large background of personal experience of the relation between public and private practice of medicine, from both points of view.

The greater detail given for Great Britain may be further justified by the fact that this country appears to have, in some respects, approached, though slowly and with many mistakes, more nearly than most countries to a solution of the difficult problems of adequate treatment and prevention of disease, especially in their bearing on the interrelation between private and public practitioners of medicine. (By "public practitioners" I mean those who are engaged in some form of medical practice at the expense of the general public or of some section of it, and not at the expense of the individual patient.) In making this statement I remember the gaps, the overlappings, and the inco-ordinations of existing medical activities. On these more will be written in my general survey of the entire subject in a concluding volume. In this volume I give, in the main, an objective statement of present arrangements.

But although I have described British arrangements in greater detail than those of other countries, the expert will at once see that it has been impossible to give more than an outline of some features of the medical work in Britain. I have, however, selected, as in my sketch of conditions in other countries, those in which there is the greatest likelihood or actual experience of friction between the private practitioner of medicine and the authorities and societies which have organised the practice of medicine or some parts of it in a communal setting.

The table of contents and the chapters themselves show that I have devoted many pages to a description of the various authorities utilising medical skill, and to their activities. It is only with such knowledge that we can begin to understand the relation between the private practitioners of medicine and these authorities, which is the subject of this and the two preceding volumes of the series.

It may appear to some that too much space is given to the official side and too little to the difficulties and feelings of the private practitioner. On consideration it will, I think, be plain, however, that the trend of events—some of them inevitable—can only be comprehended by the method adopted in these pages: and further examination will show that the reactions of private practitioners to the many developments of public medicine are in no instance left in doubt. Happily for Britain, these reactions can be summarised in extracts from the proceedings and resolutions of the British Medical Association, which (pp. 42 and 43) represents the views of the majority of private practitioners.

In this British report I have permitted myself occasionally to express opinions *calamo currente* more freely than in Volumes I and II. This could scarcely be avoided since, as already indicated, I have been personally concerned in most of the problems discussed in this volume. I have, however, postponed a statement of any reasoned judgment on British developments—their advantages, defects, and inco-ordinations—for a final volume. In that volume I hope to sum up the international position and to set out, so far as is practicable, the teaching of experience and sober judgment on the momentously important relation between the private and public practice of medicine.

Some remarks should be made on the form of the present report. The earlier sections for England, Scotland, and Ireland, respectively, contain a study of various branches of private and public medicine for each country. Then a number of detailed local studies are given in which, for the information of administrators, I have given somewhat full particulars on many points of detail.

The examples given illustrate types of local administration in England and Scotland. The description of London itself, with its many intricate medical problems, presenting almost overwhelming difficulty in securing to a reasonable extent individual medical responsibility for each sick person throughout each illness, could not be excluded. In large communities one must necessarily suffer some loss of continued personal responsibility, while gaining in less stinted and more elaborate institutional arrangements.

As a contrast to the metropolis, may be studied the details concerning rural administration in Gloucestershire, Cambridgeshire, and the county of Durham—all of which include large areas sparsely populated; and for Scotland the contrast between Glasgow and some rural counties is equally suggestive.

Swindon supplies an almost unique example of the organisation of medicine; for a large majority of its entire population receive medical care through a single self-governing association.

Brighton and Cambridge illustrate advanced public health and medical administration, which is now functioning almost entirely without friction with private practitioners. These are towns not too large to endanger the sense of individual medical responsibility, the risk of the loss of which is perhaps the greatest danger in publicly organised medicine.

Ireland is a striking illustration of a relatively poor country, which for more than half of its population and for nearly a century has had medical attendance at the expense of communal funds.

I have acknowledged in each chapter my indebtedness to the local health officers of the areas visited by me. I also owe sincere thanks to other colleagues and friends who have read every chapter of the book and have thus helped to ensure its accuracy. I am personally responsible for all expressions of opinion, and for any errors in detail which may have evaded the vigilance thus exercised.

ARTHUR NEWSHOLME

July 1931

TABLE OF CONTENTS

CHAPTER III

CHAPTER IV

GENERAL MEDICAL SERVICES IN ENGLAND (*contd.*)

CHAPTER V

CHAPTER VI

CHAPTER VII

CHAPTER VIII

PART III
SCOTLAND

VOLUME ONE : ERRATA AND OMISSIONS

Page 118 (Norway). There is now the same limit of income for compulsory and voluntary insurance; at present it is 5,200 kr., but it is proposed to reduce it to 5,000 kr. When the income limit is exceeded, the person affected loses all rights, including his past subscriptions.

Page 159, line 21, *for* Angestelle *read* Angestellte.

Page 159, line 22, *for* 6,000 marks *read* 3,600 marks.

Page 159, lines 21–22, delete words within parentheses.

The author wishes to acknowledge with thanks the help given him in Vienna by Dr. Foramitti, the head of the Government Public Health Medical Service, and Dr. Leonhartsberger, a member of his staff.

LIST OF ABBREVIATIONS IN VOLUME III

B.M.A. British Medical Association.
D.M.O. District Medical Officer (Poor Law).
G.M.C. General Medical Council.
L.C.C. London County Council.
L.G.B. Local Government Board (now Ministry of Health).
M.A.B. Metropolitan Asylums Board.
M.O.H. Medical Officer of Health.

PART I

ENGLAND AND WALES

CHAPTER I

GENERAL METHODS OF GOVERNMENT

A SHORT statement—

1. Of methods of control of public health matters; and
2. Of the conditions of entry into and retention in the medical profession is desirable for a complete understanding of the relation between the individual or private and the communal or collective practice of medicine, whether concerned with the treatment or the prevention of sickness.

Great Britain is a democratic country, governed, except in the case of the House of Lords, whose power is limited, by popularly elected representatives of the adult population. This government is exercised in part by local authorities, and in part by central authorities for the whole country. Both of these are directly controlled by Parliament consisting of two Houses. Of these the House of Commons is elected—usually at intervals of four to five years—by adult male and female suffrage, while the House of Lords is on a hereditary basis.

These statements apply to England and Wales, to Scotland, and to Northern Ireland. The rest of Ireland is now in the position of a self-governing dominion under the British Crown, and I shall not discuss its medical affairs in full, except so far as they are concerned with the general dispensary treatment of disease at the public expense, one of the oldest organisations of the kind, and with its midwifery practice, both of which present special features.

Scotland presents some peculiarities in its local government; but the main facts given hereafter apply equally to England and to Scotland.

The following scheme shows the relation between central and local governing authorities in England and Wales. The central authorities printed in italics in the scheme are common to England and Scotland; the local

26 INTERNATIONAL STUDIES

authorities of Scotland differ in certain particulars from those of England, though since April 1930 these differences have almost disappeared (page 443).

Local authorities derive their authority from Acts of Parliament, which must be approved by both Houses of Parliament and by the King. The powers of local authorities may be extended in particular towns or counties which have gone to the expense and trouble of securing additional local powers from Parliament. This is a troublesome and limited procedure, though in the past much public health reform has been thus initiated by pioneer local effort.

The chief link between local and central administration is through the Civil Service, which is composed of permanent pensionable officials. These officials are responsible to the Parliamentary Minister at the head of each of the Ministries or Boards indicated in the scheme (page 27), and the Minister himself may be the object of a vote of disapproval from the House of Commons. Thus, theoretically at least, and sometimes in practice, Parliament controls the policy and the finance of the Central Government.

Some further indication of the help given to local finance from the Governmental Exchequer will be given later. The cost of local education, of police, of some forms of public health medical work, etc., has been paid in proportions approximately equal out of central funds (derived from taxes) and local funds (derived from rates); in poor-law administration a smaller proportion (about 3 per cent.) of expenditure is borne by national funds. The sharing of expenditure by the Central Government Departments gives these departments a large "say" in local expenditure.

The Home Office, in relationship to medicine, is chiefly concerned with factory hygiene and hours of work, with the police, and with medical work in prisons; the Privy Council is the central department concerned with medical research; the Ministry of Health is concerned with public health, destitution, the work of the Midwives Board and sickness insurance; the Board of Education with the medical care of school children; the Board of Agriculture

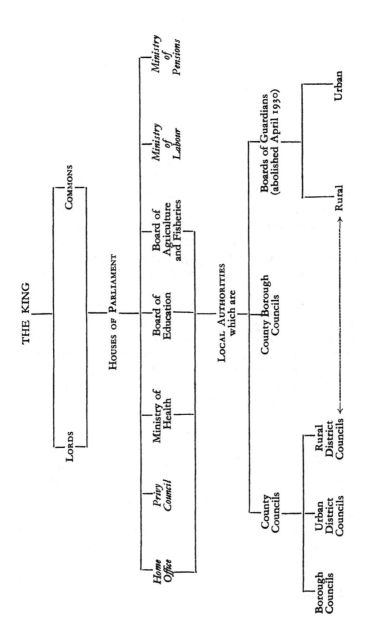

with diseases of animals communicable to man; the Ministry of Labour with unemployment and hours of work; and the Ministry of Pensions with ex-sailors and ex-soldiers. Furthermore, the Board of Trade is responsible to some extent for the health of seamen. The Post Office Department is responsible for the medical care of post office servants, through local doctors.

Local Government

The Public Health Act of 1872 divided the country into urban and rural sanitary districts. The rural representatives elected by the people acted as the board of guardians (of the poor) until 1930 (see page 29). The larger urban units were named boroughs, and they, like other urban as well as rural districts, were governed by representatives elected by direct voting of the ratepayers in each district.

In 1888 county councils were created for the government of larger areas, as set out below: and at the same time the largest boroughs were renamed county boroughs, and it was enacted that, although they were situate within the geographical area of an administrative county, sometimes of more than one county, their administration was to be independent and stand on an equal footing with that of the county council, being only subject to the supervision, and in some respects to the financial control, of the Ministry of Health.

All the authorities named (county councils, county borough councils, borough councils, urban and rural district councils, and, prior to 1930, boards of guardians) are elected by the people for a definite period, usually for three years, one-third of the council retiring each year to secure continuity of work.

The duties and powers of these local authorities are derived from Acts of Parliament; and it is their duty to exercise such powers as are conferred or are made obligatory on them by Parliament and, in the main, these only. Sanitary authorities may make additional bye-laws on certain subjects, but these must come within the general scope of legislation and must be confirmed by a central government department before they can become compulsory. Boards of guardians, in their regulation and administration of poor-law relief, have hitherto been much more controlled from London than are sanitary authorities and county councils. Now that their duties are handed over to the larger local authorities central control will become less detailed.

The local government machinery of the country has been built up on the PARISH, of which there are 12,850 in England and Wales. As modern conditions became more complex, small parishes were combined for poor-law administration, UNIONS being created, which provided a more satisfactory unit for the provision of residential institutions, etc. Parishes and Unions and the Guardians of these have existed longer than Public Health Authorities, and the history of public medicine is largely concerned with them.

BOARDS OF GUARDIANS, prior to 1930, were 635 in number, and were elected separately from representatives on sanitary authorities. In rural districts their members sat as members of the rural district council. Their function was the administration of relief for destitution, including medical aid. Under the Local Government Act, 1929, they have ceased to be separate authorities, their duties being taken over by county councils and county borough councils, with local relief committees for executive work. Under this Act the work of relief to the destitute will be transferred to the new Public Assistance Committee and to the Public Health Committee of the larger authorities. The intricate connection between workhouses and infirmaries in most areas will retard the ultimate aim, which is administrative separation between medical and other forms of aid, medical aid becoming entirely a public health procedure. When this is completed the association of medical aid with the inhibitions proper to methods of financial aid will cease.

The authorities concerned in *public health administration*, with their number in 1921–24, in England and Wales are seen below:—

LOCAL PUBLIC HEALTH AUTHORITIES

County Borough Councils   82

Municipal Boroughs	253	
Urban Districts	782	County Councils 62
Rural Districts	663	
Metropolitan Borough Councils	29	

The councillors forming public health authorities are elected by the people for a period of three years. The chairman of a municipal or a county borough is called the Mayor. He is elected by the council, and has no special privilege or power, but much dignity and influence. The councils of municipal and county boroughs (as also of counties) elect aldermen, who may be equal in number to about one-third of the councillors. This forms a convenient method of giving honour to special councillors, of retaining their services when not re-elected by the people, and, in some instances, of co-opting other non-elected persons from without the council.

As already indicated, COUNTY BOROUGH COUNCILS, unlike other municipal borough councils, have no administrative connection with county councils, unless joint arrangements are made voluntarily for special purposes (e.g. for the provision of an institution for crippled children).

The COUNTY COUNCILS are not directly concerned in the many branches of sanitary administration, though they can in some particulars exercise a minor degree of supervision over the urban and rural authorities within their area. From our present point of view, their importance consists in the fact that, outside the county boroughs, they are the local authorities concerned in administering:—

Elementary and Secondary Education,
The Care of Lunatics and Mentally Deficient Persons,
Venereal Disease Schemes,
Tuberculosis Schemes,
The Care of the Blind,

Supervision of Midwives and Maternity and Child
Welfare Schemes (in part),
Milk, Diseases of Cattle, Food and Drugs Acts,
Rivers Pollution Acts.

These statements need some modifications in detail according to local circumstances, as will appear hereafter.

EDUCATION AUTHORITIES, of which there are 317 in
England and Wales, in most instances are a special and
almost autonomous committee of the county borough
council or the county council: but where the population
of a borough in 1901 exceeded 10,000, or of an urban
district exceeded 20,000, it was legally entitled to educational control apart from the county council. Thus a
number of separate education authorities were created
within county areas. Education authorities are partially
responsible for the health as well as the mental improvement of all children attending school (compulsory ages
5–14) and, as will be seen hereafter, their work is closely
interlocked with that of private medical practitioners.

There remain INSURANCE COMMITTEES appointed under
the National Insurance Act. These are described on
page 115.

The public administrative arrangements special to
London will be described when describing the special
medical services of the metropolis (p. 380).

EXPENSE OF LOCAL GOVERNMENT

The cost of the various social measures of local government, and of local government in general, is defrayed from
two sources. There is a third source if national insurance is
included, for the personal contributions of employers and
of the employed supply at least two-thirds of its funds.
Apart from this instance, official social services are paid
for out of rates and out of taxes.

1. Rates are a local tax based on the annual value of individual holdings of buildings or land. Agricultural land is
now exempt from this taxation, and there are a number of

other exceptional partial exemptions. The local rate is the source of the local authority's funds, and is the only levy which a local authority can exact. This levy has no legal limit, and the owner or occupier of a house—rented, for instance, at £100—may find himself called upon to pay a local rate which may possibly be only £25, but may exceptionally exceed £100, per annum. The scale of valuation of properties has varied greatly in different localities, but recent changes are reducing this and are standardising the basis of local taxation (i.e. rating).

2. Local rates are aided from the National Exchequer, which has received the various taxes imposed in every locality by the Central Government. For instance, large sums are handed over to local authorities from liquor duties and from customs and estate (death) duties, as well as from the proceeds of the income-tax. Local authorities receive grants in aid for education, police, maintenance of lunatics and of certain other poor-law services, for roads, and for some of their special public health services. It is with these last-named grants and with educational grants, which, except those for destitution, are nearly half the total cost of the services in question, that we are specially concerned. But it will be noted that all these centrally dispensed grants towards local expenditure carry with them some measure of "say" on the part of the central governmental department in the spending of the money thus handed over.

The Home Office, Whitehall, pays one-half of the *approved expenditure* on local police. Local education authorities are bound to conform to certain patterns and standards imposed by the Board of Education in order that their 50 per cent. grants may be received. Boards of guardians hitherto have been even more rigidly supervised by the Ministry of Health, though even thus there has been great difficulty in preventing lavish local expenditure, especially on the part of local boards of guardians who financially are the least competent to pay the cost.

In public health matters the same difficulties do not

often arise; many local sanitary authorities need stimulation to spend judiciously rather than to be curbed in spending. But even here the Ministry of Health exercises some control; for each item in the year's expenditure of each local authority is subject to audit by a Government Auditor, who can disallow any expenditure contrary to definitely enacted law, and can make the implicated officials or members of the authority individually and collectively responsible for the disallowed amount. Furthermore, no local authority can borrow large sums of money for capital expenditure without the express sanction of the Central Government.

GRANTS IN AID

There remain the special public health grants inaugurated in the years 1912–18. Prior to this, the only local services of a personal and partly medical character which received direct governmental aid had been poor-law medical work and the beginnings of medical inspection of school children, with some treatment of minor complaints in scholars.

In 1912 tuberculosis schemes were promoted by the Local Government Board (see p. 219), capital sums were given by the Exchequer towards the cost of building tuberculosis sanatoria and hospitals, and from that date 50 per cent. of approved yearly local expenditure on the treatment of tuberculosis was paid by the Central Board.

In 1914 similar schemes, with 50–50 grants, were inaugurated by the Local Government Board for promoting maternity and child welfare work (for details see p. 184).

In 1916, in view of the national urgency of the problem, it was made obligatory on all councils of counties and county boroughs to prepare and carry out schemes for the gratuitous diagnosis and treatment of venereal diseases, the Government paying 75 per cent. of all approved local expenditure for these purposes.

Recently block grants have replaced the special grants for these particular forms of public health work, and in his circular explaining the change under the Local Government

Act, 1929, the Minister of Health drew attention to "two cardinal defects in the modern system of percentage grants": (1), they are stated to have impaired in some degree "the proper independence and vigour of local government", and to imply a continuous central control of details of affairs which ought to be local; and (2), these grants, "while they produced dramatic efforts and results in places where the local authorities were able and willing to levy rates to meet their share of the costs", often did not succeed in securing in other areas "a reasonably adequate provision and maintenance of the aided services". The circular claims for the consolidated grants now to be given, that the distribution of funds will have due regard to the relative needs of the inhabitants of each local area, and the ability of its inhabitants to meet these needs out of the rates.

In regard to child welfare work, and to anti-tuberculosis and anti-venereal work, the giving of governmental grants under the plan which has now ceased, undoubtedly expedited and extended these important branches of public health work. As administered, these grants in recent years have had some tendency to stereotype activities and shackle the administrative experimentation which is needed for further advance. Greater elasticity on the side of advance, combined with a rigid enforcement of minimum requirements, would be conducive to originality and progress. But one cannot entirely avoid some apprehension in regard to the cessation of central grants proportionate to local expenditure. It is doubtful if the old methods tended to stereotype activities more than the new block grants will. There is real risk that advances and new efforts by local authorities will be reduced by the absence of equivalent grants from national funds. Experimentation can, of course, be made by a local authority at its own expense; but such developments will not give a claim to increased block grants, when the first period of these grants ends; for future grants, the Minister of Health has announced, will be given on the basis of need, not of expenditure. Thus a "needy" authority, according to formula, may receive larger grants than a less needy authority which has done its work vigorously and progressively.

DEMOCRATIC CONTROL

It must be remembered that both locally and centrally public health medical administration is on an essentially democratic basis. It is the representatives of the people, whether elected for the local or central government, who govern, while the permanent officials—in theory at least—merely carry out the behests of their representative masters. So far as the Central Government is concerned, the control exercised by Parliament is dual: (1) the laws, to the carrying out of which all local authorities are limited, are enacted by Parliament; and (2) Parliament passes the financial estimates for the work of each Department. Evidently, however, this leaves a vast range of executive detail in local and central government unregulated outside the Department concerned, except when complaint respecting it is voiced in Parliamentary questions or debates. Within this range much control is exercised by means of Departmental Regulations and Orders. The Minister of Health, as head of the central department concerned with public medicine, is liable to a vote of censure by Parliament; but the contingency is remote, as it would probably imply the fall of the entire Cabinet. Short of this the Minister himself is largely bound by precedent in finance and law; but within these limits he can check or impede the efficiency of administration or secure important reforms.

Locally, the councillors and, until recently, the guardians elected on the various local authorities can very effectively retard or hasten sanitation and the personal public medical services in their area. The medical officer of health, the tuberculosis medical officer, and the medical officers engaged in maternity and child welfare work, or in medical inspection and treatment of school children, cannot carry out their work or extend it beyond the financial limits imposed by the budget of the local authority. Hence at every step, each year, the medical officer is first and foremost an educator of his local authority; and in the writer's view this is far and away the most important direction in which educational work is persistently needed. In Britain this educational work is so advanced that there is rarely any recurrent struggle year by year as to the main items in the personal or impersonal branches of public health work. On the minimum side a large mass of good work is being done in every area. Sometimes it is temporarily stinted; but the partial financial partnership between central and local authorities prevents this from becoming serious. On the other hand, each advance needs to be made the subject of missionary educational work on the part of the medical officer proposing it, and he is fortunate when for such an advance he can quote a guiding statement from the central authority. In these matters the general public outside the local council may be an indifferent, a reactionary, or a stimulant influence, and the wise and efficient medical officer is he who gradually improves the education of the public, and especially of voluntary social workers, as well as of the officially elected representatives with whom he has chiefly to work.

CHAPTER II

THE ORGANISATION OF THE MEDICAL PROFESSION IN THE UNITED KINGDOM

THE GENERAL MEDICAL COUNCIL

The position of the medical profession in its relation to the general public is governed by the Medical Act of 1858, which is described as "An Act to regulate the qualifications of practitioners in medicine and surgery". In the preamble to this Act it is stated to be enacted because "it is expedient that persons requiring medical aid should be enabled to distinguish qualified from unqualified practitioners".

By this Act "The General Medical Council (G.M.C.) of Medical Education and Registration of the United Kingdom" was formed, its members being one representative each from the various universities and colleges in the United Kingdom conferring degrees and diplomas of practice, and six direct representatives of the Central Government.

In 1886 the Government representatives were reduced to five; and three new elective members were prescribed, elected by direct vote of the medical practitioners of the United Kingdom.

The Act conferred wide powers upon the G.M.C. for supervision and regulation of the standard of professional knowledge of medical students. It also provided for the maintenance of an official register by the G.M.C., entry on which is guarantee of eligibility to practise in the United Kingdom and in any part of the British Empire with which there is reciprocity.[1] Such registration also confers the

[1] The King in Council has power to decide the colonies and foreign countries the medical practitioners of which can be admitted on the British Register. Only those colonies and foreign countries are included which give equal privileges to practice to registered practitioners of the United Kingdom.

exclusive right to demand and recover in any Court of Law "reasonable charges for professional aid, advice, and visits, and the cost of any . . . appliances, etc., supplied" by the doctor to his patient. No other person is thus entitled to recover medical or surgical charges in any Court of Law.

A qualified medical practitioner is not bound to register his name on the official register; but if he fails to do so he cannot hold any official medical appointment. Similarly any medical certificate required by any Act of Parliament is invalid, unless the person signing it is registered under the Medical Act.

The Medical Act does not prohibit the practice of medicine by unqualified or unregistered persons, but distinctly prevents such persons from recovering debts by legal process, and makes them ineligible for appointment to public medical work. An unqualified practitioner must not, moreover, use any name or title implying that he is registered or legally recognised as a medical practitioner.

More rigid restrictions apply to midwives and dentists. Those already in practice when the Midwives Act, 1902, or the Dentists Act, 1921, was enacted might continue to practise after registration; but dentists thus registered were not entitled to use a name suggesting that they had a diploma. They might call themselves "dentist," but not "dental surgeon". Apart from these, no person not on the register can now practise dentistry or midwifery or recover fees.

The G.M.C. is not intended to act as the guardian of medical practitioners, but to maintain, in the interest of the whole community, a high standard of professional education and of professional conduct.

In the performance of these duties the representatives of the various medical examining bodies, and, until quite recently, all the five Government representatives, have been qualified medical practitioners.

The main disciplinary clause of the Medical Act, 1858, is Section 29, which states:—

If any registered medical practitioner shall be convicted in England or Ireland of any felony or misdemeanour, or in Scotland of any crime or offence, or shall after due inquiry be judged by the General Council to have been guilty of infamous conduct in any professional respect, the General Council may, if they see fit, direct the Registrar to erase the name of such medical practitioner from the Register.

The G.M.C. may restore a name thus erased after an interval prescribed by them, if they think fit. There is no appeal to Higher Courts against a decision of the G.M.C. Their verdict as to what constitutes in a given case "infamous conduct in any professional respect" cannot be upset.

The use of the word "infamous" in the enactment is unfortunate. A better phrase would be "serious misconduct in a professional sense", and this is what is meant by "infamous" conduct.

The employment of an unqualified medical assistant, and the issuing of untrue, misleading, or improper certificates have been held to be infamous conduct in a professional sense. Advertising or touting for practice comes in the same category, as does also habitual drunkenness; and adultery, while attending medically or being the recognised family doctor of the family affected by the offence, is similarly punished on conviction by erasure of the offender's name from the Medical Register. The G.M.C. sits as a judicial body, hearing evidence for and against the alleged offender.

Prosecution may be initiated by the G.M.C. or by any person aggrieved, or a case may be presented for adjudication by the British Medical Association or a medical protection society.

The interests of the medical profession are protected by various voluntary associations. Medical defence societies protect their members against actions for neglect or malpractice or libel. There are also larger associations of general or special practitioners of medicine, as the Society of Medical Officers of Health, of Poor Law Medical Officers, etc. The most important of these voluntary organisations is the British Medical Association (B.M.A.).

THE BRITISH MEDICAL ASSOCIATION

This is a voluntary organisation and has no statutory powers. It fulfils, however, important functions in securing combined action of the majority of the medical profession on important medical problems, and in obtaining an adequate hearing of the medical side of current events from public authorities, both central and local.

In 1929 the B.M.A. comprised 34,979 members, of whom 22,080 lived in England, Wales, and Scotland, and 1,020 in Ireland. This is about 60 per cent. of the total medical practitioners, and a somewhat higher percentage of those engaged in general medical practice.

There are many branches of the B.M.A. in the United Kingdom, and in Australia, New Zealand, and South Africa, and representatives from these branches are elected on its Central Council.

In the negotiations preliminary to the initiation of the National Insurance Act, the B.M.A. took a chief part, and the Government accepted their terms. Although at first the B.M.A. was averse to the project of medical practice on a contract basis, and characterised such work as degrading to the medical profession, the terms they have secured in successive readjustments of their contract with the Government have led to a vast change in their outlook. Thus at the Annual Meeting of the B.M.A. in 1922 the following resolution was passed:—

The measure of success which has attended the experiment of providing medical benefit under the National Health Insurance Acts system has, in the opinion of the Representative Body, been sufficient to justify the profession in uniting to ensure the continuance and improvement of an insurance system.

The attitude of the B.M.A. to various kinds of medical work is set out in subsequent chapters. Among these reference may be made especially to the problems of the relation of the private practitioner to maternity and welfare work (pp. 163, 192), to tuberculosis work (p. 225), to venereal disease work (p. 231), to pathological work (p. 214), and to school medical work (p. 209), a statement of which is set out in its appropriate connection; and the B.M.A.'s attitude to encroachments on private medical practice by hospitals and otherwise is given on page 42.

It is convenient to detail here other pronouncements of the B.M.A. on the general relation between private and public medical practice, as in this way one can give most succinctly a clear indication of the trend in the medical opinion of the majority of private practitioners, as expressed through their Association. The present position, I think, is one of increasing cordiality between private and public medical services, though there continues to be some misunderstanding on points of detail. In the attempt to adjust matters, the B.M.A. and local authorities alike are increasingly taking a broad and statesmanlike attitude, and this augurs well for the future.

ATTITUDE OF THE BRITISH MEDICAL ASSOCIATION ON PROBLEMS AFFECTING THE RELATION OF THE MEDICAL PROFESSION TO THE PUBLIC

1. DOMICILIARY MEDICAL ATTENDANCE

It will be found (p. 114) that the majority of practising doctors in Great Britain are engaged in contract medical work for about one-third of the total population, thus providing the domiciliary medical attendance which is within the competence of an average practitioner, on the basis of payment at so much per insured person on the doctor's list or panel, whether the insured person falls ill or not. This plan, in the interest of patient and doctor, is safeguarded by two conditions: each insured person chooses his own doctor and places his name on the doctor's panel; and, after giving notice, each patient can change his doctor. Correspondingly, the doctor can accept or reject a given patient.

Before and since 1912, when this immense contract system was initiated, other "encroachments" on ordinary private medical practice have occurred not only in the work of voluntary hospitals, but also in the official midwifery work, in antenatal medical care, in infant consultations, in school clinics, in tuberculosis and venereal disease clinics. It is not surprising, therefore, that the B.M.A., acting as the chief organ of the British medical profession, has voiced its apprehensions and its desire to stop or at least control the current of events. In doing so they have not always, I think, paid adequate attention to the important considerations: (1) that prior to the initiation of these special services many patients in the above-mentioned groups were being ignored or neglected because advice from private doctors was not sought; (2) that this would almost certainly have continued had no public provision been made; and (3) that in all these groups, under the new arrangements, patients are brought under early treatment, and thus multitudes are prevented from becoming ill, who apart from the new arrangements would never have seen a doctor, or only at a belated stage of illness.

In 1927 the following resolution was passed by the B.M.A.:—

The Representative Body, viewing with considerable concern the insidious inroads continually being made on private medical practice under the auspices of the State, voluntary bodies, and others, and being of opinion that this is not only detrimental to the interests of the individual members of the medical profession, but ultimately to all classes in the community, instructs the Council to watch all such developments and actively to interest itself in safeguarding private practice amongst all groups in the medical profession and to develop through the Branches and Divisions closer co-operation with the local medical profession for that purpose.

This resolution was judicious and moderate in so far as it deprecates interference with private medical practice. No public authority desires to intrude on medical care already attainable and attained.

Next year a more specific resolution was adopted, stating that—

Domiciliary attendance should, in the best interests of the patients, be provided by private practitioners in the area concerned, and not by a whole-time medical officer.

To the resolution words were added which expressed realisation of the impossibility of this in certain areas, as, for instance, when "no practitioners are willing to undertake the domiciliary work on suitable terms". The resolution expresses a view with which there will be fairly general agreement. There is no wish on the part of any public authority to take over medical care when, as said above, this is already attainable and attained.

With the proposed extension of the principle of the above resolution to poor-law patients, which is quoted below, one can only agree if and when insurance practice is extended to the dependents of the insured (pp. 93, 297). In 1924 the Representative Body of the B.M.A. resolved that—

The principle of free choice of doctor should as far as possible be recognised in the domiciliary attendance on poor-law patients.

2. PART-TIME OR WHOLE-TIME MEDICAL APPOINTMENTS

In 1911 the following resolution was adopted by the B.M.A. :—

In every form of public medical service (other than that of medical officers of health) the system of part-time appointments of medical practitioners should be maintained, as far as such appointments can be made consistently with the requirements of the service.

This resolution, even though modified by recognition of the governing condition of "requirements of the service", is drastic; and it is doubtful if in 1931 it would again be passed in the above form.

With the growth of public medical services whole-time medical appointments have greatly increased.

It is agreed by all that medical officers of health should not be engaged in private medical practice; and the same agreement holds for the assistant medical officers of health. These number more than their chiefs.

Many of these assistant medical officers of health may have allotted to them special duties, especially tuberculosis and

maternity and child welfare work; more often they engage
in such special work during part of their time, the rest of
which is devoted to general and especially to epidemiological
work.

When tuberculosis medical officers and medical officers for
child welfare work are limited to their special work, almost
universally these are now whole-time officers; and in practice
it has been found that part-time appointments are relatively
unsatisfactory. From the point of view of the chief M.O.H.
of a county or a county borough—the two chief types of
public authority concerned—whole time appointments must
necessarily appeal; for by means of these (a) the work in
different sections of the administrative area is rendered more
nearly uniform in quality, (b) the work of necessary supervision of work is facilitated; and (c) the difficulties arising
from the part-time officer having urgent non-official medical
calls are avoided. These remarks are subject to further
considerations, which will be debated in my concluding
volume.

Similar remarks apply to school medical appointments
(see also p. 209).

In the Public Assistance Medical Service it is nearly
universal for the district medical officer attending the sick
poor in a given district to be also a private practitioner. In
rural and smaller poor-law infirmaries part-time medical
appointments are also common; but for large infirmaries,
now called public assistance hospitals, whole-time medical
superintendents, with whole-time assistant medical officers,
are nearly always appointed. This is often associated with
the appointment of a part-time medical and surgical staff of
consultants, thus greatly enriching the service.

Venereal disease clinics are commonly manned by a
member of the staff of the voluntary hospital at which the
official clinic is held; and he usually engages also in private
practice. This has usually worked well; but some local
authorities have appointed whole-time V.D. medical officers,
who have proved very successful in their work. There
cannot be said to be any principle involved in the differing

practice. At all V.D. clinics private practitioners are welcomed, and consultations respecting private patients are
invited.

It will be remembered that in the final decision as to
whether a given official appointment shall be whole-time or
part-time, the public lay authority concerned is supreme. Its
members are willing to listen to representations made either
by the B.M.A. or by the M.O.H. of the authority.

3. RELATION OF THE MEDICAL PRACTITIONER TO THE
   M.O.H.

In his personal relationship a medical practitioner in any
administrative area is concerned with the M.O.H. in his
duty—

    to notify births in default of the parent;
    to notify cases of the chief infectious disease, including
      tuberculosis;
    to certify accurately the cause of death of patients dying
      under his care.

He is entitled—

    to secure the aid of the M.O.H. in the diagnosis of
      doubtful cases of infectious disease;
    to avail himself of officially provided means for aiding
      diagnosis—

      by bacteriological tests,
      by X-ray examinations,
      by consultation with the medical officers of official
        clinics.

Collectively the B.M.A. has done much to assist medical
officers of health in their work. In evidence of this a number
of resolutions of its Representative Body may be quoted.

First comes their endorsement of the principle of whole-
time service by the medical officers of health (1911).

In 1923 this has been followed by a general statement of
what they regard as the right policy of association between

preventive and curative medicine. They (the B.M.A.) state they are—

in general agreement with the view of the Consultative Council on Medical and Allied Services as stated in that part of paragraph 6 of its interim report which recited :—

"Preventive and curative medicine cannot be separated on any sound principle, and in any scheme of medical services must be brought together in close co-operation. They must likewise be brought within the sphere of the general practitioner, whose duties should embrace the work of communal as well as individual medicine."

They then state that they are prepared to advise local authorities :—

(1) That where private general practitioners place their opinions before local authorities on any proposed scheme of medical survey or inspection and treatment, their representations should have due consideration by the local authority, in order that it may be ascertained how far it is practicable or desirable to give effect to their view.

(2) That those engaged in general practice must either be prepared to accept responsibility for the treatment of such of their private patients as are discovered by medical survey or otherwise by the local authority to be in need of treatment, or they should agree that treatment be undertaken by the local authority without regarding such medical provision as an encroachment on their practice. To this end persons found to be in need of treatment should in the first instance be referred to their private medical practitioner, or, if they have no regular medical attendant, they should be advised to consult a private medical practitioner.

(3) Private practitioners should assist local authorities by intimating their willingness or otherwise to undertake the treatment of patients discovered in the manner stated to be in need of treatment.

The significance of the words "in the first instance" under (2) will be appreciated. I regard it as carrying with it the implication that, as no socially-minded doctor can be complacent over untreated disease, the local authority is justified and, indeed, under an obligation to treat cases which otherwise would be neglected. It may also be regarded as implying that some public authority or voluntary charitable organisation must treat all patients who cannot afford to pay a private practitioner. Of course, this treatment may conceivably be arranged for with a private practitioner, and paid for out of private or public funds. More can be said on this after discussing medical insurance.

It should be noted further that the B.M.A. takes due note of the obligations and powers conferred upon local authorities by Acts of Parliament (a) for medical survey or inspection, and (b) for treatment; and advises medical practitioners to express their willingness to undertake the treatment of patients found by the medical officers of local authorities to need treatment.

The statement of policy of the B.M.A. goes on wisely to enunciate:—

(4) That private medical practitioners should be able to refer to clinics and centres, for advice and treatment, patients who would thus be most appropriately provided for.

(5) That payments or charges, if any, made in respect of medical treatment should be either voluntary or of such a character as will not deter persons from seeking advice and obtaining early treatment.

Further recommendations of the B.M.A. as to centres and clinics are stated on pages 158, 163, 193, 209.

In a final section the above-quoted report states that for the purpose of a better understanding:—

(a) Private general practitioners or consultants accepting offices under local authorities must realise that the duties of these offices require to be fulfilled strictly in accordance with the conditions of the appointments and in priority of all other engagements.

Paragraph (a) quoted above deals with one of the great difficulties in employing private practitioners for public clinics. At out-patient departments of voluntary hospitals patients are often kept waiting for hours, to their serious economic loss; and this evil it has been difficult to avoid to a minor extent at official clinics served by private practi-

tioners. At venereal disease clinics this evil has been particularly great, though it occurs also at maternity and child
welfare centres.

(*b*) Health policy is settled by local health authorities, not only
on medical grounds, but after due regard has been given to the
closely related questions of administration and finance, local
conditions and other relevant considerations.

(*c*) The M.O.H. should so far as possible secure the co-operation of the local medical profession in the discharge of his duties.

(*d*) The final decision on health policy must always rest with
the local and central authorities.

(*e*) It is the duty of the M.O.H. to ensure that effect is given
to the decisions of those authorities.

In reading the previous paragraphs one realises that great
advance has been made towards securing the co-operation
between private and public medicine.

Although the matter is discussed elsewhere, it may be said
here that two facts have largely conduced to this end:
(1) it is realised that much of the medical care given by
public health and education authorities was previously
neglected; and (2) the private practitioner reciprocally
benefits under the new conditions—(*a*) by obtaining the
advantage of expert consultations, and (*b*) by the discovery
and reference to him of many cases which formerly were
neglected.

The B.M.A. has given valuable help in improving the
standard of remuneration of medical officers of health.
Joint conferences of the Society of M.O.H. and the B.M.A.
have agreed on what should be the minimum salary to be
given to health officers of various grades and for communities of differing population. Their decision has been
placed before the associations of local authorities and the
Ministry of Health. The support of the Ministry has been
obtained, and most local authorities have accepted the scale.
The medical and public health journals have refused to
accept advertisements of appointments in which a salary
below the scale has been offered, and have warned all
medical practitioners against applying for them. The general

result has been an elevation of the standard of public health and medical work.

Two further illustrations may be given in which dispute as to the relation between professional and non-professional work may arise.

4. ADMINISTRATION OF ANÆSTHETICS

Should anæsthetics be allowed to be administered by a lay (i.e. non-medical) person?

On this point the Representative Body of the B.M.A. has very definite views. In 1927 they passed the following resolution:—

(1) No person other than a registered medical practitioner should administer any anæsthetic for medical or surgical purposes, except that a registered dentist who has received special instruction in the administration of anæsthetics may administer anæsthetics for dental purposes only.

(2) Where a general anæsthetic is administered, it is undesirable that any person should act both as operator and administrator in the same case where this can be avoided, but it must be recognised that cases occur in practice in which this responsibility may justifiably be undertaken.

More recently a Special Committee of the B.M.A.[1] emphasises the fact that prolonged chloroform inhalation during parturition may lead to delayed poisoning, and that in some cases light anæsthesia during the second stage of labour is not always successful. "In the very numerous cases in which it can be carried out it is a very humane and a safe proceeding," and the delay in labour and the risk of post-partum hæmorrhage have both been minimised by the use of pituitary extract. They are of opinion, however, that "the midwife should not administer anæsthetics, opium, pituitary extract . . . except in so far as she may be acting under, or carrying out the instructions of, a medical practitioner."

In the United States a fully qualified nurse who has had special training in this work often gives the anæsthetics

[1] *Interim Report of Departmental Committee on Maternal Mortality*, 1930, p. 119.

needed in major surgical operations; and the practice has justified itself. It would be unwise to extend the permission to other nurses; and in Great Britain even the above practice is looked at askance.

The almost complete disallowance stated as above is, I think, unwise; in an emergency a surgeon having to undertake a serious operation without a medical colleague would not hesitate to instruct a nurse to administer the anæsthetic under such supervision as he could give.

In childbirth a more definite case arises calling for gradual relaxation of the present prohibition. A—perhaps minor—reason for the too frequent and socially detrimental one-child families is believed to be the experience of unnecessary shock and suffering experienced by primiparæ, which might have been greatly alleviated by judicious intermittent administration of chloroform, as is commonly done by doctors in middle and upper class practice.

Under present conditions the midwife in attendance at a confinement is authorised to give up to, say, 30 grains of chloral, 60 grains of bromide, or one drachm of tincture of opium without medical supervision. Sometimes chloroform is also indicated either (1) to produce full surgical anæsthesia, as when forceps are applied, or version, or Cæsarean section is needed, or (2) to relieve pain in natural labour.

A Committee on Anæsthetics in Confinements appointed by the Royal College of Physicians of London has recently reported to the Ministry of Health,[1] and its recommendations represent the views of the chief obstetric consultants in London as well as of the College. In this report the reader is reminded that "full surgical anæsthesia can only be safely induced by a specially trained anæsthetist or medical practitioner", and that it is not permissible to give an anæsthetic solely for the relief of pain in labour until the second stage has definitely commenced. In a natural labour chloroform in practice is the only anæsthetic which can be used to

[1] *Interim Report of Departmental Committee on Maternal Mortality*, 1930, p. 116.

relieve pain. Its "intermittent administration can be made by an unskilled person under the direction of someone who has had expert training"; but it must only be given for a limited period. The Committee recommend that arrangements should be made for the giving of chloroform in the lying-in wards of hospitals, all medical students and midwives being instructed in the "intermittent method" of administration of chloroform. They go further and urge that:—

Some responsible body, such as the Central Midwives Board, should be asked to draw up the necessary regulations as to the increased training for the midwives, and stringent rules as to how far a midwife could give chloroform on her own responsibility.

Such rules would require very careful consideration, but the first and most important one would of necessity be one which placed a very definite limit on the length of time a midwife might administer an anæsthetic without informing or sending for a doctor.

The desirability of intermittent anæsthesia in the later stages of normal confinements, especially of primiparæ, being accepted, it must be recalled that more than half of the total confinements are attended by midwives. It follows that unless institutional attendance in parturition can be greatly extended, midwives should be enabled to acquire the skill and experience to administer chloroform to a definitely limited extent.

A complete medical service for this purpose would be too costly; and the risks of uterine inertia and hæmorrhage from too prolonged anæsthesia should be capable of avoidance by regulations corresponding to those already restricting midwives in other respects.

5. DENTAL SERVICES

Dentistry is a branch of medicine which happily is in the hands of qualified dentists who are now legally protected from competition by unqualified persons. These can no longer hold themselves out to be "dentists" or "dental surgeons".

This outlawing of unqualified dentists led to some

scarcity of dentists, especially for the care of children's teeth; but it is doubtful whether this now continues. A more frequent complaint is that the average income of the dentist is inadequate in view of his long period of training. It is but fair to add that dentists have shown much public spirit in fostering the formation of public dental clinics, especially for school children. In most areas some curative treatment for dental caries and defects in school children is given at the public expense, and increasingly this is being extended to secure similar skilled aid for expectant and nursing mothers, and for toddlers, as well as for tuberculosis patients.

School dentists have been appointed on a large scale (p. 201), some whole-time, some part-time officials. In school dental clinics nurses are employed to make preliminary surveys of teeth, and to scale teeth. In a few instances the more competent nurses have been allowed to undertake extractions of temporary teeth. On this much controversy has arisen. The practice of permitting specially trained nurses to take part in the surgical work of dentistry has been deprecated and often forbidden, and the policy illustrated by it is in abeyance. I am not clear that this is wise. Multitudes of children's teeth still are neglected because of the expense of dental staffs, or because of the difficulty in securing dentists. Given that a dentist supervises the minor dental work done by a specially trained nurse, much more work could be done, and the health of children greatly improved. From the point of view of public policy, it is unwise to use highly skilled workmen for work that can be satisfactorily done by workmen of less skill, always assuming that the work of the latter is adequately checked and controlled. The same principle is involved in much of the minor surgical work undertaken at school clinics by school nurses. This may include the treatment of chilblains, of festering minor wounds, of eczema, impetigo, etc. A vast amount of treatment of minor ailments is being done by school nurses, of minor but really injurious conditions which except for their efforts would be neglected.

CHAPTER III

GENERAL MEDICAL SERVICES IN ENGLAND

A. Voluntary Hospitals

The multiform medical services in England need next to be considered in their relation to individual private medical practice. Below is given a scheme of the chief organisations concerned; this is not quite exhaustive. One important omission is noteworthy. Neither in this nor in any other chapter have I given detail concerning the institutional treatment of the feeble-minded and the insane. This omission has been found necessary, in part because some choice of material was necessary in giving illustrations of the relation between the private and the institutional treatment of disease, but chiefly because in regard to the care of the feeble-minded and insane few, if any, differences of opinion arise. There is general agreement that the institutional treatment of mental diseases must be undertaken mainly by public authorities commanding the community purse.

SCHEME OF PUBLIC MEDICAL SERVICES

I. Voluntary Hospitals and Dispensaries

These are intended for the poor who are not in receipt of official public assistance, though the latter also often benefit, especially when exceptional medical skill is required.

The chief form of this charity consists in the provision of *Hospital Beds* in general hospitals, in hospitals for special diseases, and in maternity hospitals. It comprises also—

Treatment in Out-Patient Departments

Many *General Dispensaries* exist in towns, supported by voluntary contributions. Some of these undertake the domiciliary treatment of those obtaining "letters" of recommendation.

There are also a few *Provident Dispensaries*, supported in part by subscriptions of the charitable, in part by weekly payments of the beneficiaries. Since the passing of the National Insurance Act, 1912, these dispensaries have been largely superseded.

II. THE PUBLIC ASSISTANCE MEDICAL SERVICE

This consists in *Domiciliary Treatment* for those certified by the official relieving officer to be eligible for assistance; and *Infirmary Treatment* under similar conditions.

Vaccination against smallpox for all applicants. This hitherto has been administered as a part of the Poor Law Medical Service, but since April 1930 it is placed, like the entire Poor Law Medical Service, in the hands of the larger public health authorities.

III. PUBLIC HEALTH MEDICAL SERVICES

The chief constituent services are:—

A. *Hospital Provision* for the chief infectious diseases; also provision of *Nurses* for some patients treated at home.

B. *Pathological Service* varying in extent.

C. *Maternity and Child Welfare Service.*
Provision and supervision of midwives.
Maternity homes and hospitals.
Antenatal and Postnatal consultation.
Consultations for infants and pre-school children.
Hospital beds for some sick children.

D. *Tuberculosis Service.*
Tuberculosis dispensaries.
Nurses for home visits.
Medical officer to visit home cases in consultation, etc.

Sanatoria for adults and for children, including residential institutions for the treatment of non-pulmonary tuberculosis.

Hospitals for "observation cases" and for other cases of tuberculosis.

E. *Venereal Disease Service.*

Clinics free to all applying.

Consultations with private practitioners, domiciliary or at the clinics.

Hospital treatment as required.

Diagnostic facilities for all practitioners.

Supply of arseno-benzol preparations to practitioners.

IV. School Medical Service

Medical inspection of scholars.

School clinics (treatment of minor and of some special ailments).

Hospital treatment.

Orthopædic hospitals, massage, etc.

V. Insurance Medical Service

Domiciliary and office medical attendance on the insured.

Occasional special benefits: dental, ophthalmic, etc.

General Observations on Medical Aid.

Public provision of medical aid in England, especially in earlier days, has been commonly associated with material relief of general destitution, and must be considered partially in this setting. Material relief has been derived from three chief sources: the personal help rendered in all ages by charitably disposed persons; similar voluntary help given by groups of charitable persons organised into committees and societies, who solicit and collect funds from the general public for their special object; and official bodies for local or central government, carrying out similar work for the necessitous. Historically it is broadly true that official bodies in the initiation of their work and during a large part of their existence have acted only or chiefly when voluntary activities have been painfully inadequate.

These different activities have continued side by side; their respective spheres of work have seldom been defined and delimited; and in the aggregate they have not completely fulfilled the needs of the people from the point of view of the curative and still less of the preventive possibilities of social and personal medicine. On the other hand, voluntary and official activities have often wastefully overlapped. In most areas there has been no systematic registration of collective charitable work.

The present position of the official Public Assistance Services of England is the outcome of long years of growth, usually not associated with logical or scientific study of the services needed and, in part, already given. New demands often have been met by new organisations unrelated to existing organisations which might have been utilised, and by the development of which wasteful creation of new social machinery might have been avoided. This is true of the chief forms of Public Assistance which are supported out of local rates and national taxes. They are the following:

Local Authorities

1. The Poor Law (Public Assistance) Service   Board of Guardians.[1]
2. The Public Health Service   Public Health Authorities.
3. The School Medical Service   Education Committees of Public Health Authorities.
4. The Insurance Service   Insurance Committees.

[1] The Boards of Guardians in April 1930 ceased to be separate authorities, being replaced by special committees of county councils and county borough councils (see page 29).
The organisation of Public Health and Education and Insurance authorities is further described on pages 30–31.

Existent official medical relief work comes under these four headings. It comprises (*a*) *general medical care* of the poor; (*b*) *medical care, chiefly institutional, of certain forms of sickness,* given by public health or educational authorities as part of the policy of prevention of disease; and (*c*) the *insurance medical service.*

I have grouped the Insurance Service as a form of Public Assistance; it is partially so in virtue of the contributions of the State to its cost, even if we assume that the still larger compulsory contributions of employers are an indirect addition to the workers' wages and not public assistance like the State grant.

All the above four services are still largely indebted for their current efficiency to voluntary organisations, and especially to voluntary hospitals. Were it not for the aid thus given out of voluntary charitable funds the rates and taxes required for these services, and especially for public assistance and sickness insurance, would rise to a marked extent.

VOLUNTARY HOSPITALS

It will probably, therefore, be well to describe, first, some of the more important agencies for giving voluntary medical aid. Of these, hospitals are the most important, but non-residential dispensaries and nursing associations have also played an important part in ameliorating the lot of the sick and poor.

As stated in my *Public Health and Insurance* (Johns Hopkins Press, 1920):—

Hospital services have grown in a manner which is characteristic of the Anglo-Saxon: first largely under voluntary management, and as examples of Christian charity; afterwards continued in the same way, but followed by official provision of hospitals on an even larger scale, the two systems working side by side. The extent to which the more satisfactory institutional treatment is replacing the domiciliary treatment of disease may be gathered from the striking facts that in England and Wales one in every nine of the deaths from all causes in 1881 occurred in public institutions, and in 1910 one in every five; while in London the proportion increased from one in five in 1881 to two in five in 1910.

Since then the proportion of total deaths occurring in institutions to deaths at home has further increased.

The facts as to pulmonary tuberculosis are even more significant. In the year 1911, in England and Wales, 34 per cent. of male and 22 per cent. of female deaths, and in London 59 per cent. of male and 48 per cent. of female deaths, from pulmonary tuberculosis occurred in public institutions; and in this instance also the proportion of institutional deaths in recent years has still further increased. The significance of these facts, not only for the treatment but also for the prevention of many diseases, and especially of tuberculosis, is seldom appreciated at its full value. Increasing aggregation of the people in towns has greatly enhanced the difficulties of housing; and were it not for the supplementary housing provided by hospitals, and the special medical and surgical skill rendered in them, much of the lowered national death-rate which has been experienced would not have occurred. Hospitals, in fact, have furnished a partial—alas! only a partial—solution of housing difficulties, besides being centres for the highest professional service.

Voluntary hospitals have been pioneers in this great highway of medical and hygienic progress, though rate- and tax-supported hospitals have entered more and more into the field. This does not imply diminished activity of voluntary hospitals, but there has been a rapid increase of call for hospital beds, to meet which recourse to the local and national funds of the country has been required. Dr. F. N. K. Menzies gives the number of beds in London provided by public assistance (poor law) authorities as about 80,000, and states that the institutional treatment of nearly five-sixths of the sick in London is undertaken out of public funds. Under the recent reorganisation of local government the London County Council will be responsible for eight times as many sick beds (including provision for the insane) as all the voluntary hospitals of London. In the early history of voluntary hospitals, specially those of ecclesiastic origin, the ideal was one of charity and care rather than of treatment and of cure. In mediæval times a *hospital* was literally a place of *hospitality*, and the name denoted a residential school,

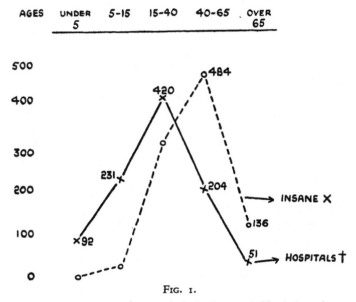

FIG. I.

Proportion of Insane in Asylums and of other Patients in Hospitals not being Asylums per 1,000 Total Population, England and Wales, at each Age Period.

* In Asylums and Homes for Insane.
† In Hospitals and Nursing-Homes, including Naval and Military Hospitals.

or an asylum for the aged, or a place for the sick without discrimination. Now more and more hospitals are becoming also chief centres for prevention of disease; in part, by prevention of its protraction and of its secondary consequences, medical or other; even more by preventing infection as in tuberculosis and syphilis and in acute infectious diseases, such as typhus and smallpox. They are, furthermore, an important means for teaching patients a better way of life; and they are indispensable in preparing physicians and, in part, nurses for their life-work.

It has to be remembered that hospitals are not convalescent homes. These are an essential complement for the full efficiency of hospitals, which must be omitted from my necessarily brief sketch.

The need for more active preventive work is shown by the age-distribution of hospital patients in England, as derived from census figures in Fig. 1. Of every 1,000 hospital patients at all ages, 420 are aged 15–40, while of every 1,000 at all ages, 484 patients in asylums and homes for the insane are aged 40–65. In both instances the main stress on hospital or asylum accommodation is between the ages of 15 and 65, the chief working years of life. What an immense scope for preventive medicine is here revealed!

In 1911 an official return was obtained for England and Wales, showing the accommodation in voluntary hospitals, in isolation hospitals for infectious diseases, and in poor-law infirmaries. Its results are summarised below. The return did not include tuberculosis hospitals and sanatoria, convalescent homes, nursing-homes, or hospitals for mental diseases. It included 2,664 institutions with 178,105 beds, which is equivalent to 4·9 official and voluntary beds per 1,000 of the population in 1911.

	Number	Beds
General hospitals	594	31,329
Special hospitals	222	13,654
Fever hospitals	755	31,149
Smallpox hospitals	363	7,972
Poor-law infirmaries	700	94,001

The three last-named are official, the two first voluntary, hospitals; and it is noteworthy that more than 75 per cent. of the total accommodation is in official hospitals. This proportion would have been greatly increased had the beds in lunatic asylums been included.

This is shown by the following estimate of hospital provision in England and Wales of recent date:—

	Number of Institutions	Number of Beds
Voluntary hospitals, general and special	847	50,460
Isolation and port sanitary hospitals	1,046	38,200
Tuberculosis hospitals and sanatoria	463	22,655
Institutions for lunatics and mental defectives	441	139,122 [1]
Poor-law institutions	713	120,235

[1] In the year 1927, out of 138,293 total insane patients under treatment in England and Wales, only 14,646 were under private medical care.

A relatively small part of accommodation for tuberculous patients and for the insane is in institutions not provided by public authorities; but allowing for this, the extent to which total official provision preponderates over total voluntary provision for the institutional treatment of disease is evident.

In 1921, after the Great War, the voluntary contributions and bequests to non-official hospitals in London and the rest of England and Wales proved inadequate for their support, and the Government came to their aid with a grant of half a million pounds sterling, a Commission being appointed to apportion this sum and to investigate the general problem. It was understood that no further Government assistance would be forthcoming; and in the apportionment of the grant the principle was adopted of disbursing *pro rata* against fresh money from other sources raised or in sight. The final Report of the Voluntary Hospitals Commission, 1928, gives the bed accommodation in 1924 of *voluntary hospitals* as 13,880 in London and 36,799 in the rest of England and Wales, which is equivalent to 1·33 beds per 1,000 of population. (The total beds in the 30 public assistance hospitals of London have some 19,000 beds, while the 130 metropolitan voluntary hospitals have nearly 14,000 beds. These figures do not include special mental hospitals or hospitals for infectious diseases.)

For London more detailed statistics as to voluntary hospitals are given in the reports of King Edward's Hospital Fund for London. This fund is derived from voluntary contributions. It was established in 1877, and it annually disburses large sums, apportioned with judicious care, according to the needs and merits of each voluntary hospital.

The Report of the King Edward's Hospital Fund gives statistics for 136 hospitals in and near London having 15,040 beds.

These in 1926 had 202,600 new in-patients,
and in 1927 had 212,100 new in-patients.

The estimated population of London in 1926 being 4,615,400, the in-patient rate per 1,000 of population was 43·9, and the beds in voluntary hospitals were in the proportion of 3·17 per 1,000 of population.

In 1926 1,645,000 new out-patients attended these voluntary hospitals, or 356 per 1,000 of population.

The total attendances of out-patients numbered 7,553,000 in 1926 and 7,902,000 in 1927, representing in 1926 a rate of 1634 per 1,000 of population. (For comments on out-patients, see page 86). Metropolitan hospitals draw patients from outside London; but even allowing for this, the extent to which sickness is treated by voluntary charitable agencies is striking.

In 1926 the average stay of each in-patient in hospital was 21·9 days. Each out-patient on an average made between four and five attendances.

Twelve of the metropolitan hospitals have medical schools attached to them, and the following table shows in percentages the proportion of beds in these hospitals devoted to different diseases, and the proportion of out-patient attendances in each group:—

TWELVE VOLUNTARY HOSPITALS WITH 5,267 BEDS, AND AT
WHICH 3,698,710 OUT-PATIENT ATTENDANCES WERE MADE
IN 1927

	Percentage Ratios	
	Beds	Out-patient Attendances
General surgical	33·8	27·6
General medical	33·4	18·4
Gynæcological	5·2	1·5
Maternity	4·4	—
Ear, nose, and throat	4·3	4·1
Ophthalmic	3·0	2·9
Isolation and septic	4·9	12·2
Orthopædic, skin, and observation	3·6	—
Accident	2·6	—
Venereal	1·1	—
Private and staff wards	3·7	—
TOTAL..	100·0	
Massage, electric and rays		21·5
Dental		4·6
Skin		3·4
Ante- and postnatal maternity and infant welfare		3·2
Tuberculosis		0·6
TOTAL..		100·0

The funds of the King Edward's Hospital Fund are
distributed to all hospitals within 11 miles of St. Paul's
Cathedral, many of these being, in fact, national hospitals.
In 1927 one in eight of the in-patients in the general
hospitals of London came from other parts of the
country. The sum thus disbursed by the Fund to hospitals, convalescent homes, and tuberculosis sanatoria
(voluntary) in—

$$1897 \text{ was } 56,826$$
$$1907 \text{ was } 123,750$$
$$1917 \text{ was } 190,000$$
$$1926 \text{ was } 284,754$$

These funds were derived in 1926 from voluntary sources chiefly as follows :—

	£
Annual subscriptions	23,192
Donations	27,319
League of Mercy	15,000
Legacies	37,064
Income from investments	166,435
British Charities Association	15,000

Voluntary hospitals also receive large sums from the Hospital Sunday and Hospital Saturday Collecting Funds and from Contributory Schemes.

Hospital Sunday Fund, 1926	London	Provinces[1]
	£	£
Collections from congregations on Hospital Sunday	37,920	56,188
Legacies, special donations, etc.	49,129	142,917

[1] Fifty-nine provincial towns.

The Hospital Saturday Fund receives money from an annual street collection and from gifts of workers in workshops and factories. In 1926 the sum collected was £109,769, of which £15,917 was devoted to dental work, £10,715 was for surgical appliances, and £566 for ambulances.

The following table shows for the metropolitan hospitals the proportion of each source of income to total expenditure or income :—

1927. TOTAL GENERAL FUND

Total income	100·0
Voluntary Gifts :	
Subscriptions and donations	28·6
Central Funds	10·2

For services rendered:

Patients	24·1
Public authorities	7·5
Fees and other receipts	0·7
Income from investments	18·4
Legacies	10·2
Other extraordinary income	0·3

The *high proportion of total income derived from payment for services rendered* may be noted. These sums are derived from patients, from public authorities, and from special fees; they represent considerable departure from the position of

METROPOLITAN HOSPITALS

Hospitals	Number of Beds	Percentage of Ordinary Income (excluding Legacies) derived from Payments for Services Rendered		
		Total	From Public Authorities	From Fees, Patients, and their Societies
12 teaching hospitals with medical schools	5,267	26·4	5·3	21·1
varying from ..		18·9	St. Bartholomew's	
to ..		44·8	King's Col. Hosp.	
7 General hospitals with 150 or more beds, but no teaching school .	1,471	37·3	10·0	27·3
14 General hospitals with 70–149 beds ..	1,561	30·9	3·9	27·0
6 Hospitals for women .	437	47·3	1·8	45·5
8 Children's hospitals .	916	18·4	2·5	16·1
8 Maternity hospitals .	497	35·7	10·3	25·4
9 Ophthalmic hospitals	262	36·6	7·6	29·0
3 Throat, nose, and ear hospitals	138	65·7	2·4	63·3

a charity. This does not mean that voluntary subscriptions and donations have declined, but that services rendered in these hospitals are being paid for to an increasing extent. Thus the percentage of income of the hospitals subsidised by the King Edward's Hospital Fund for London derived from subscriptions and donations was about 31 per cent. in 1913 and 29 per cent. in 1927. In 1913 the sum derived from these sources was just under half a million sterling,

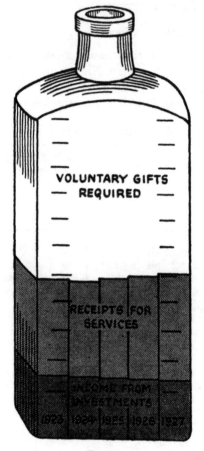

VOLUNTARY GIFTS
— REQUIRED —

RECEIPTS FOR SERVICES

INCOME FROM INVESTMENTS

1923 1924 1925 1926 1927

FIG. 2.

while in 1927 it had risen to £926,000. Subscriptions had nearly doubled, but their proportion to the total hospital income had not increased.

The proportion of their total current income received by voluntary hospitals for services rendered varies greatly according to the type of voluntary hospital. In the statement on page 65, extracted also from the Report of the King Edward's Hospital Fund, some of the variations are shown. The statement gives also the number of beds in different types of metropolitan hospital.

Smaller hospitals, including some special hospitals, are not included in the above statement.

The diagram (Fig. 2) on page 66 of a medicine bottle taken also from the same report shows the total general fund expenditure of 136 hospitals aided by the King Edward's Hospital Fund, and the proportions of income from investments and from receipts for service during each of the five years 1923–27. The unshaded part of the bottle shows the gap remaining to be filled up by voluntary gifts.

FINANCIAL SUPPORT OF VOLUNTARY HOSPITALS

A vast amount of hospital provision in England and Wales under voluntary management and supported by voluntary contributions is being given, and these hospitals are rendering admirable and in some measure irreplaceable services; but there is an almost complete lack of effective co-ordination of the services in different voluntary hospitals. The King Edward's Hospital Fund, through its large contributions to all metropolitan voluntary hospitals, is able effectively to act in the direction of uniform bookkeeping, and to some extent in adjusting work; but even in London there is much redundancy along with local inadequacy of voluntary hospital provision. The voluntary hospitals, especially the larger hospitals having medical schools attached to them, are too closely aggregated in Central London, and this is one reason why (see page 98) public assistance hospitals are serving identical purposes in most of the outer-ring areas of London. Even were the voluntary hospitals distributed according to population, they would now be utterly inadequate to meet the needs of London if unaided by the larger-scaled work of public assistance hospitals.

In the provinces this is even more true. Many large

voluntary hospitals are supremely good; but there are smaller voluntary hospitals, and still more cottage hospitals, manned by physicians and surgeons who, while doing much good work, cannot give service which is much higher in quality than that of the general practitioners from whom they were elected.

Prior to the Great War voluntary hospitals succeeded in maintaining themselves by subscriptions and legacies; and "hospital letters" were usually given to subscribers proportional to the amount subscribed. These, when signed by the subscriber, gave the recipient a partial priority to out-patient or in-patient treatment in the hospital concerned. One can visualise the experience of tired and anxious women trudging to one well-to-do home after another to beg a "hospital letter," often to find that the subscriber's letters had been exhausted. This system happily is now becoming obsolete; the growth of hospital contributory schemes, in particular, has put it out of action. Admission to a hospital bed, of course, is conditional on the patient really needing this provision in the opinion of the hospital doctor.

SYSTEMS OF PAYMENTS IN VOLUNTARY HOSPITALS

1. We need not detail the growth of the practice of having paying wards or private rooms in which the charge made covers the basic expenses of the hospital, including the services of its residential staff.

These beds are now very numerous, and, in addition, there have sprung up a multitude of privately managed hospitals and nursing-homes where somewhat high charges are made, in addition to the charges of the attending physicians and surgeons. Nursing-homes, even when good, are usually inferior to a well-organised hospital.

In London 80 hospitals already provide special pay-beds to the number of 1,055 (R. G. Hogarth, November 7, 1928). The greatest demand, hitherto, has been for beds charged at not more than 3 to 4 guineas a week (i.e. about 15 to 20 dollars).

These charges imply that the services of the hospital medical staff are given gratuitously.

2. Some hospitals attempt to secure from each patient a promise of payment at a reduced charge for maintenance in hospital, the charge being assessed by the hospital almoner according to the earnings and size of family of the patient. In some instances payment by instalments is promised, with unsatisfactory results.

In many hospitals patients attending the out-patient departments are charged a sum which may merely cover the cost of medicines, or more than this. Large sums are collected in this way. Evidently this practice puts the out-patient department to some extent in competition with the private practitioner.

The sums thus obtained are irregular in amount, and the system is not altogether satisfactory.

3. Some form of provident provision for contingent hospital treatment is made. A number of systems on this principle are in actual working. Their conditions may be briefly indicated.

The Hospital Saturday Fund is partially of this character, and may be mentioned first. Founded in 1873, its income is mainly derived from the sums collected weekly or otherwise systematically in workshops and business houses. In return for the sums contributed to hospitals, "letters" entitling suitable persons to treatment in the hospital are often given. The method is not so efficient in raising funds as the more systematic contributory schemes outlined below, and the "letter system" is decidedly objectionable.

Hospital Contributory Schemes

Before remarking on the general arrangements characterising these schemes, a few outstanding illustrations are given. In this chapter the Sheffield, Birmingham, and Metropolitan schemes are specially noted. In the chapter on Brighton (page 354) the Sussex scheme is outlined.

Such schemes have long existed in certain towns, but

only in recent years have they become general. Now such schemes number at least a hundred.

THE SHEFFIELD SCHEME is on the principle of a weekly contribution by workers of 1d. in the £ of their wages (that is 0·4 per cent. of wages), this sum being deducted from the weekly wages by the employer with the consent of the workers. The employer, in paying the aggregate amount to the Joint Hospitals Council, adds one-third to the total of the employees' contributions. The system has worked admirably in the great factories and foundries of Sheffield, and the secretary informs me that during the past three years much progress has also been made in obtaining contributions from shopkeepers and small employers. The number of the last-named already enrolled is 2,500. These are allowed to be enrolled for an annual payment of £1, their employees paying the usual rate of contribution. The pooled sums are distributed by a committee on which all the voluntary hospitals of the city are represented. An ambulance service is also supplied from these funds.

The population of Sheffield in 1928 was 515,000.

Its four voluntary hospitals had 15,433 in-patients and 549,836 out-patient attendances during the year, and 1,583 patients were sent to its convalescent homes. Of the in-patients about one-fifth came from districts outside the city; and contributions are therefore asked from workers employed in these districts. The growth of the contributions is remarkable. In 1920 the amount distributed to the four voluntary hospitals was £20,373; in 1928 it had become £90,939. The last-named sum is about 60 per cent. of the total expenditure of these hospitals.

They also received during 1928 £3,466 from the Hospital Sunday Fund, £6,145 from direct payments by patients, £4,851 from Approved Insurance Societies, and £3,143 from Public Authorities.

These figures are given as illustrating the fact that individual charitable contributions, excepting legacies, do not now bulk as largely as in the past in the total income of these hospitals. The expenses of administration of the above scheme amount to about 4d. in the £ of the total receipts. They would be much greater if employers did not act as collectors of the 1d. in the £ of wages, thus playing the same part as in the scheme of national sickness insurance.

HOSPITAL SAVINGS ASSOCIATION

The Voluntary Hospitals Commission appointed by the Government to consider the temporary collapse of voluntary hospital finance after the Great War in their final Report (1923) made the important remarks quoted below as to future support of these hospitals.

It is noticeable that in certain areas where recovery has been most marked some system of mass contribution has been established. In reviewing the sources of income upon which the voluntary hospitals can rely, receipts from legacies are necessarily a problematical element. As regards subscriptions, some few hospitals have received princely benefactions from individual contributors; but the percentage of income derived from large subscriptions is scarcely likely to increase. The interest of the middle-class subscribers has been, we think, remarkably well maintained, having regard to the fact that the proportion of these subscribers who benefit directly from the existence of the voluntary hospitals is comparatively small. But it would be a mistake to look for a considerable increase of income from this source. The only quarter whence any substantial growth of income may be looked for in future would be from contributions from the industrial classes. The permanence of the voluntary system depends upon its ability to meet the needs of the people, and nothing is so certain to imperil its continuance as the growth of long waiting lists. Excluding London, whose position as the consultant centre for much of south-east England, is quite exceptional, most of the hospitals which are prosperous, and which are keeping pace with the growing demands upon them, are those which draw revenue from mass contribution schemes. We are convinced that the future of the voluntary system depends in a large measure on its success in securing in one form or another the continued support of the small contributor. It must be recognised, however, that the framing of any scheme of mass contributions calls for the exercise of great care to avoid the acceptance by the hospital of liabilities which cannot be discharged, or the creation in the minds of contributors of expectations which may not be fulfilled. At the same time the effect of such a scheme upon the government of the hospital and the relations of the medical staff must also be taken into consideration. It is hoped that those local voluntary hospital committees which have not turned their attention to this problem will make a real effort, in conjunction with the hospitals, to establish, under adequate safeguards, such schemes wherever circumstances permit. We have not in the past pressed this conclusion upon local committees because we realised the manifest risks and difficulties which the system entails. But the experience of recent years has convinced us that this is the main source of new income, and while the dangers are real we do not believe them to be insuperable.

This recommendation led to the foundation of the Hospital Savings Association, the first council of which consisted of the chairmen of some of the large metropolitan voluntary hospitals with other representative men. The scheme was assisted in its initiation by a grant from King Edward's Hospital Fund.

CONDITIONS FOR CONTRIBUTORS

The main objects of the Association are to secure regular contributions towards the support of hospitals and to relieve contributors and their families from hospital charges when they need treatment.

The work of the Hospital Savings Association is done in district groups, each with an unpaid secretary, whose duty is to secure recruits, and to ensure that no prospective contributor earns more than the income limits laid down. These limits are as follows :—

	Per week
Single man or woman	£4
Married couple, without children under 16 ..	£5
Married couple, with children under 16	£6

The regular contribution is 3d. per week, or 12s. per annum in advance. Young persons under 18 may join a Group *in their places of employment* for a weekly contribution of 2d. to cover themselves, but not dependents.

There is no entrance fee, but 1d. is charged for a new card, and 1d. for each renewal card.

The contribution covers the following dependents: wife (or, alternatively, a dependent relative acting as housekeeper) and children under 16; also parents and grandparents, and brother and sisters (under 16) when living with and wholly and permanently dependent upon the contributor.

A long list of hospitals is given at which contributors presenting their vouchers, if accepted for treatment by the hospital, are relieved from—

1. Inquiry at hospital as to means;
2. Any payment in respect of maintenance as an in-patient in an ordinary ward (subject to ten weeks' limit at certain special hospitals); and
3. Any payment as an out-patient (including medicines ordinarily supplied).

If treated at a voluntary hospital not on the list, or at an infirmary supported out of public funds, he will be reimbursed (within certain limitations), normal payments which he has been called upon to make towards the cost of his maintenance, for a period not exceeding ten weeks.

The arrangement for paying charges made on a contributor at hospitals not on the list of the Association holds good also for the charges made in public assistance hospitals.

The following statement sets out the limits of the work of the Association:—

(a) The Association does not deal with diseases for which local authorities provide treatment, such as tuberculosis, once it has been diagnosed; nor does the Association deal with cases of venereal diseases, for which free clinics are provided, nor with cases of infectious disease removed by order of the medical officer of health.

(b) The Association deals with hospital treatment in the ordinary acceptation of the term. It does not, for instance, deal with ordinary maternity cases, or with cases undergoing treatment in a mental hospital or asylum, or in a nursing-home, nor with any cases of treatment at home.

Trivial cases, or cases which can equally well be dealt with by the private doctor, are not intended to be dealt with at a hospital, and this again impresses the desirability of procuring a doctor's letter of recommendation when first attending the hospital.

Although chiefly restricted to hospital treatment—

Assistance is given in meeting the cost of dental treatment and dentures, as well as of convalescent-home treatment, surgical appliances, spectacles, and ambulance service. These benefits are given only within the limit of a fund specially set aside for this purpose, and if this limit is exceeded the scale of benefits must be curtailed.

Dental assistance is reserved for contributors themselves; and no benefit is given where the treatment has commenced within 52 weeks of joining. In no case is simple dental treatment, such as ordinary extractions, provided for.

Payments to Hospitals.—When the Hospitals Savings Association was first started each patient admitted into a voluntary hospital was paid for at the rate of 2½ guineas (52s. 6d., or about $10.50) per week, and 7s. 6d. ($1.50) for each out-patient treated. Now a smaller weekly payment is made; and then at the end of the year surplus funds are distributed to the hospitals *pro rata* to the total paid to each on the weekly basis.

Payments to the authorities concerned with public assistance hospitals for treatment are made on the basis that they shall be reimbursed approximately what, on the average, they might expect to collect from patients whose income is within our limits.

The scale is as follows:—

	Per week	
	s.	d.
For the first six weeks' maintenance:		
For a Contributor	15	0
For an Adult Dependent	10	0
For a Dependent Child	5	0
For the next four weeks' maintenance:		
For the Contributor	10	0
For the Adult Dependent	7	6
For the Dependent Child	2	6

It may be noted that 136 voluntary hospitals come within the scope of the great work of King Edward's Hospital Fund for London, and at these hospitals the total annual expenditure is a little over 3 millions sterling, while the

651,713[1] contributors of the Hospital Savings Association in 1930 paid £320,714 towards the cost of hospital treatment whenever needed by the sick among them. Of this sum—

£264,376 was paid directly to voluntary hospitals;

£37,900 was paid to public assistance hospitals; and

£23,557 were refunds of hospital payments made by contributors.

In addition, £69,700 was paid for extra-hospital benefits to hospitals not on the Association's list, such as convalescent home treatment, dentures, spectacles, ambulance, etc.

The growth of the scheme is shown by the fact that in 1925 the total funds distributed by the Hospital Savings Association amounted to £65,215, in 1930 to £395,532.

It will be noted that 67 per cent. of the total contributions were paid to voluntary hospitals and between 9 and 10 per cent. to public assistance authorities. The proportion of in-patient treatment given in these hospitals does not correspond to these payments, but is roughly in the ratio of five days' maintenance in voluntary to three in public assistance hospitals.

It is distinctly understood that the contributions do not involve or imply a contract of treatment, and that all hospitals accepting the vouchers of the Hospital Savings Association retain their complete freedom to reject or receive patients on medical grounds alone. During 1928 roughly some 10 per cent. of the in-patients in metropolitan hospitals, and about 8 per cent. of the out-patients at these hospitals, were contributors to the Hospital Savings Association.

No statistics are available as to contributions under this scheme from employers of labour; it is probably much less than one-third of the total amount reached in Sheffield.

On this point we may quote a recent speech of Sir Alan

---

[1] Probably there are 3 million workers in London whose weekly earnings would bring them within the income-limits laid down by the voluntary hospitals.

Anderson (November 28, 1928), who is chairman of the Hospital Savings Association:—

Industry is beginning to do its part. The Group Secretary is doing his, and doing it splendidly; the wage-earner is doing his. What of the employer? He gives generously out of his private purse to hospitals; but the individual employer is being steadily replaced by the limited company, and the board of a limited company hesitates to give its shareholders' money even to charities which each member of the board would support as a private employer. I venture to suggest that our Association enables the limited company to accept obligations which none of its shareholders would wish to ignore, and to give direct and material help to those whom it employs. The employer can help materially. He can give facilities which will greatly ease the Group Secretary's work; and, when the men so decide, he can collect the contribution through the pay-roll, as the Great Western Railway and many other companies are doing. I look forward to the time when it will be a matter of civic pride for every company or firm to see that, by the joint efforts of employee and employer, neither the employee nor his family will be a charge on charity when he goes to hospital. That is the ideal; in one sense it will cost nothing, or will actually save money. If to-day the sick are healed by public charity, it will cost no more to heal them to-morrow out of the profits of their own work. If to-day the sick are not healed because too many people are asking for too much charity, then our plan of self-reliance will prevent not only sickness and suffering, but great economic waste. Our figures show the actual number of cases in each group treated at hospital, and the statistics of the King's Fund tell us the cost. Take one example; it is a company employing some thousands of workpeople, and practically all of those whose wages are within our income-limits are contributors. During the last twelve months they paid up £5,200—a splendid help. Now we know exactly how many out-patients went to hospital, how many in-patients, and for how many days the hospitals kept them. There were 2,671 out-patients and 629 in-patients from that one body of workpeople and their families; and by using the averages supplied by the King's Fund we find that those patients cost the hospitals of London about £7,000. From that £5,200 received from the employees certain expenses have to be deducted, for dental benefit and other things that are not only essential to health, but reduce the call on hospitals. But, speaking broadly, one may say that if the employer added 1d. per week to the worker's 3d. industry would have relieved the charitable public of the whole financial burden of healing the worker and his family. That example is typical; it gives the measure of the deficit to be made good either by charity or by industry. I do not believe that shareholders would deny that a contribution on that scale—which, incidentally, would not be subject to income-tax—was a proper charge against their profits, or would question that health for the worker and his family contributed to a healthy Profit and Loss Account for the business.

THE BIRMINGHAM SCHEME was initiated in 1927, under the direction of a Management Committee comprising representatives of the Voluntary Hospitals Council, the Birmingham Voluntary Hospitals, the Birmingham Hospital Saturday Fund, the Birmingham Hospital Officers, and the Birmingham Chamber of Commerce. The existent Hospital Saturday Fund had already standardised contributions in the factories and workshops at 2d. per head per week, and included 4,219 contributing firms with 260,000 workers. In 1926 the income thus derived reached £67,000. The present extended contributory scheme in its first year raised £141,000 in contributions, and the total membership in 1929 had become 366,857, and the total amount collected £187,323. The population of Birmingham is close to a million.

The following items give the chief points in the scheme:—

(a) Employees in factories and workshops join the industrial section of the scheme, viz. the Birmingham Hospital Saturday Fund.

(b) Employees in municipal, professional, and commercial offices, banks, shops, warehouses, etc. (if not already contributing to the Hospital Saturday Fund) and private individuals of limited income may join the scheme and secure its benefits through the head office, High Street, Birmingham; or at any of the branch offices throughout the city and district.

(c) Domestic servants (indoor and outdoor) may be registered by their employers in the names of their occupations, instead of in the names of persons actually employed at the time. The difficulty arising from change of personnel in domestic staffs may thereby be met.

Contributors pay not less than 2d. a week. In factories, etc., voluntary arrangements can be made for deducting this amount from the wages.

It will be noted that in the Birmingham scheme there is no limit of income for eligibility to be included in the scheme. The practice in this respect varies in different towns. Those who join the Birmingham scheme are, however, warned that—

Contributors who are regarded by the hospital authorities as not coming within the definition of the phrase of "limited income" will, if accepted for treatment, be called upon to make some additional payment towards the cost of their maintenance and treatment, in accordance with the present practice of the hospitals.

Thus the hospital almoner decides as to whether additional payment shall be required from contributors to the scheme who receive hospital treatment.

The scheme safeguards itself against guaranteeing treatment in any case in the following words:—

Membership of the scheme does not of itself ensure admission to any hospital: patients will continue to be admitted in accordance with the discretion of the medical staffs, the accommodation available, and the present practice of the hospitals.

There are 15 voluntary institutions included in the Birmingham scheme, including several special hospitals, but the majority of patients are treated in two large general hospitals. From a financial statement furnished by Mr. Place, the secretary of the Hospital Contributory Scheme, the following interesting summary is derived:—

STATEMENT OF COST IN 1928 AND 1929 £

	£
Total cost of all patients treated in hospitals	645,836
Total cost of contributory patients	326,566
Amount paid from scheme for contributory patients, or about 64 per cent. of cost.	215,366

The hospitals received in the same period £142,400 in the shape of grants from public authorities, in fees, and for private-ward patients. Some of this would go to reduce the proportion of the cost of contributory patients which the contributory scheme does not defray.

THE OXFORD SCHEME

At Oxford a scheme has been initiated, which shows that the principle of contribution can be applied in an agricultural district. Contributors pay 2d. a week, and are entitled to treatment in the Radcliffe Hospital. Non-contributors are expected to pay towards the cost of their treatment. In this scheme also no limit of income is exacted, but it is made clear that treatment on this basis is only intended for those who cannot otherwise afford adequate treatment. Captain Stone states that 60 per cent. of the total income of the hospital is furnished by these contributions. This hospital undertakes the treatment of acute cases sent from poor-law infirmaries, and links up its work with that of rural cottage hospitals.

The preceding examples show that, in certain particulars, no uniform practice is followed. Thus some schemes adopt an income limit, others do not; though in the latter case the contributing patient may be asked to make an additional personal payment if he is found to be well-to-do. In none of the schemes is an absolute promise given that hospital treatment will be forthcoming. Whether it will be given or not depends on the stress of applicants for treatment, and on whether, in the judgment of the medical staff of the hospital, the case is one which ought to receive hospital treatment. Subject to these conditions there is a moral but not a legal contract that the contributor will receive hospital treatment as needed.

The organisers of contributory schemes usually deprecate the view that the contributions constitute an insurance for hospital treatment. The contributions are inadequate to guarantee the cost of this. It is emphasised that the primary object is to secure mass contributions towards hospitals from which contributors as well as more necessitous persons will receive benefits.

The formation of contributory schemes is rapidly becoming general throughout the country; and the movement shows what can be done by well-organised voluntary effort.

This voluntary action is now doing much to make good the chief defect of the national sickness insurance system, which fails to provide consultants and hospital treatment.

Some local contributory schemes are industrial in organisation, as, for instance, the employees of a railway company. Most of the schemes are, however, organised on a local basis. Captain Stone (in *Hospital Organisation and Management*, 1927) states that in 57 schemes contributions are collected by deductions from wages. This evidently is economical of effort, as the employer can deduct the voluntary 2d. or 3d. along with the statutory sum under the National Sickness and Unemployment Insurance Acts (page 111). In most districts employers contribute liberally, but further efforts are needed to ensure a steady proportion between the amounts contributed respectively by employer and employee. The amount contributed by the employee may be 1d., 2d., or 3d. a week. There is difficulty of collection from employees when they are not collected in large industrial establishments, as, for instance, shop-assistants and domestic servants.

THE ALTERED POSITION OF VOLUNTARY HOSPITALS

These contributory schemes raise new medical and administrative problems. The workers contributing these large aggregate sums—even though the amount never suffices to pay the entire expense of treatment—will inevitably begin to claim through their associations some share in the government of the hospitals concerned. In some instances, in smaller towns, this has already occurred. Working-men, members of hospital (especially of cottage hospital) committees, have not always been wise in their appointment of medical staff and in other details of hospital management. This difficulty can only gradually be overcome; and a similar difficulty arises occasionally in the management of official hospitals by elected committees representing the rate-payers. If there is interference in medical care, and especially in the teaching of medical students and nurses, harm will result; but with the spread of intelligence and public spirit this risk will decrease.

Fear has been expressed that contributory schemes may scare away charity. To combat this it can be pointed out that (*a*) the contributions do not cover the entire cost, and that (*b*) a large number must always remain for whom gratuitous treatment is required. There is no essential difficulty in combining charity and providence.

From what has been written it is clear that the rôle of voluntary hospitals has been greatly modified and extended. They remain, as always, invaluable treatment centres for the very poor, and their utility has become more general; their physicians and surgeons give priceless unpaid services to an extent which is marvellous. These hospitals are the chief laboratories in which advances in diagnosis and treatment are tested, and in which almost miraculous triumphs are being secured both by medicine and surgery; and they are the schools in which the physicians, and to some extent the nurses, of the future are trained for their life-work.

But the very advances in scientific treatment obtainable in these hospitals impel conscientious private practitioners to press for the admission of an increasing proportion of their own patients into hospital wards. Many patients, not very poor in the ordinary sense, secure admission also without private medical introduction. Although not necessitous, they cannot afford surgeons' fees for an operation, or the high charges in nursing-homes. For them modified charges are needed and are being slowly and still too scantily arranged. These may vary from payment of the expense of lodging in the hospital, to an amount which still fails to recoup the hospital for the average upkeep of each occupied bed. Sometimes more than this can be paid.

The working of the National Insurance Act has led to further encroachment on hospital beds, with but little addition to hospital funds[1]; and local authorities (see

[1] Captain Stone (*op. cit.*, p. 207) quotes the statistics of a large hospital for 1925, showing that of the total male admissions to its wards 57·1 per cent., and of the total female admissions 35·6 per cent., were of insured

pages 157, 206, 219, 234) have made terms with voluntary hospitals for treating cases of tuberculosis, venereal disease, and maternity and infantile ailments, for which they regard themselves as partially responsible. In addition, much work has been thrown on voluntary hospitals through the Employers' Liability and Workmen's Compensation Acts. The Education Act of 1918 imposed upon all education authorities the "duty" of treating the children under their care in lieu of the previous "power" to treat them and led them to secure and pay for the help of voluntary hospitals in this work.

The essential fact is that hospitals have ceased in large measure to be charitable institutions. An early departure from the strictly charitable position consisted in the payment of large subscriptions by employers of workmen on a large scale. On the strength of these subscriptions treatment for their employees was expected almost as a right.

In recent years workers themselves have contributed on what in the aggregate is a colossal scale, with a partial claim on hospital treatment. It is beside the mark to regard these changes as constituting abuse of hospitals. They represent an evolutionary development which is in the public interest.

England in this respect is approximating the same position which already exists in American hospitals, in which the majority of the patients occupy pay-wards or pay-beds. The difference is that in England, in the majority of instances, treatment will be secured by collective voluntary insurance. True the voluntary insurance payments to secure this, so far, do not cover the cost; but extension of voluntary insurance is competent to secure this end for a large proportion of the population.

PRIVATE PRACTITIONERS AND VOLUNTARY HOSPITALS

The conditions outlined in previous paragraphs affect private medical practice momentously. On the one hand the

persons. For Guy's Hospital, London, Dr. H. L. Eason, C.B., states that 40 per cent. of patients of insurable age attending this hospital were insured persons; 9.4 per cent. of the total ordinary income of 118 metropolitan hospitals was contributed by public authorities.

family doctor is able to call to his aid experts in the serious contingencies and in the circumstances of difficult diagnosis which arise in the general practice of medicine. Such cases are seldom rejected by hospitals, except when (as frequently happens) no bed is available.

As to In-patients.—A patient may be admitted to a hospital bed consequent on an interview in the out-patient department, or he may be admitted on the initiation of his private doctor, or owing to an unexpected emergency or accident. A large proportion of the total cases of illness can be more satisfactorily treated in a hospital than at home. The ever-increasing use of hospitals is evidence of this; and there is no reason to think that the "peak point" has yet been reached.

Decade by decade the position of voluntary hospitals as hospitals for the destitute has been steadily undermined. Poor-law infirmaries, prior to April 1930, were the only hospitals which are strictly hospitals for the destitute; and even for them the definition of destitution legally accepted had come to mean only inability to provide the special medical care needed for health.

The increasing practice of accepting or even exacting payment from patients in voluntary hospitals has substantially changed their position. A system of "finance by begging" (Osler, 1913) is gradually giving way to the practice of taking pay from patients or from public authorities, often from both. The table on page 65 shows that in the majority of hospitals a third, or even a half, of their ordinary income may be thus derived.

It is unfortunate, and is detrimental to both patients and doctors, that usually the private doctor loses touch with his patient when he is admitted to hospital. Sometimes this is due to the private doctor's own inertia. He may be indolent or overworked, or he may not care to visit his patient in the hospital when no fee attaches to the visit. At some hospitals the medical staff have arranged for keeping contact with the practitioner who sent the patient into hospital. Thus at some great hospitals in London the

private practitioner is supplied with an abstract of the
in-patient notes of his patient, including X-ray and pathological reports. This abstract is written by a resident medical
officer, and checked by the visiting physician or surgeon
concerned.

Such a practice could be made general in the out-patient
department, and if the reforms suggested on page 86
are adopted it would become so. I reserve to a concluding volume discussion of the moot point as to whether
and to what extent private doctors can continue to treat
their patients while they are in a hospital. The point
arises also in subsequent chapters as related to official
tuberculosis institutions and maternity hospitals (pp. 158
and 220).

Several further points need consideration: (1) As to the
position of the visiting staff of general and special hospitals
when the hospital receives payment for patients.

Many voluntary hospitals receive payment from public
health authorities for patients sent to them by these authorities. Those patients may include cases of surgical tuberculosis,
venereal disease, minor operations for school children,
etc. In London (p. 65) 7·5 per cent. of the income of
metropolitan voluntary hospitals is derived from this
source. But the visiting medical and surgical staff of these
hospitals are almost always honorary officers, and the
attitude of the British Medical Association and of a majority
of the medical profession is that their services should not
be given gratuitously for such patients. The same problem
arises in a less acute form under the hospital contributory
schemes described in preceding paragraphs. The B.M.A.
recommends that a certain proportion of the payments
received—say 10 to 20 per cent.—by the hospital for such
patients as the above should be handed over to the staff
(not to the individual member of the staff who has treated
a given case), and that this should be divided among the
staff or used for new apparatus, for research, or otherwise
as the staff may decide. These medical payments are undoubtedly advisable, and the advantages in professional

prestige accruing from a position on an honorary medical staff do not veto this conclusion.

(2) Should the family doctor have the right to continue to treat his patient when admitted to a hospital, perhaps subject to consultation with the regular staff of the hospital? The discussion of this point is reserved, as is also (3) the more general problem of the future relation between voluntary and public assistance hospitals, as bearing on private medical practice.

As to out-patients, for even well-to-do patients, the family practitioner rightly arranges for treatment in a hospital or other institution and for expert diagnostic tests when special knowledge and skill and special appliances are required, which he in his individual capacity cannot supply. In a much larger proportion of his cases, when the patient, although competent to pay the doctor's own fees, cannot afford a consultant's fee or the cost of a radiographic or other examination, the private doctor who wishes to do the best possible for his patient arranges for a consultation at the appropriate department of a general or at a special hospital. In such cases, when he sends an explanatory note to the hospital consultant, the latter, although an unpaid officer of the hospital, is generally willing to send back a considered diagnosis. When a verbal message or merely the doctor's card is sent, no communication may be received; and in such instances the private doctor must be held in default. If a satisfactory report was expected, at least all preliminary information should have been furnished.

The out-patient departments of voluntary hospitals are still very largely abused. As nearly all the wage-earners in the population are insured, these departments ought to be used chiefly and almost solely for consultation between the hospital and the private doctor. If hospital authorities would agree to this, there would be immediate relief of the strain on hospital doctors. In some hospitals this has already been done, as, for instance, at the London Hospital (one of the metropolitan general hospitals with a medical school attached to it). At this hospital it is stated that, practically speaking, out-patients are only seen when they come with a letter from a private practitioner, to whom a letter concerning the patient is sent in due course.

Figures as to the influence of national sickness insurance on the number of out-patients differ in various towns. One would have expected insurance to reduce out-patients to a very large extent; often, however, they have increased beyond the increase of population, in part, doubtless, owing to the personal desire of the poor to obtain those expert facilities for diagnosis and treatment which richer persons can afford, and which are not provided at present in national sickness insurance medical work. But it may be that in other instances the fact that the "panel" doctor is paid, whether the patient is well or ill on a capitation basis, has some influence.

From the view-point of the patient, there is need to restrict the number of out-patients so that each may receive adequate attention. It is a scandal that out-patients may sometimes be kept waiting for many hours before they obtain a medical interview, and that then this interview may be hurried. The aggregate economic loss of working hours for workers and indirect loss for mothers which is tolerated in present arrangements at many hospital out-patient departments must be colossal, and would go far to pay for the increased cost of prompt and unhurried consultations. The loss of wages alone would often suffice to pay for satisfactory medical advice.

The B.M.A. on the Problem of the Out-Patient

Since the above paragraphs were ready for publication, the Council of the B.M.A. has issued a useful report (*Brit. Med. Journ. Supplement*, February 21, 1931) on this subject. The Report classifies out-patients as: (1) casualty cases; (2) ordinary chronic cases; (3) consultation cases, including those retained for special treatment; and (4) discharged in-patients. The second of these groups is probably responsible for the great bulk of unjustifiable demands on the services of the hospital staff, and the report properly advises sending such patients back to a private or insurance or public assistance doctor. The report mentions a real difficulty in securing this in every case owing to "the existence of practitioners who are quite willing that patients of the chronic variety, particularly contract patients, should go elsewhere for their treatment".

They give, in conclusion, the following summary and recommendations:—

1. That a large amount of the work at present undertaken at the out-patient departments of voluntary hospitals is unnecessary and can be reduced.

2. That the volume of work at present undertaken at the out-patient departments is such that the best use cannot be made of the services of the members of the hospital staffs.

3. That there is considerable wastage of public money and of professional time and skill.

4. That the existing internal and external checks at present employed are not sufficiently stringent.

5. That further checks and safeguards should be established at all voluntary hospitals before treatment is undertaken at the out-patient department.

6. That the primary object of the out-patient department should be for consultation.

7. That while there should be adequate opportunities for consultation purposes between the private practitioner and members of the visiting medical staffs at out-patient departments, practitioners should not countenance the use of that department by their patients, except in the ways laid down in this memorandum.

8. That the casualty department should be available in any emergency.

9. That only such treatment should be given at the department as cannot in the best interests of the patient be obtained elsewhere under the usual arrangements as between private practitioner and private patient, or under contract arrangements.

10. That cases admitted for treatment at out-patient departments should be reviewed at regular intervals by the medical staffs.

11. That no person, except in cases of emergency, should be accepted for treatment as an out-patient at a voluntary hospital unless he brings a recommendation from a private medical practitioner, a provident or other dispensary, a public clinic, or from a public assistance medical officer of a local authority.

CHAPTER IV

GENERAL MEDICAL SERVICES IN ENGLAND (*continued*)

B. OFFICIAL MEDICAL ASSISTANCE FOR THE NECESSITOUS

FROM the remote past, and particularly during the eighteenth and nineteenth centuries, gratuitous medical aid has been given by medical practitioners, either in the course of their daily personal medical work, or through organisations such as dispensaries and hospitals. In 1687 the Royal College of Physicians of London authorised its members to give medical aid gratis to the poor. At that time a struggle was going on as to the relative spheres of the physician and the apothecary, and policy as well as philanthropy may have actuated this increased provision of gratuitous medical service for the poor. The history of hospital and dispensary provision need not be pursued here; but at an early stage clear-sighted philanthropists recognised that medical relief is relatively free from the abuses liable to be associated with monetary gifts. The Rev. Dr. Chalmers, of Glasgow, in the first decade of the nineteenth century enunciated this difference very clearly :—

An ostensible provision for the relief of poverty creates more poverty. An ostensible provision for the relief of disease does not cause more disease. The human will is enlisted on the side of poverty by the provision which is made for it. No such provision will ever enlist the human will on the side of disease.

This important distinction during many decades failed to receive adequate recognition, especially in the official relief of the poor, a fact which goes far to explain the imperfections of its medical side during the nineteenth century. The modern system of poor-law administration from which England has only very gradually emerged was initiated in 1834, and the Annual Report of the Poor-Law Commission for 1841 included the following significant paragraph, which illustrates our point:—

We entertain no doubt of our being able ultimately to establish a complete and effective system of medical relief for all paupers, yet its very completeness and effectiveness, however beneficial to those who are its objects, may have an influence, which ought not to be disregarded, on other classes of society. If the pauper is always promptly attended by a skilful and well-qualified medical practitioner . . . if the patient is furnished with all the cordials and stimulants which may promote his recovery . . . this superiority of the pauper . . . will encourage a resort to the poor rates for medical relief.

Here it is suggested plainly that medical treatment for the necessitous, in view of the social consequence of acting otherwise, should be kept on a lower plane of efficiency than treatment for other sections of the population. At the present day this suggestion would be repudiated by all, and in theory at least the universal standard is accepted that every sick person, whether able to pay fully, partially, or not at all for treatment, ought to be treated with equal skill and care in essentials.

We need not blame the poor-law system for its earlier and less humane view. Similar distinctions contrary to the principles of Christian charity have only broken down very gradually in the regulation of conditions of industrial work, of domestic sanitation, and of other departments of communal life. Even now in some communities medical treatment for the poor is far from reaching the ideal, but the general wish is to attain to it. This wish is not actuated solely by humanitarian sentiment; it is powerfully stimulated by the realisation that its fulfilment is in the economic interest of the community. Such a large share of destitution is due to sickness that the two problems of sickness and destitution cannot be successfully treated in isolation from each other. In England "one-third of the paupers are sick, one-third children, and one-quarter either widows encumbered by young families or certified lunatics". And we know that the widows and children dependent on public assistance most often have become so as the result of sickness and death of the breadwinner.

The boards of guardians have always been strictly regulated in their activities by the Central Government; and the general principle adopted has been one of more or less limitation of relief, so as not to curtail private charity and thrift. Furthermore, as we have seen, it has been held that the condition of the person relieved shall compare unfavourably with that of self-supporting families, a principle of deterrence which, however legitimate for the able-bodied destitute, constitutes a fundamental social blunder when applied to children and to sick persons. In respect to both of these it has gradually been abandoned.

A person must be destitute before he becomes eligible for official relief. Personal merit rightly does not enter into the question of the bestowal of this relief. The poor-law authority under general law has had no option but to give the needed relief when the need for it is proved, and thus during several centuries no person in Great Britain has needed to continue to suffer from protracted hunger or from lack of lodging. But this beneficent provision had within it no influence in preventing destitution. In strict accordance with the law the former guardians and the present public assistance committees can only relieve existent destitution: they cannot spend the ratepayers' money in action which might prevent a person from becoming destitute.

Happily in recent decades destitution has been interpreted to *include the lack of material resources to satisfy any existent or threatening physical need, as, for instance, the need of medical care.*[1]

[1] The fuller definition, officially accepted, is that given by Mr. Adrian, Legal Adviser to the Local Government Board, in his evidence before the Poor Law Commission, as follows:—

"Destitution when used to describe the condition of a person as a subject for relief, implies that he is, for the time being, without material resources (i) directly available and (ii) appropriate for satisfying his physical needs— (*a*) whether actually existing, or (*b*) likely to arise immediately. By physical needs in this definition are meant such needs as must be satisfied (i) in order to maintain life or (ii) to obviate, mitigate, or remove causes endangering life, or likely to endanger life or impair health or bodily fitness for self-support."

The realisation that a person may be specifically destitute in respect of need for costly medical care, while not absolutely so in other respects, has opened the way to rapid improvement in the poor-law medical service during the present century. In later paragraphs are given some particulars of the more modern medical arrangements under the poor-law.

These from 1930 onward will be administered by public assistance committees of the large public health authorities.

The fact that destitution, general or specific, as, for instance, the inability to pay for medical care, must exist before public assistance can be given, means that the aid given has its minimum capacity for being restorative in character, and possesses relatively little power to prevent later destitution. Disease is treated when already well-established. Not only so, but in practice medical treatment under the poor-law and the associated monetary grants have not been so administered as to conduce to a better life. Thus the patient with delirium tremens was not disciplined, the prostitute with gonorrhœa or syphilis was not restrained from spreading infection, the consumptive patient in a crowded bedroom was not treated in conditions which held out the prospect of recovery and avoided serious risk to others.

These defects were not, of course, special to poor-law arrangements, though in the circumstances of the necessitous they were especially serious. In wider circles preventive medicine failed to become effective. In the case of the necessitous, however, there existed exceptional but neglected power to enforce reform by making it a condition of the weekly money allowance associated with medical aid; and this power was seldom utilised.

In some instances the giving of relief was made conditional on admission to the poor-law infirmary; but this was not consistently utilised as a specific means of securing reformed habits or the prevention of infection.

General dissatisfaction with poor-law administration led to the appointment of a Royal Commission on the Poor

Laws, which reported in 1909, recommending the abolition of directly elected boards of guardians, and their replacement by committees of the great local authorities elected for all purposes of local government. This reform has been accomplished in 1930.

The details of the defects of poor-law administration on its medical side were fully revealed in the reports of the Royal Commission. It was shown how defective was the medical care and nursing given, especially in the smaller poor-law infirmaries, even though there had been slow improvement decade by decade; and detailed investigation showed that the whole system of poor-law medical provision was inadequate and needed to be continuously supplemented from without. It was, in short, "a cripple supported on two crutches, the general (voluntary) hospitals on one side, and gratuitous medical work on the other" (McVail). These props were inadequate, for general hospitals were unequally distributed, private charity was spasmodic and erratic in its incidence, and the willingness of doctors to do gratuitous medical work varied greatly.

The public assistance medical service has two branches—domiciliary medical attendance, and institutional treatment—for those who cannot be satisfactorily treated in their homes. Notwithstanding the serious defects indicated above, this dual service is the most complete public medical service in existence in the British Isles, for it provides both domiciliary and institutional treatment, unlike voluntary hospitals or the National Sickness Insurance Act. Poor-law medical provision, nevertheless, was regarded by the people with distaste, and was only accepted by the majority of the poor when other possibilities had been exhausted. This distaste has broken down to a considerable extent for infirmaries for the sick; though these have been utilised less than was desirable, owing to the persistence of the antipathy of the poor to receive help from a source which implied serious loss of social standing.

ADMINISTRATIVE MACHINERY FOR RELIEF

Prior to April 1930, poor-relief including medical aid was under the control of boards of guardians elected directly by the ratepayers of each parish or union of parishes. The number of these boards is given on page 29. Since the above date the elected local authorities of counties and county boroughs, which are larger units than most parishes or unions, carry on the relief work through a special public assistance committee, while certain parts of the former work of the Guardians, including hospital provision and care of children, is or may be transferred to the public health and education committees of the councils.

Medical relief, as we have seen, may take the form of domiciliary or of institutional treatment. I do not propose to describe the provision for the insane, as no problem of encroachment on private practice is involved in their care.

HOME TREATMENT OF THE SICK POOR

There is a parochial medical officer (D.M.O.) for each parish or union, more for very populous unions. In England they number over 3,400. They are paid a salary for attending the sick poor in their homes, the salary varying from a few pounds to £100 per annum, or perhaps more. The D.M.O. has security of tenure of office. He can only be removed from office with consent of the Ministry of Health after inquiry. He is also eligible for a pension on retirement. These appointments are held by private practitioners in the district: and the appointment, although usually held at a salary which is inadequate for the amount of work done, is sought after as forming a useful introduction to more lucrative practice. Often well-established doctors in rural districts retain the position to avoid competition from new-comers. In a few towns whole-time medical officers attend the sick poor in their homes. This is exceptional, and the appointment of whole-time physicians for clinical work outside hospitals is strongly opposed by the British Medical Association.

In Bermondsey, Lambeth, and Rotherhithe, divisions of London, the assistant medical officers of the public assistance infirmary act also as district medical officers, and it is claimed that while good domiciliary medical aid is given, the selection of patients for institutional treatment can thus be more satisfactorily made than by private practitioners.

With the increasing utilisation of poor-law infirmaries by those seriously ill, and since the advent of the Sickness Insurance Act, the work of the D.M.O. has declined. Very often he is also public vaccinator for the union, and in this capacity is required to undertake the primary vaccination and sometimes the revaccination of all applicants, irrespective of social or economic position. He is paid a fee for each vaccination by the public assistance committee.

Thus in every parish throughout the country any person unable to pay a medical fee is entitled to free medical attendance. Even the prior investigation by the relieving officer, the lay official concerned to make the necessary inquiries for the public assistance committee, can be dispensed with in emergencies.

This domiciliary work sometimes has been carelessly performed and has fallen into disrepute. When the work is well done, it is admirable. When district nurses are available it can minimise the stress on institutional provision otherwise inevitable. In one union in London with a quarter of a million population, the number of daily home visits required were stated by the D.M.O. to average four. In addition, he has one hour's surgery work daily for these patients. There can be no doubt that (a) a doctor is still needed for the sick poor living at home; and that (b) the D.M.O. is often needed to protect the infirmary against the admission of patients who can satisfactorily be treated at home. The practice in this respect varies greatly. The medical superintendent of one infirmary informed me that he always accepted the certificate of any private practitioner without the intervention of the D.M.O.; another superintendent was emphatic that although some doctors' certificates could be implicitly trusted it was necessary in other instances to have the check of the D.M.O. or of an assistant medical officer sent specially from the infirmary.

In an address as President of the Poor Law Medical Officers' Association (July 1925) I outlined the position in the following words:—

Whatever plans are evolved for future administration of medical aid to the sick poor, the preliminary duty devolves upon the public of expressing their indebtedness to the district medical officers who for many decades have tended the sick poor in their homes. While agreeing that the standard of medical work, like that in ordinary general medical practice, has varied within wide limits, there can be no hesitation in stating that these officers, in the main, have rendered invaluable service to those most in need of it, generally for remuneration which has been quite inadequate, often disgracefully so. As you know, the post of district medical officer has been frequently offered and accepted at a figure which was a direct temptation to neglect of the sick; and it is no defence of this inadequate remuneration to remember that the doctor accepting it often did so in order to avoid the competitive intrusion of a rival doctor into his district. Even now there is needed some standard of payment for domiciliary medical attendance on the sick poor, based on records of work done and on amount of travel required in doing this work; and it is unfortunate that the lamentable deficiency of records and of statistical summary of records in nearly every union through the country makes this, in the absence of reform, almost impracticable.

The circumstances of the work of district medical officers have changed with the great increase of institutional treatment under the Poor Law. There has been great increase in the work of the district medical officer in regard to certification, but reduction in the actual amount of continuous domiciliary attendance.

Institutional Treatment of the Insane

I have not included in my survey treatment of the insane and feeble-minded at the public expense, as almost no difficulties arise in the adjustments between private and public medical practice; but it is convenient to insert here some of the chief figures as to the treatment of mental disorders in England and Wales. On January 1, 1930, the

number of notified insane under care was 142,387, of whom
14,537, or nearly 10 per cent., were private patients maintained at no cost to public funds. In the year 1929 the cost
of lunacy provision for rate-aided cases was £8,441,037.
Of this sum £1,766,428 was recovered from various sources,
including £651,815 from relatives.

Patients are admitted to mental hospitals unconditionally
in respect of finance; their ability or that of their relatives
to contribute is settled after their admission to the mental
hospital or to the public assistance hospital to which they
may have been sent in the first instance. Where contributions to cost are assessed, these are collected by an officer of
the public assistance authority.

Institutional Treatment of the Sick Poor

The slow development of infirmaries for the poor is the
best illustration of the prolonged process of escape from
the earlier deterrent views as to the treatment of the sick
poor. Workhouses (poor-houses) preceded infirmaries; sick
wards were a later development. Even when treatment was
given, it remained the general rule to transfer patients needing skilled surgical treatment to voluntary hospitals. In
1864–65 there was public agitation anent the neglect of the
sick poor in workhouses and their sick wards, led by Dr.
Rogers and other reformers; and from 1867 onwards reform
advanced. A chief feature of this reform was the more
general provision of infirmaries for the sick poor in separate
wards and to a steadily increasing extent in separate institutions from the workhouses with which they had previously
always been combined.

In London the Metropolitan Asylums Board was formed
to provide for the treatment in hospitals of mentally
defective and crippled children, of fever and smallpox
cases, on a uniform basis for the whole of the metropolis.
The provision of lunatic asylums has rested chiefly with
the London County Council.

In the last 20 or 30 years urban boards of guardians,
especially in the larger towns, have provided infirmaries

which in completeness of structural arrangements compare very favourably with the best voluntary hospitals. If we omit the institutions in which the old, the infirm, and decrepit, who are not necessarily ill, continue to be treated along with other patients suffering from serious disease, the improvement is marvellous; and there is little doubt that the mixed institutions which remain will ere long disappear. This separation involves difficulties, as many workhouse inmates being old and feeble are intermittently ill and require careful medical care and nursing.

The medical staffing of public assistance infirmaries or hospitals has greatly improved. Prior to the Great War it was often inadequate to the work. Now, in the larger institutions, there is always a whole-time medical superintendent with whole-time medical officers competent for all ordinary medical and surgical work. Many of these institutions also have a visiting staff of physicians and surgeons for consultative work. London infirmaries all have a staff of specialists who can be called in at any time by the medical superintendent.

Comparisons of the medical and nursing staffs of official and voluntary hospitals may be somewhat misleading. The superintendent of a public assistance hospital cannot refuse patients in urgent need of hospital care, while at a voluntary hospital cases can be selected; and it is a general practice to transfer incurable post-operative and other cases including various chronic diseases from the wards of voluntary hospitals to a public assistance hospital. The differences in utilisation of voluntary and official hospitals are rapidly diminishing as the demands for hospital provision increase and voluntary hospitals become more and more unequal to meet it.

The nursing staff of infirmaries was formerly most inadequate and inefficient. In earlier days nursing was entrusted to able-bodied women who were paupers residing in the workhouse, and only gradually were these replaced by trained nurses.

Dr. C. T. Parsons, in the *Lancet* (March 10, 1920), gave

a table for metropolitan infirmaries showing that the number of beds varied in that year from 7·1 to 13·4 for each nurse, whereas in metropolitan voluntary hospitals the number of beds varied from 2·0 to 2·6 per nurse. The difference is not completely explained by the greater proportion of bed-ridden chronic cases (e.g. paralytic, helpless senile, rheuma-toid arthritic cases) in the infirmaries; these often need more nursing than acute cases. Improvement has steadily occurred. Thus, at the West Middlesex Hospital at Brentford (until 1930 under the Poor Law), there are 140 nurses for 400 beds. Untrained women are now never employed as nurses, the nursing staff is more adequate, and public assistance hospitals have become the chief training centres for nurses in Britain.

Public assistance hospitals have come into use also very largely for accidents and for acute illness, especially when the beds in available voluntary hospitals are full. In fact, the two have become complementary to each other: and the notion that public assistance infirmaries can be ear-marked for chronic and incurable patients and voluntary hospitals for acute cases and cases requiring special skill has proved to be untenable. Before the recent transfer of the management of poor-law infirmaries to the public assis-tance committees of public health authorities occurred, the word "poor-law" had been dropped, and that of in-firmary changed to hospital, in order to decrease the prejudice arising from the association of these hospitals with poor-law administration.

Now that these official hospitals are open to all who need hospital treatment, either gratuitously or on payment assessed according to the patient's means, there will cease to be undesirable inhibitory influence to their use.

Notes on some Public Assistance Hospitals

(1) *The West Middlesex Hospital.*—This hospital serves the thirteen parishes comprising until 1930 the Brentford Union. The population of these parishes has swarmed over from London, and in 1921 it numbered 291,438 on an area of 23,062 acres. The hospital has 400 beds, with a staff of

140 nurses, of whom 90 are probationers. Its whole-time medical superintendent, Dr. Basil Cook, has four assistant medical officers (whole-time). The staff of visiting consultants comprises an electro-therapeutist, a radiologist, a consulting surgeon, a consulting physician, a consulting gynæcologist, and a consulting aural surgeon.

In the year 1929 the patients admitted numbered 3,294, as compared with 2,003 in 1921. Dr. Cook, in a recent report, makes the following remarks which summarise the distinction between an official and a voluntary hospital:—

The difference between the work in a voluntary hospital and a poor-law hospital is not always appreciated. The former refuses to admit cases when all its beds are full. We cannot refuse cases, and if all our beds are occupied extra beds have to be erected down the centre of the ward when necessary.

There are also cases of an infectious or undesirable nature, such as puerperal fever, erysipelas, measles, as well as epilepsy, mental cases, etc., which are altogether refused admission by voluntary hospitals. We cannot select our cases, and we are compelled to make provision for nearly every class of disease.

The rapid increase in the surgical work of official hospitals is shown by the following figures for this hospital:—

Year				Number of Operations
1896–97	..	..	..	.. 30
1914 ..	..	..	..	.. 111
1929 ..	..	..	..	.. 452

(2) *Lambeth Hospital.*—This hospital serves a large section of inner London on the south side of the Thames.

(3) *Lewisham Hospital.*—This hospital serves a wide area in the south-eastern suburbs of London.

The Lambeth Hospital (A) serves a population of 312,000, the Lewisham Hospital (B) of about 223,000. A has 902 beds staffed by trained nurses, and 610 further beds for the infirm; B has 427 beds. A had 767 in-patients, not including the infirm, while B had 4,927 patients in 1927. At A 1,899 operations and at B 1,228 operations were performed in the operation theatre in the year. In A 451 and in B 337 infants were born in the year. Only a small minority of the patients paid a share of the cost of maintenance in each hospital. The maximum charged in A is 35s. a week. Each hospital has a resident medical superintendent and a whole-time resident staff of five to eight doctors, some appointed for two years only. There are also paid non-resident consultants for each hospital.

Each of these hospitals has a pathological laboratory, special departments for massage and electric treatment, and an out-patient department which acts as a receiving ward and is utilised for the treatment of minor ailments.

These institutions emphasise the absurdity of the contention sometimes advanced that official hospitals should be utilised mainly for "remainders"—for patients who are scarcely suitable for voluntary hospitals; though we can agree that when both voluntary and official hospitals are within reach, the aim of the voluntary hospital should be to secure a rapid succession of cases needing expert investigation, of acute cases, and of cases requiring major operations. The adjustment between voluntary and official hospitals is in process; and local needs will determine the result. Doubtless voluntary hospitals, especially the larger hospitals, in which the teaching of students is undertaken, will be able to continue to select their patients, while official hospitals cannot do so when there is need for hospital treatment; and voluntary hospitals will continue more largely than official hospitals to be centres not only for teaching but also for research. For teaching there should be no insuperable difficulty in making the invaluable clinical material of public assistance hospitals available for medical training, and tentative efforts in this direction have already been made. The experience of Aberdeen is especially interesting (p. 490). Public assistance hospitals are already the centres for the training of the majority of midwives and nurses.

The examples already given of highly efficient official general hospitals, now controlled by the great public health authorities, are not exceptional. There are many such in Britain, and their number and standard of work steadily increase. Their increase in number and accommodation is in sharp contrast to the relatively stationary accommodation of voluntary hospitals, whose beds form a decreasing proportion of aggregate hospital provision. This is not surprising, as the majority of the patients applying for treatment in voluntary hospitals are legally entitled to relief in an official hospital. It is becoming increasingly evident that, with steadily growing demands, voluntary hospitals cannot deal with more than a relatively small percentage of the necessitous sick. Both voluntary and official hospitals now admit an increasing proportion of patients who pay partially or entirely for their maintenance in hospital.

The changes roughly indicated above have arisen in part because of the obligatory duty of public assistance committees to admit all patients in need of hospital treatment. Their increasing use for the treatment of patients suffering from the results of street emergencies and accidents has conduced to the same end. And perhaps even more the increased use of hospitals has arisen because of the growth of medical science, necessitating a vast increase in utilisation of the special resources of a hospital. The private practitioners are primarily responsible for this increased use of hospitals; for it is their realisation that the expert surgeon or physician or pathologist, or all of these, are needed for their patient that has necessitated the increase of hospital beds. Voluntary hospitals have not failed in their work; but they could not keep pace with the demands. Hence many patients day by day are denied admission, and sent instead to public assistance hospitals. This trend is increased, especially in London, by the fact that these hospitals are fairly well distributed throughout outer as well as inner London; while most of the voluntary hospitals are centrally placed.

The distinction between public assistance hospitals and voluntary hospitals was breaking down even before the Great War, so far as concerns the kind of patients admitted and the financial conditions. A pioneer example is that of Bradford (its estimated population in 1927 was 293,200). A Scottish example is quoted on page 490.

For the following statement as to Bradford I am chiefly indebted to Dr. J. J. Buchan, the M.O.H. of this city.

Bradford at the end of the war had a large war hospital of 1,500 beds, which had developed from the small nucleus of a workhouse infirmary of 250 beds by reconstruction and rebuilding, in the course of which the whole of the workhouse attached to the old infirmary had been included. For the destitute a permanent workhouse had been built elsewhere.

Before the war the City Council had been considering how to meet the deficiency of voluntary hospital beds, and now the Board of Guardians were faced with the reversion of a large hospital of which they could not make full use. Negotiations followed in which it was agreed that this hospital should be let by the Guardians to the City Council on the undertaking that it should be conducted as a public general hospital for the city, receiving on behalf of the Guardians such of the sick poor as required hospital treatment, but without making any differentiation of patients on other than medical grounds.

Some opposition to the city running a general hospital arose, but this was overcome. Evidently the relation of the Bradford Royal Infirmary—a voluntary general hospital— to the proposed new institution was involved. The City Council undertook that the new hospital would be conducted as a large general hospital, and that it should have not only a resident but also a consultant and specialist staff. For this purpose about half of the staff of the Royal Infirmary were asked to serve also on the staff of the new hospital, and this having been arranged harmony was greatly helped. The staff, unlike that of the Royal Infirmary, were paid. Each consultant as a rule received £500 per annum, being required to spend on his work in hospital at least eight hours weekly during at least three sessions. In fact, this minimum is often greatly exceeded by the staff. One surgeon performed nearly 1,000 major operations in 1930, although his salary was only as above. At both the Royal Infirmary and at the New Municipal Hospital, paid resident house physicians and house surgeons are appointed for a limited time only. The choice of patients between the municipal and voluntary hospitals is determined by the local reputation of the staff of each hospital, as judged by the general practitioner who sends his patient for hospital treatment. The known specialisation of members of a hospital staff is always an important determining factor in the distribution of patients. The voluntary hospital may, furthermore, refuse a case which will occupy a bed for a long time, and so on. In short, the sorting of patients takes place without any definite laying down of rules.

The Relation of the General Practitioner to the Public Assistance Hospital

As already stated, the general practitioner is himself largely, perhaps chiefly, responsible for the greater resort of patients to hospital. It is his increased knowledge and his conscientious regard for his patient's welfare which sends so many patients into hospital, even though by so doing he deprives himself of much medical interest and some income. As Dr. Nockolds, the superintendent of the Lewisham Hospital, has put it (*Lancet*, July 16, 1927): "It is the general practitioner who overcrowds our wards and who sends in patients at all hours of the day and night. . . . It is the needs of the general practitioner which have to be met. . . ." And he adds: "A larger number of poor-law hospitals throughout the country will have to adapt themselves to the needs of the local practitioners, as it seems doubtful whether the increased accommodation needed for the future will be entirely met by increased voluntary hospital accommodation."

A facile method of allowing private practitioners to send their patients to hospital without prior consultation is open to abuse. Sometimes dying patients are sent, or patients who ought to be retained at home because of hæmoptysis or hæmatemesis; or patients with acute abdominal disease are sent without any intimation that morphia has been administered, or patients are sent without intimation that they are infectious. A mental case may be sent as neurasthenia, and so on. At Lambeth Hospital these difficulties have led to a system of examination of patients before admission by one of the infirmary assistant medical officers (p. 94); but in Lewisham direct admission on the certificate of a private medical practitioner is allowed.

Official hospital provision—as also that of voluntary hospitals when obtainable—often relieves the hard-pressed practitioner of responsibility, with which, single-handed or even when helped by a confrère, he could not successfully cope. Many operations are beyond his competence; and in a still larger number of cases the home nursing and comforts available do not give the patient a fair chance of recovery.

Cases of inoperable cancer, of rheumatoid arthritis, hemiplegia, etc., need hospital care for prolonged periods, which cannot be provided in voluntary hospitals. Such cases go far to explain the statement sometimes made that the treatment given in public assistance hospitals is commonly belated and is treatment only of "end-products". There are, however, other instances in which the private practitioners are blameworthy. Here are a few instances recently given me by the medical superintendent of a public assistance hospital:—

1. A patient admitted on Saturday had been suffering since the previous Tuesday with violent abdominal pain. When sent in by the patient's doctor, he was certified to be suffering from "paratyphoid". Within an hour a perforated gastric ulcer of five days' standing was stitched up, and the patient recovered!

2. Sometimes patients are admitted with a history of diarrhœa of 6 to 8 months' duration, for which they have been treated medicinally. They have never been examined *per rectum*, and on admission an inoperable carcinoma is found.

3. A boy, aged 10 years, was admitted having been certified as suffering for four days from bronchitis. Diphtheritic membrane covered the pharynx, and tracheotomy was necessary at once.

4. Midwifery offers the widest range of unnecessary complications, followed by loss of life or injury for life, in the experience of both official and voluntary hospitals.

Thus the doctor attending the patient uses forceps in a case in which forceps are not indicated; through his inexperience or otherwise, the patient is badly lacerated and septic; and sometimes the doctor has not, after all, succeeded in delivering the child.

The superintendent giving me this information adds: "No one who has not worked in a poor-law infirmary can have any idea of the appalling inefficiency of some panel doctors in a poor locality."

In quoting these exceptional instances of *mala praxis*, I must protest against wide generalisations based on occasional incompetence. But the instances of inexperience and incompetence are so numerous in the aggregate as to give institutional doctors a deep desire that their services could be obtained at an earlier date, when they would have a reasonable prospect of saving patients from permanent injury or death. They also indicate the need for the provision of ample consultative facilities for poorer patients in their own home, when an inexperienced practitioner is in doubt or difficulty.

SUMMARY

The poor-law (now municipal and county) official medical service, as already stated, more completely meets the need of the necessitous than any other medical service. It is unique in that potentially—and already in fact to a certain extent—it provides for the treatment of the sick poor at home or in hospital in every parish in the land; and that it constitutes a complete acknowledgment on the part of *the people* that—in the absence of other provision—they *are responsible for the medical care of the sick poor.*

As it is now an accepted principle that the necessitous sick must be treated in accordance with the nature of their illness, and not with skill or care which varies with the degree of ability to pay, there is no reason to doubt that all requiring this succour will receive it to a fuller extent than has hitherto been realised. The increasing adoption of payments for treatment assessed in proportion to means, both in voluntary and in official hospitals, brings this end more quickly within reach.

A few figures may be added showing the increase of poor-law relief given in England and Wales when 1914 is compared with 1928. In 1914 the proportion per 10,000 of the estimated population receiving relief was 208, 154 in 1920, and 347 in 1928; while the rates collected per head of the estimated population were as follows:—

RATES COLLECTED PER HEAD OF POPULATION

	1914	1927	Percentage Increase
	£ s. d.	£ s. d.	
For relief of the poor and purposes connected therewith ..	0 6 5	0 19 2	+199
For all other purposes .	1 12 6	3 2 6	+ 92

The increased *per capita* expenditure is, in part, accounted for by the exceptional prevalence of unemployment. In so far as it implies increased use of beds in official hospitals and asylums it represents increased provision out of the communal purse for common needs rather than a greater amount of destitution.

CHAPTER V

GENERAL MEDICAL SERVICES
IN ENGLAND (*continued*)

C. THE ENGLISH INSURANCE MEDICAL SERVICE

THE immediate aim of sickness insurance is to ensure maintenance and help in sickness. This, apart from association and combination of large numbers, is usually impracticable for wage-earners. The value of such co-operation is evident; and insurance from the view-point of medical practice is as acutely interesting and important as it is from that of the insured and of the social student. We assume, then, that no objection can be raised to provision by mutual insurance against a most serious and almost universal contingency in life, and that dissension will be limited to the methods of application of the principle. Every member of the community is concerned that he himself and every other member of the community has an adequate and, if possible, an equal opportunity of maintaining and recovering health; for social efficiency and individual independence of charitable aid depend chiefly on health. For education and health there is no difference in social opinion as to the necessity of communal provision, though action in regard to education has outpaced efforts for the improvement of health. This is especially true as regards the efficient diagnosis and treatment of sickness in workers, and the measures of personal hygiene which should form part of medical practice.

Sickness insurance had a firm hold on English workingmen before 1911, when the first National Insurance Act (referred to hereafter as N.I.A.) was passed.

Wage-earners had formed friendly societies, some with and some without geographical limitations in their membership, for ensuring money benefits and medical attendance during illness. In 1815 the membership of these societies was 925,439. In 1904 they numbered 5,700,000. As a rule the members of these older societies were the more thrifty workers, while those most liable to become a burden on public funds held aloof. This may be regarded as justifying the departure in 1911 from the voluntary system of insurance, compulsorily bringing within its scope from 12 to 13 million employed persons.

The voluntary system had virtues which can only be acquired slowly by a compulsory system. Each club or society was concerned with the health of its members. A sick member was visited by other members of the society, not in the capacity of spy—though that element may have existed—but as mutually interested in each other's well-being. There was a strong element of local and club patriotism which made it a point of honour to "go on the club" as seldom and to stop on it for as short a time as possible. This identification of self with the communal interest is a plant of fragile and slow growth in a compulsory system, in which societies with an immense clientèle are the rule, and the friendly society atmosphere has faded; and in which there exists too often a vague impression that the State is a separate entity, whose funds may be drawn on to an unlimited extent without affecting the financial welfare of each member of the community.

The weak point of the old friendly societies was their medical arrangements. Doctors in working-class districts were alive to the fact that they would often fail to receive payment for their medical services, unless some arrangement were made on a contract basis. The system of contract medical service for such people was not objected to so much as its detailed management, and oft-times doctors were in effect competing with each other for appointment by these societies, after the fashion of a "Dutch auction". A contract was made by each society with a local doctor, who usually received annually 3s., 3s. 6d., or 4s. (4s. nearly equals a dollar) for each member of the society, and for this the doctor was required to give ordinary medical attendance and medicines. Competition between doctors in a district sometimes led to even lower terms of service; disputes between doctors and the secretaries of the societies were frequent, and in various ways doctors were placed in a lamentable position of servitude to the petty tyranny of these secretaries. The system was taken advantage of by persons who ought not to have exploited an inadequate medical payment; while this underpaid work tended to be scamped. There was seething discontent among the club doctors themselves, which was voiced by the British Medical Association, who expressed their agreement with the following statement made in the *Report of the Royal Commission on the Poor Law* (Majority Report, Part V. chap. 3, para. 235):—

Largely, no doubt, owing to the close competition of its own members, medical men have contracted to give their services to the friendly societies at a lower rate than was desirable from any point of view. Some concordat on this question of remuneration is of pressing importance.

The National Insurance Act dealt with sickness and unemployment. In its sickness or "health" section it followed somewhat on the lines of previous German legislation, and, like its prototype, it adopted the principle of compulsory insurance. The defence for such compulsion, in a matter which concerns family welfare and not immediately outsiders, lies in the consideration that this insurance is concerned not with each individual as such, but with him as a member of the social community, the integrity of which is endangered by neglect to provide for a chief contingency in life.

Compulsion on the part of the State necessarily meant some responsibility on its part for the working of the scheme; and in Great Britain the State bears part of its cost, besides controlling its main features.

The Act was termed "National", but it is not strictly national. No scheme can be regarded as such which applies only to a third of the total population. Nor has the title "Health", as applied to its sickness section, been justified hitherto by the working of the Act. There were, and are, great potentialities of preventive medicine in the mere fact that more than half of the general practitioners in the country are treating one-third of its population on a capitation basis.

In experience the directly preventive possibilities of such attendance have been almost entirely undeveloped; though it is true that prompt and continued attendance in sickness by a private practitioner constitutes hygienic work of a secondary kind. This treatment is not adequate, in the sense that it does not include specialist or institutional treatment. In practice it is an improved form of the former "club practice". It is free from the petty tyranny which sometimes occurred when the individual doctor had to deal with the individual friendly society or club or its secretary. For every registered practitioner can participate; every insured person has a free choice of doctor; doctors do not dispense their own prescriptions, except in remote country districts; and to some extent doctors participate in administering the scheme. Even limited as the National Insurance Act is, it is a definite medical gain that medical and hygienic aid to the extent indicated is accessible without let or hindrance to all the wage-earners of the community.

The National Insurance Act was hastily prepared, imperfectly considered, passed through Parliament with very inadequate discussion, and became law in conditions which were chaotic and promised ill for its success. In the words of the *Report of the Royal Commission on National Health Insurance*, 1926:—

The original Act was in many respects complex with a complexity which in practice yielded no adequate compensating advantage.

That its working has been relatively successful during the last sixteen years constitutes a triumph for the able executives who have been responsible for its gradual moulding into practical shape. This has been aided by several amending Acts passed as the defects of the Act of 1911 emerged in its working. That this relative triumph has been extremely costly to the finances of the insured and of the community, and that excessive expenditure still characterises the English insurance system is an undoubted fact. This will emerge more clearly when we have sketched the contents and working of the Act.

SCOPE OF THE ACT

At present some 15 million employed persons come within the scope of the National Insurance Act, or about one-third of the total population. It forms part of the industrial system of the community, and its present smooth working as between employers and employed is the best guarantee of its permanency.

But its industrial character differentiates sickness insurance from public health services, the operations of which are truly national in character. Even in the industrial population a large number are excluded who, though earning a mere pittance—much below the income-limit named below—are not in the employment of any master. (But see also p. 130.)

The National Insurance Act applies, with a few exceptions, to all persons, men or women, over the age of 16, who are employed in manual labour, and to all other employed persons whose rate of remuneration does not exceed £250 (about $1,250) a year.

RATE OF PAYMENTS

Insured persons and their employers pay their respective weekly contributions as shown in table on page 112. These sums now include pensions.

Thus each week the employer must place stamps in the insured employee's book to the value of 1s. 6d. for men, of which sum he has deducted 9d. from the insured man's wage: and stamps to the value of 1s. 1d. for women, of which he has deducted 6d. from the insured woman's wage.

The stamps placed by the employer weekly on each insured person's card represent also the payment for the benefits of the Widows', Orphans', and Old-Age Contributory Pensions Act. Old-age pensions become available at the age of 65, and sickness insurance payments then cease. The State is a partner in insurance against sickness, and pays part of the total expenditure. At present the State pays one-seventh of the total cost of the benefits and of the administration of the benefits by Approved Societies and Insurance Committees for men, and one-fifth of this cost for women; and, in addition, the whole cost of the central administration of insurance. The higher proportion for

	Amount Payable			
	By Employer		By Employed Person	
	For Men	For Women	For Men	For Women
	d.	d.	d.	d.
For Health Insurance ..	4½	4½	4½	4
For Pensions	4½	2½	4½	2
TOTAL	9	7	9	6

women includes the maternity benefit. The magnitude of the scheme may be gathered from the statement that in the first fifteen years of the working of the N.I.A. employers and employed had contributed over 300 millions sterling. The State contributes over two-ninths of the cost of the insurance medical service.

Before considering our chief subject, that of Medical and Maternity Benefits, the machinery of the National Insurance Act(N. I.A.) must be outlined.

CONTROL OF INSURANCE.

This is in the hands of three authorities: the Ministry of Health, which is the chief controlling authority, and of Insurance Committees and Approved Societies.

The *Approved Societies* were the societies who already had working schemes of sickness insurance, and other societies who took up sickness insurance work on the passage of the N.I.A. The original Approved Societies were: (1) Friendly Societies, and (2) Trades Unions. The first of these specialised in sickness insurance; the second, when they engaged in it, did so along with their arrangements for unemployment insurance.

The new societies comprise collecting industrial insurance societies, previously engaged in life insurance and in burial insurance, who took on the new task with avidity. Many new societies were created for this purpose. The new societies differ from most of the old in the fact that the democratic representation of the insured is most tenuous and negligible though supplied in theory. It would carry us too far afield to discuss this unfortunate development. But the power of the Approved Societies, especially of those whose members may number hundreds of thousands, is not without its sinister side. They control vast sums of money; they are highly centralised, with practically no representative control; they have a large staff of officials who can exercise much political pressure; and there is definite fear that a political control may develop—if it does not already exist to some extent—which is inimical to the public welfare. Meanwhile this gigantic financial influence is being exerted, so far as one-half of the insured population is concerned, by societies in which there is "complete lack of any real opportunity for membership control". (*Minority Report Roy. Commission on Health Insurance*, p. 304.)

According to a recent return of the total insured population—

22·7 per cent. are insured with Friendly Societies having branches.
23·8 per cent. are insured with Friendly Societies with only centralised administration.
9·9 per cent. are insured with Trades Unions.
0·8 per cent. are insured with Employers' Provident Funds.
24·8 per cent. are insured with Industrial and Collecting Societies.

There are about 1,000 Approved Societies for sickness insurance in Great Britain. Of these 969 have no branches and 31 have branches, which number as many as 7,000. The number of members in a society may be under 50 or more than 2 millions. It is stated that in England 65 per cent. of the total number of societies comprise only 2 per cent. of the total insured persons, while 76 per cent. of the insured persons are included in only 2·5 per cent. of the societies.

The insured population in Great Britain now comprises about 9½ million men and over 5 million women. The persons insured range from the age of 16, when compulsion begins. At the age of 65 an insured person ceases to pay contributions and to be entitled to sickness and disablement benefit; but he remains insured and entitled to medical benefit. The employer of an insured person aged over 65 must pay the employer's contribution.

There are some local societies, but, as a rule, there is no such geographical distribution of the insured. Hence there is almost insuperable difficulty in utilising insurance sickness statistics for medical or public health investigations. The members of a given society may be distributed all over the country, and the volume and intricacy of the book-keeping and correspondence implied in this fact can be imagined. Some societies are chiefly occupational in grouping, with resultant segregation of lives of high or low rates of sickness.

It will have been noted that a flat rate of payment is required for all ages, young and old, and irrespective of greater or less risk of sickness in different localities and occupations. The payments and the benefits under the Act are the same, whatever may be the worker's wage. In respect of its flat rate of contributions and unvarying sickness money allowances, the British differs from most foreign insurance schemes.

It would conduce immensely to the efficiency of the British scheme if a National Society could be formed with local branches in each county and county borough; much of the present inordinate book-keeping would be avoided, the number of paid officials could be reduced, and it would become possible to utilise the national and local experience of sickness as a means of detection of excessive sickness, with a view to remedial measures. Such a territorial arrangement would not, of course, obviate territorial differences of sickness experience. The North would continue to have more sickness than the South, and industrial towns more than rural districts. The vested interests involved are gigantic, and there seems to be no early prospect of this much-needed reform. *Local Insurance Committees* were provided for in the N.I.A., one for each county and for each county borough in the country. The main function of these committees has never been allotted to them, owing to the force of circumstances, which compelled the Central Government from 1912 onwards to undertake negotiations with the medical profession on a national basis for medical work. This unavoidable national bargaining has meant "blanketing" of these committees, and the *Report of the Royal Commission on National Health Insurance*, 1926, recommended their abolition, and the transference of their remaining duties and powers to special committees of the county and county borough councils, possibly with a proportion of co-opted members.

These committees owed their existence to the fixed determination of the medical profession that under the N.I.A. they would not allow themselves to be controlled by Approved Societies.

The British Medical Association was equally determined at that time not to allow the medical arrangements of sickness insurance to be organised by public health authorities.

In England and Wales there are 146 local insurance committees, and in Scotland 45.

Three-fifths of the members of each committee represent insured persons, elected by Approved Societies; one-fifth are appointed by the council of the county or county borough. Two medical members are elected by the local medical committee, one medical member is appointed by the local council, and several members are appointed by the Minister of Health, including among them two women.

It will be seen that the Minister of Health forms the intermediary between the Approved Societies and the organised doctors. Theoretically each local insurance committee might make arrangements with the local doctors as to terms of medical practice; but right from the initiation of the N.I.A. a national flat scale of medical payment has been settled for the whole country. The local insurance committee receives and publishes lists of doctors and druggists who will undertake the necessary prescribing and dispensing, and settles disputes as to medical and pharmaceutical work. Each committee has, for administrative purposes, to keep two registers of the insured population of its area. In one the insured persons are arranged in order of Approved Societies; in the other in order of doctors. As there are many removals, deaths, and new entrants into insurance, these registers are constantly changing and it is a laborious task to keep them up to date. Each committee has also to furnish each doctor with a list of the insured persons for whom he is responsible and to keep this list up to date. Committees also arrange for the pricing of over 54 million prescriptions annually, and they distribute about nine millions sterling in payment of an enormous number of small accounts of doctors and chemists. The cost of this administrative work of the local insurance committees amounts to nearly 5 per cent. of the cost of medical benefit.

The local insurance committee must confer under certain circumstances with three other local committees.

In each area the local doctors elect a *Local Medical Committee*, representing all the practitioners in the area, and the insurance committee are expected to consult this committee on general questions affecting the administration of medical benefit. This medical committee is purely consultative.

The N.I.A. of 1913 provided for the appointment of a *Panel Committee* in each county and county borough area. This may or may not be identical with the local medical committee. Similarly, a *Pharmaceutical Committee* is required to be consulted on questions as to the supply of medicines and appliances for insured persons.

A sub-committee of the local insurance committee investigates complaints of neglect, etc., made by insured persons. This sub-committee contains an equal number of representatives of the insured and of doctors, and has a neutral chairman. In 1928 there were only 299 such cases in England and Wales. The hearing of complaints is private. In experience it is found that the doctor receives a fair and even a lenient hearing in these inquiries. If grave neglect has been found the case may be referred to the Ministry of Health. This happened in 42 cases in 1928, monies in various amounts which were due to the offending practitioner being withheld in punishment. The Minister, in taking this disciplinary action, is advised by an Advisory Committee including insurance practitioners.

BENEFITS

For the payments made by him under the heading of insurance, the insured person is entitled after a minimum period to—

(*a*) Money Benefits
{
Sickness Allowance.
Disablement Benefit.
Maternity Benefit.
}

(*b*) Medical Benefits.

In the Irish Free State there is no medical benefit, and a fee is necessitated for each sickness certificate. In that country it is stated that claims for sickness benefit are more frequent than in England or Scotland for equal numbers insured.

The Sickness Benefit is 15s. a week for men and 12s. a week for women during incapacity for work by reason of sickness, beginning on the fourth day of incapacity and continuing for 26 weeks.

Disablement Benefit to the amount of 7s. 6d. a week is given to both men and women after the right to sickness benefit has lapsed. It is paid for an indefinite period, so long as incapacity continues, until the insured person becomes eligible for a pension at the age of 65.

Maternity Benefit consists of the payment of £2 (about $10) on the confinement of an insured woman or the wife of an insured man. A married employed woman receives an additional £2 on confinement.

Additional benefits are given by some societies (p. 136).

MEDICAL BENEFIT

When the National Insurance Bill was before Parliament in 1911 it was provided that medical benefit should be administered by each friendly society for its own members; but the medical profession succeeded in replacing this arrangement by *ad hoc* independent committees for this purpose.[1]

These local insurance committees cannot select or reject doctors wishing to be placed on the local list known as the "panel". Every registered practising doctor is entitled to be placed on the list. In Great Britain there are some 38,000 practitioners on the Medical Register, of whom probably two-thirds are engaged in general medical practice. In England 14,300 and in Wales 976 out of some 18,000 general medical practitioners are doing medical work under the N.I.A. Every patient also is entitled to choose his own doctor from the local list.

The medical arrangements, it will be seen, are territorial; the arrangements for the monetary benefits of insurance unhappily are not.

The provision of medical attendance and treatment in the homes of the people for a third of the people constitutes the second great step in domiciliary treatment of the people by statutory provision. Previously this provision had been confined to the necessitous sick.

[1] Further information on sickness insurance, and especially on its medical side, is given in *Memorandum on the English Scheme of National Insurance, with Special Reference to its Medical Aspects*, by G. F. McCleary, M.D., 1929; *Report of the Royal Commission on National Health Insurance*, 1926 (Cmd. 2596); and *Medical Insurance Practice*, by R. W. Harris and L. S. Sack (British Medical Association, 3rd ed., 1929).

Scope of Medical Treatment

No limitation of treatment is stated in the N.I.A.; but it has been ruled that the treatment which a practitioner is required to give to his patient comprises all proper and necessary medical services other than those involving the application of special skill and experience of a degree or kind which general practitioners as a class cannot reasonably be expected to possess. In view of the fact that every doctor has statutory right to appear on the panel, and that an insured person is only entitled to one medical attendant, the Insurance Regulations stating this limitation appear to be in accord with the intention of the legislature.

It is sometimes difficult to determine whether a given attendance comes within the limits of the above definition. The following illustrations of decisions on this point may be cited:—

Ruled to be within the doctor's obligations:—
  Fracture of leg,
  Curetting of uterus,
  Reduction of dislocated elbow under an anæsthetic.
  Removal of needle from foot.
  Taking blood for Wassermann test.
  Vaccination.

Ruled to be outside the doctor's obligations:—
  Passage of Eustachian catheter.
  Intravenous injection of novarsenobillon.
  Removal of tuberculous glands in neck.
  Application of radiant heat and ionisation.
  Removal of appendix.
  General anæsthetic for tonsillectomy.
  Operation for hæmorrhoids.
  Testing of eyes for refraction.

The treatment to be given does not include attendance in labour (parturition) or within 10 days after labour in respect of any condition resulting from labour.

If any doubt arises on the range of general practitioner treatment the point is referred to the local medical committee, and if this committee and the local insurance committee fail to agree, it is submitted to three referees appointed by the Minister of Health, two of the referees being doctors.

Emergency treatment must always be given to the extent of the practitioner's capacity, even though the patient is not on his list. The range of general practitioner service may vary according to local custom; thus a differing standard of skill may be necessary according to distance from a hospital.

CHARGING INSURANCE PATIENTS

Some doctors offer to treat their insurance patients for special conditions outside the general practitioner scope. This is admissible in cases in which special skill is required, e.g. extraction of cataract. In border-line cases the panel doctor may be open to suspicion and disputation may arise. To avoid this the insurance Regulations require the panel doctor, if he treats one of his insurance patients for a condition which does not come within his contract, to give notice within two days to the insurance committee that he has done this, and to supply all necessary particulars concerning the treatment he has given. If the committee decide that the treatment in question fell within the scope of the practitioner's obligations, they can recover the amount from him and repay the patient.

If specialist treatment is needed it is the panel doctor's duty to advise his patient how to proceed. He cannot charge for the administration of a general anæsthetic, even when the operation is performed by a specialist.

REMUNERATION OF PRACTITIONER

The method of remuneration of the practitioner for his services under the N.I.A. has been the subject of much controversy. It might be based (1) on the *actual work done* by the doctor for his individual patient; and this method has been adopted in some European countries. It involves minute account-keeping and encourages excessive charging on the part of a minority of doctors to the detriment of the majority if their contributions depend on the total pool available.

(2) *A whole-time service* by special insurance doctors in each area was threatened in 1911, when doctors refused to contract for treating insured persons on the basis next mentioned. The possibility of this led to a dramatic collapse of opposition and acceptance of

(3) *The capitation basis*, which gives a fixed sum annually for every insured person placing his name on a doctor's list. This is the universal system in Great Britain; and, as already seen, the British Medical Association commend it and recommend its continuance (p. 40).

Theoretically it interests the doctor in the maintenance of his client's health; but this interest is still in most cases undeveloped, though it need not continue so.

A modification of this scheme has been suggested, which would give a higher rate of payment for the first 500 on a doctor's list and less for further clients. This has been defended on the assumption that 1,000 patients do not give twice as much trouble as 500, but the only saving would be in travelling. In England at present doctors are not allowed to have more than 2,500 insured persons on their list.

The towns of Manchester and Salford adopted a plan which appeared attractive, but it was abandoned in 1927-28. Under this plan the money due for the medical benefit of the insured was pooled, and payment was made to each doctor in accordance with the work done by him. The system involved much more book-keeping than the capitation system; it was associated with excessive expenditure on drugs, and it has now been abandoned.

Over two-thirds of the doctors in practice in England are engaged in insurance medical practice. In industrial areas the proportion may be nearly 100 per cent. In the county of Devonshire it is 54 per cent., in Kent 61 per cent., in Birmingham 65 per cent., and in Sheffield 66 per cent.

The method of distribution of the capitation payments is

fully described on page 129 *et seq.* of Harris and Sack's Guide.

The amount of remuneration for each insured patient was settled in 1912 on a national basis at 7s. 6d. per annum per insured person. This national method of settlement has been continued to the present time. In 1924 a Court of Arbitration settled the present capitation fee of 9s.

The average number of persons on a single insurance doctor's panel in England and Wales is 930.

A panel of 1,000 implies an annual gross income of £450 (about $2,250). There is no expense for drugs. These are separately paid for out of insurance funds, pharmacists being employed for this purpose. The family of the insured person equals about 1·5 persons on an average, and generally the insurance doctor secures the independent private care of these. The insurance remuneration cannot, I think, be regarded as unsatisfactory, especially in view of its monopolistic value. The financial position of doctors since the N.I.A. was enacted has greatly improved, even when allowance for the increased cost of living is made. Prior to that they did much unpaid work; "bad debts" were common, and special collectors were needed. Now for one-third of the population there is certainty of payment for services rendered.

As early as 1913 the National Funds had to be drawn upon to provide for the excess of cost of medical benefit beyond the estimated cost. In 1920 weekly contributions of employees and workers were increased with the same object and to provide for the fact that the limit of non-manual workers brought within the scope of the N.I.A. was increased from £160 to £250.

COMPULSORY ALLOCATION

Sometimes patients are refused admittance to a doctor's list; and it may occasionally be necessary to assign a patient to a given doctor. This is carried out by a special subcommittee of the local insurance committee. No extra payment is given in such cases.

Pharmaceutical Arrangements

These are somewhat similar to medical arrangements, as all registered pharmacists can be placed on the list of persons entitled to dispense medicines for insured persons.

Total Cost of Medical Benefit

In 1928, in England and Wales, 15,276 doctors were in insurance practice, and medicines and appliances were supplied as part of the medical benefit at about 9,000 chemists' shops. Some 13,900,000 persons were entitled to this benefit, and it cost over 9 millions sterling. Insurance doctors received £6,831,300, and £2,241,780 was paid to chemists. Thus on an average each insurance doctor was paid £447 in 1928. Each insured person represented an average cost per annum of 9s. 10d. for medical attendance, and of 3s. 3d. for drugs and appliances.

In addition, £300,000 was paid to country doctors on account of extra mileage; and £10,000 was set aside to enable country doctors to attend courses of post-graduate study, and for the maintenance of telephones, branch surgeries, and motor-cars. The working of the N.I.A. has reduced the inadequacy of medical service in sparsely populated areas. Doctors also received £190,000 for emergency medicines and appliances supplied by them, and in country districts for medicines dispensed by them.

Excessive Prescribing

Excessive prescribing not infrequently occurs. This may come under any one of these categories:—

(1) Without giving a bottle of medicine a doctor consulted by an insured patient for a slight ailment may fail to satisfy his patient unless he enters into a tiresome explanation with him. In a similar case in his own family the same doctor would give hygienic advice, but no drug. To change public opinion in this respect will be a slow educational

process. Prescribing a bottle of medicine for its psychological effect may be defended in special cases where it is needed in order to secure confidence and hope of recovery in the patient.

(2) There are some doctors who insist on giving the most recent vaccine treatment, or on the administration of a new drug, of the kind concerning which a wise physician of the last generation, referring to the short life of most of such drugs, advised his students: "Make haste to prescribe them, or you will have lost your chance of doing so." No exact line of reasonableness can be drawn in such cases, but the doctor may reasonably be asked to consider the interest in economy of the rest of his insurance patients, while not denying his present patient what has been proved to be useful.

(3) In recent years, especially under the pressure of economic distress, doctors have often prescribed extract of malt or cod liver oil as nutriments and not because of any specific indication for them. Is this justifiable? Or does it introduce a non-medical consideration into a medical prescription? A most difficult question to answer fairly, unless one has regard to the limitation of total insurance funds available and to the medical welfare of all the insured on the doctor's panel, as well as that of the individual patient. Of course, every under-nourished person should be supplied with adequate nourishment; and there are State provisions to this end for the necessitous, not through a medical prescription. In similar circumstances one might, if this practice were justifiable, legitimise the giving of milk or butter out of insurance funds.

Investigations into excessive prescribing have been made by medical committees; a national formulary to save trouble and expense has been compiled; and it may be hoped that all insurance practitioners ere long will realise that an essential part of their duty to the insured is to educate them out of their present extravagant belief in the need for and efficacy of unnecessary drugs.

CHANGE OF DOCTOR

The doctor can remove a patient from his list, in which case he must at once send the insured person's record card to the insurance committee. The removal then becomes operative within 14 days, or on acceptance by another doctor, whichever occurs first. This change is subject to some possible limitation by the Allocation Scheme; this is obviously necessitated by the inevitable residuum of undesirable patients.

An insured person may at any time apply to another doctor to be accepted on his list, and if he is accepted this doctor at once becomes responsible for his treatment. But this does not hold good if he is already on the list of a doctor in the same district. In this case both doctors must agree to the transfer in writing on the medical card, or failing this the insured person must give to the insurance committee 14 days' notice of his wish to transfer.

MEDICAL CERTIFICATION

The medical certification of incapacity for work is the pivot on which the whole of sickness insurance revolves. Some 20 millions sterling are distributed annually in Great Britain in sickness and disablement benefits, chiefly on the strength of these certificates. Doctors sometimes fail to realise that each medical certificate is a cheque drawn on the Benefit Funds of sickness insurance. Their position is difficult. It would be still more difficult were they the direct employees of the Approved Societies, and thus became the official guardians of the funds of these societies, as well as the medical attendants of the insured. But this very freedom from irksome interference carries with it a moral responsibility.

The insured can change their doctor if dissatisfied with him, and the rules governing this throw light on the natural unwillingness of the doctor to be very severe in his limitation of certification.

Evidently the doctor has a strong motive to avoid being

severe and even to be complaisant in certification, either
in regard to certifying incapacity to work or capacity to
return to work. It is not suggested that there is collusion
between doctor and patient except in a relatively small
minority of cases. This notion can be dismissed. It is,
furthermore, likely that practitioners, as their sense of the
hygienic aspect of their work increases, appreciate more
highly the value of rest in the treatment of disease, and the
risks of a curtailed period of convalescence. This will
account for some of the increase of incidence of sickness
in the insured in recent years. But neither this nor repeated
epidemics of influenza offer a complete explanation. The
facts are intriguing. The Government Actuary examined
the sickness and disablement experience of a representative
group of Approved Societies during the period 1921-27
(Cmd. 3548). The results showed that claims for sickness
benefit had increased between 60 and 100 per cent. in the
space of six years. The claims of men for sickness benefit
rose by 41 per cent., of unmarried women by 60 per cent.,
and those of married women by 106 per cent. For disablement benefit the corresponding increased percentages were
85, 100, and 159. If the same results be stated in terms of
persons claiming sickness benefit each year per 100 in each
group the following comparison emerges :—

	1921	1927
Men	14	23
Unmarried women	12	21
Married women	19	38

The increased expenditure has been most marked in the
case of married women under 45 years of age, and in the
words of the official circular (Memo. 324, A.I.C.), "an
important contributory factor has been the payment of
claims in respect of pregnancy and post-confinement". The
circular just quoted reminds doctors that money insurance

benefits can only be paid to a pregnant woman who is *incapable of work*; furthermore, no monetary benefit is payable during the puerperal period of four weeks, during which time married women are prohibited from engaging in remunerative work, but they receive the maternity benefit (p. 164).

The factors producing increased certification are multiform. The following quotation states one factor to which importance must be attached. It is taken from the presidential address of Mr. F. Lewis, the president of the National Conference of Friendly Societies (representing a voluntary and state membership of 13¼ million persons), given September 18, 1930.

A large proportion of the insurance practitioners were giving to insured persons treatment and attention that was commendable, but there were too many medical men whose treatment of insured persons was perfunctory and negligent, and some who were willing to do almost anything in order that they might secure a cheap popularity and a long panel list, even to the extent of assisting persons to obtain benefit to which they were not justly entitled.

A resolution was subsequently adopted by the Conference to the effect that—

There was a general agreement that a varying and sometimes inadequate standard of medical certificates had had a substantial effect on the sickness claims ratio.

A similar view from a different angle is well expressed in the following extract from a recent issue of the *National Insurance Gazette*:—

The average doctor takes the view that his patient engages him and that his sole duty is owed to that patient. That is the doctor's traditional attitude, and it was entirely correct in former times. It is only partly correct under the National Health Insurance system. The first part of the proposition is true, but the second part is not. The patient engages the doctor, but the whole body of insured persons pays the doctor's fees, and therefore a duty is owed to that body. The individual patient does not pay the doctor's bill. The whole body pays, and we put it to the doctors, as honest men, that a duty is owed to that body.

Steps are being taken which will help to reveal the identity of those doctors who habitually over-certify; as also to ascertain for the information of each local insurance committee which particular doctors habitually indulge in over-prescribing. It is, however, highly improbable that the sudden and most remarkable increase of sickness certification which occurred can be due to a similar sudden and remarkable increase of medical laxity of certification. Lowered morale of workers is often quoted, "many of these having become certificate hunters in search of easy money". The increased popularity of the Act is adduced; as is also the lowered vitality due to unemployment and malnutrition; while some assume that societies have become more lax in their administration.

Representatives of the B.M.A. and of Approved Societies have been called into conference. The former rightly emphasise the unlikelihood that suddenly increased laxity in certification of sickness can have been largely responsible for increased sickness and disablement expenses. But it is not doubted that there is need for greater exactitude and moral responsibility in medical certification by a section of practitioners. Great improvement is likely to accrue from the educational work of the B.M.A. among its members. The following circular issued by the Ministry of Health in July 1926 to insurance practitioners in England and Wales indicates the official anxiety caused by the recent excessive experience of sickness.

CERTIFICATION OF INCAPACITY FOR WORK

The Minister has noted with much concern the abnormal increase during the last two months in the number of insured persons receiving sickness and disablement benefit, and the resulting heavy expenditure incurred by many Approved Societies. Information available from other sources does not indicate the prevalence of any marked epidemic or exceptional outbreak of sickness which would account for this increase in the number of cases of certified incapacity, and it is significant that the ratio of expansion is not uniform throughout the country, and that its geographical distribution corresponds closely with the incidence of unemployment due to the dispute in the coal trade.

The results of the examination of a large number of cases referred to referees, and in particular the high proportion of claimants who sign off in preference to presenting themselves for examination, suggest strongly that large numbers of insured persons have succeeded in obtaining, or continuing to obtain, medical certificates although they were not in fact incapable of work. The Minister cannot escape the conclusion that many practitioners in the industrial areas mainly affected have failed to appreciate the danger that in times of acute unemployment there is inevitably a tendency to magnify minor ailments and to claim sickness benefit in circumstances in which, under ordinary conditions, no claim would be made. Normally the difference between sickness benefit and average earnings is sufficient to afford the employed person a substantial inducement not to leave work or to return to it as soon as he is able to do so; and doctors have, no doubt, in the past proceeded on the assumption that in cases in which there were no definite physical signs, the patient's account of his subjective symptoms might, in general, be accepted in the absence of any indication to the contrary. But in many areas this economic safeguard against ill-founded claims no longer exists, and the Minister fears that practitioners have not sufficiently realised that an increase in the number of claims in itself necessitates more than ordinary care in considering whether the statutory conditions for the receipt of sickness and disablement benefit have been fulfilled.

He therefore desires to remind practitioners that the statutory test of title to these benefits is that the insured person has been rendered incapable of work by some specific disease or bodily or mental disablement, and that strict regard must be had to this criterion in considering all cases coming before them. No practitioner is justified in allowing the economic position of the applicant for a certificate to lead him to adopt a less stringent standard than the Acts require; it should be remembered that any laxity in the issue of certificates, whether unconscious or deliberate, is extremely unfair to those doctors who have continued to take a strict view of their obligations under the Terms of Service. Moreover, it must not be forgotten that excessive indulgence to individual members of Approved Societies must thereby deprive members in general of sums which might otherwise have been used in providing additional benefits in the future.

The opportunity is taken to reissue herewith Memorandum 280A.I.C. prepared for the guidance of practitioners in interpreting the term "incapable of work".

REGIONAL MEDICAL OFFICERS (R.M.O.)

The Ministry of Health has a staff of 59 medical officers for England and Wales, organised on a territorial basis, who have important duties in controlling the certification of sickness. Their chief duty is to examine insured persons referred to them either by the Approved Societies or by insurance practitioners, and to advise as to the result of their examination. Cases may be referred for consultation, or for determination of doubtful incapacity. The practitioner is required to send particulars of each case thus referred to the R.M.O.

In 1927 the Ministry's staff dealt with 312,580 cases of persons whose incapacity for work was doubted. This is more than 2 per cent. of the total insured population. Of this number—

135,829 failed to attend for examination, chiefly because they had ceased to receive benefit.
176,751 attended for examination, of whom 125,800 were found to be incapable, and 50,951 not incapable of work.

The first number given above indicates the large numbers who return to work rather than face a consultative examination. Some of this number, however, even without the projected testing, were on the point of returning to work.

The mass of referee work was so great as to necessitate the engagement of a number of part-time medical referees.

EXTENSIONS OF SICKNESS INSURANCE, 1928

In addition to other modifications, the Act of 1928 made new classes of persons liable to compulsory sickness insurance. The additional persons thus included had a similar economic position to that of the workers already insured, but they had hitherto been left outside insurance because they were not employed under a contract of service. They include occupations such as the following: workers at piece rates, the crews of small trading vessels working on a share system, etc.

Reference may be made here to the voluntary contributors

to the insurance scheme, of which there are 231,000 in England. This includes a large number of persons who voluntarily become insured to qualify at the age of 65 for an old-age pension.

Use of the N.I.A. for Prophylaxis

The Act passed in 1911 had a National Health Insurance section, and as I have already stated, this in the main has failed to justify the inclusion of the word "health", except in the sense that all extensions of and improvements in the treatment of illness conduce to improved communal health. Provision was made in the Act for investigation into excessive sickness in districts or occupations, but this has remained a dead letter. It could not be otherwise, with the existent chaotic geographical distribution of the insured in societies.

A finding of a committee of inquiry on the part of the Scottish Board of Health was to the effect that the expression "treatment" in the Medical Benefit Regulations includes treatment for the prevention as well as for the cure of sickness; and that furthermore the word "patients" is defined in Section 3 of these Regulations as including all insured persons who are on the practitioner's list. If this finding is acted on, a hitherto neglected field of preventive medicine is open for cultivation, and new links can be forged between the practitioners of clinical medicine and the medical health officers appointed under the Public Health Acts. Already vaccination is considered part of an insurance doctor's obligations.

Under the conditions of panel medical practice, the practitioner is interested in keeping his patient well; but this motive has not in practice led to systematised, and rarely even to sporadic, preventive work by the practitioner among his clients.

Objections to Compulsory Sickness Insurance

1. An objection frequently urged is that the money allowance is inadequate. In Scotland, for instance, it is

stated that 5·9 per cent. of the insured applied for poor relief. (*Rep. R.C. on National Health Insurance*, p. 25.)

The insured person when sick or out of work cannot support his dependents on the benefit accruing to him, and he applies for relief for them. This objection merely states that the value of sickness insurance is only partial; that it is so should not decrease the desire of the insured to fill by personal thrift the gaps in the official provision. There is no valid evidence that it has this effect. But the inadequacy of the money benefit does show the need for public health and social remedies which will decrease both unemployment and sickness. Prevention as well as, and more than, provision is needed.

2. The relation of unemployment insurance to sickness insurance is unsatisfactory. The full sickness insurance allowance is 15s. a week, while that for unemployment is 18s., with 5s. additional for the wife and 2s. for each dependent child. Unemployment in circumstances in which the unemployed person is ineligible for the unemployment benefit doubtless increases claims on sickness benefit. To discuss this intricate social problem would carry us too far afield.

3. The non-inclusion of dependents of the insured in medical benefit is discussed in a concluding volume.

4. The drawbacks of sickness organisation in separate non-territorial Approved Societies have already been stated.

5. The inadequacy and incompleteness of the medical benefit for the insured are discussed later in this volume and in a concluding volume.

6. So also is the maternity benefit and the reforms needed in its utilisation and administration.

7. A very vulnerable point in sickness insurance is—

THE BORDER-LINE HARD CASES of those excluded from its benefits. Something towards removing this defect has been effected in the Insurance Act, 1928 (p. 130), but there remain vast numbers of struggling families, the head of which earns rather more than £250 a year, who are excluded from the working of sickness insurance. Through national taxes they contribute towards the expenses of the State in helping national insurance; but, although they have a hard struggle to maintain efficiency and are hard hit by sickness, they receive none of the help which the State-aided system of mutual insurance affords.

The State contribution to sickness insurance, which amounts altogether to 21·5 per cent. of the total cost, may be regarded as not in accord with the general principle that governmental expenditure should enure to the benefit of the entire community and not exclusively to a section of it. This principle has frequently been disregarded, usually when but for the exceptional help the rest of the community would suffer, as, for instance, in poor-law relief (public assistance).

8. The Views of Practitioners on the Medical Benefit

In connection with the periodic review of capitation payment for medical care of the insured, and apart from this, the views of individual practitioners on the medical benefit have been freely expressed in both the medical and the lay Press; and although I have omitted the copious extracts from letters of medical practitioners to the medical Press which I had collected, it is necessary at this point to state that there remain the most acute differences of opinion as to the value and success of medical insurance work. These differences include indictment of the "bondage" of the medical service, destruction of the self-respect of the medical profession, and many points of detail, including those already noted. Nevertheless, the vastly preponderant view of doctors as represented by the B.M.A. is that the service, although incomplete, is so satisfactory that it should be continued. (See p. 40.)

Evidence as to the Value of the Medical Benefit

The medical profession, a majority of whom (and a large majority of general practitioners) belong to the B.M.A., have repeatedly expressed a strong antipathy to the "degrading" character of contract medical work as formerly conducted. At an early stage the B.M.A. passed a resolution to the effect that the conditions of service proposed under the N.I.A. were derogatory to the medical profession and detrimental to the public health. In their experience in the domiciliary treatment of the destitute poor under boards of guardians, and still more in "club practice" in the pre-compulsory period of sickness insurance, this attitude has had ample justification. But as is seen in their evidence before the Royal Commission on National Health Insurance, 1926 (*Report*, p. 13), the B.M.A. has profoundly changed its attitude in relation to contract medical work under the N.I.A. Their official evidence states:—

The evidence as to the incidence of sickness benefit does point to the fact that the scheme has almost certainly reduced national sickness, and we are quite sure that if the immense gain to national health includes immense gain to the comfort of the individual in knowing that he can have medical attention whenever he needs it, the gain is most marked.

The Commissioners, in their report, express a similar opinion:—

We are satisfied that the scheme of National Health Insurance has fully justified itself and has, on the whole, been successful in operation.

The B.M.A. in 1922 expressed more fully their reasons for regarding with favour the continuance of medical benefit on the present lines:—

(*a*) Large numbers, indeed whole classes of persons are now receiving a real medical attention which they formerly did not receive at all.

(*b*) The number of practitioners in proportion to the population in densely populated areas has increased.

(*c*) The amount and character of the medical attention given is superior to that formerly given in the best of the old clubs, and immensely superior to that given in the great majority of the clubs which were far from the best.

(*d*) Illness is now coming under skilled observation and treatment at an earlier stage than was formerly the case.

(*e*) Speaking generally, the work of practitioners has been given a bias towards prevention which was formerly not so marked.

(*f*) Clinical records have been or are provided which may be made of great service in relation to medical research and public health.

(*g*) Co-operation among practitioners is being encouraged to an increasing degree.

(*h*) There is now a more marked recognition than formerly of the collective responsibility of the profession to the community in respect of all health matters.

Similar views have been expressed by some of the Approved Societies, although some of these are extremely unhappy on the score of lax certification of incapacity for work. (See p. 127.)

It can be accepted that for the majority of insured persons medical benefit as now administered has been a boon. For (*a*) every obstacle to early medical consultation and diagnosis has been removed; and (*b*) a serious source of anxiety—the expense of domiciliary medical attendance—no longer exists so far as concerns the wage-earner in each family.

These are important gains to set against the *alleged inferior service* under medical benefit. It is certain that some doctors—especially those with large panels—have their surgeries crowded during limited hours, and oft-times give a perfunctory interview, followed by the prescription of a bottle of medicine, not preceded by an adequate overhaul of the patient. In mitigation it may be said that persons of the same social class would, apart from insurance, receive similar treatment. This, of course, does not justify unsatisfactory contract work; and as the education of the insured improves, practitioners acting thus will lose in prestige and practice.

It is certain also that a considerable number of the insured lack confidence in the panel doctor and prefer to go elsewhere for medical advice, either to a hospital or to a non-panel doctor (see p. 86).

But I have found no reason to doubt that the majority of panel doctors give honest and competent service within the prescribed limits; and this conclusion is confirmed by the evidence given before the Royal Commission on Health Insurance.

SCHEMES OF ADDITIONAL MEDICAL BENEFITS

Approved Societies which have surplus funds in their sickness experience can give certain additional benefits. Surpluses are determined at the periodic valuation of assets and liabilities conducted by a Government valuer. The following information (*Ministry of Health Annual Report*, 1928–29) shows the number and magnitude of the chief schemes in operation in England and Wales in 1928:—

	Number of Schemes	Amount Allocated
		£
Dental	6,243	2,520,293
Ophthalmic	5,633	419,311
Hospitals	1,934	272,928
Convalescent Homes	2,190	207,444
Surgical Appliances	3,365	125,595
Nursing	422	20,660
Others	648	56,638
		3,622,869

The additional benefits which may be adopted by Approved Societies having a disposable surplus now number sixteen. They include besides those summarised in the preceding table an increase in cash benefits and treatment at approved clinics for rheumatism or other diseases.

The majority of the members of Approved Societies receive dental and ophthalmic benefits to a varying extent, half of these similarly benefit to a limited extent through hospitals and convalescent homes (note the small sums given above), and there are other minor additional benefits.

The societies providing funds for additional treatment

are not authorised themselves to provide treatment; and their participation, even to the extent of financing such treatment, is resented by the medical profession as an intrusion into the region debarred from them, at least for domiciliary medical work, by the legislature. But not all Approved Societies possess these surplus funds; others have none: and universal pooling of surpluses (also of deficits) and distribution of additional medical benefits through local insurance committees, the authorised agents of medical treatment, are impracticable.

The present separation of additional medical benefits from the general medical benefit fund is a serious evil. It is difficult to see how it can be remedied, except by a break-up, partially if not entirely, of the segregation of the finances of individual Approved Societies.

More generally the complete liberty of association in separate Approved Societies necessarily carries with it some suggestion of unfairness to a large number of the insured. This apparent unfairness may be stated to be inherent in the flat rate of payment which is the same for young and old, who have an unequal incidence of sickness. In foreign sickness insurance schemes there is no flat rate. There may similarly be said to be unfairness in women workers with little or no prospect of marriage having to pay towards a general maternity fund—also for pensions for orphans. But if we admit that these anomalies must continue, and that the advantages and easy workability of the flat rate go far to justify its continuance, there remain the anomalies due to occupational and regional segregation of societies. Local societies can scarcely represent the average experience. The agricultural worker pays something for the less healthy town worker. The gardener pays to support the drayman, or saloon barman, or worker in a dusty occupation, and so on.

In the opinion of the Royal Commission on National Health Insurance (p. 102) amalgamation into a national scheme "would create as much discontent as it would allay"; and they add "from this point of view we have come to the conclusion that a system of self-governing bodies is to be preferred and should be retained".

I cannot coincide with this view, but hold that in the circumstances of Britain the four Commissioners who signed a Minority Report are right in stating the following among other conclusions:—

.   .   .   .   .

(6) That the Approved Society system is a hindrance to the development of a complete public health policy.

(7) That it is undesirable to retain Approved Societies any longer as the agencies for the distribution of cash benefits to insured persons.

(8) That local authorities could and should take the place of Approved Societies as the bodies through whom sickness and disablement benefits should be administered.

.   .   .   .   .

(10) That in considering the cost of proposed developments of health services there should be taken into account the loss to the nation resulting from neglect to provide sufficiently for the health of all persons who are or will be employable.

(11) That an outlay which safeguards industrial well-being and conduces to efficiency should not be regarded as a burden on industry or on the community.

(12) That as the provision of a complete medical and treatment service would tend to prevent sickness and to effect a speedier and more complete cure of illness, it would result in economy of expenditure on cash benefits, and that the provision of such a service should not, therefore, depend for its finance entirely upon current contributions.

.   .   .   .   .

(14) That medical benefit should be provided for the dependents of insured persons.

DENTAL BENEFIT

The British Medical Association has urged that any form of specialist treatment should be available only on the recommendation of the patient's insurance doctor, though they agree that dental treatment may properly be made an exception to this rule. Societies are not allowed to select particular dentists for their members. These may go to any dentist chosen by them who is willing to work on the scale of fees agreed with the societies generally.

The provision of dental benefit opens up some considerations which do not apply, or at least not to the same extent, to the medical profession. The supply of dentists is scarcely equal to national needs, and the majority of the wage-earning parents are not willing or not able to pay fees which will adequately remunerate dentists for work on their children's teeth. In particular, dentists are commonly willing to hand over children to whole-time dentists employed by school authorities (pp. 208 and 274).

A National Dental Service Committee of the British Dental Association has recently reported in favour of extending the present inadequate provision for the following services:—

1. Dental treatment of expectant and nursing mothers and for children up to 5 years of age.

2. Dental inspection and treatment of all children of school age.

3. Dental treatment of adolescents.

4. Dental treatment for all persons insured under the National Health Insurance Act, and for all other adults who are unable to afford dental treatment by private dental practitioners.

5. Dental treatment as an essential element in cases of tuberculosis and of venereal disease.

6. The institution of a co-ordinated scheme for education in oral hygiene, which would be simple in its application and general in its incidence, but with particular attention to the young, with the object of preventing dental disease.

Already good, though irregular and inco-ordinated, work is being done under these headings. The committee advocate the control of the entire work under a dental section of the Ministry of Health, the formation of which they advocate. They set out a scale of salaries for wholetime dentists for local authorities. The report also emphasises the facultative provision of dental aid under the N.I.A. and the mischief accruing from its not being available for dependents, or for young people between 14 and 16, after they leave school, and before they come to the insurable age.

The report is important as showing the willingness of the dental profession to undertake important national work.

OPHTHALMIC BENEFIT has raised further difficulties. The B.M.A. urge that all ophthalmic cases should receive benefit only on the recommendation of a medical man.

This contention is made on the strength of the intimate relation between the state of the eye and that of the general health of the body. Non-medical opticians have pushed their claims, using the erroneous analogy of dental disease, but so far their claim for similar treatment has been disallowed. Mere eye-testing for refraction may ignore the fact that in perhaps 5 per cent. of the cases serious disease may be the cause of the defective vision. At the present time combined efforts are being made in towns throughout the country to organise ophthalmic clinics for the insured, where they will receive skilled guidance in treatment at reasonable terms.

A board has been set up known as the National Ophthalmic Treatment Board, the members of which have been nominated by the B.M.A., the Association of Dispensing Opticians, etc. Under this scheme—

it is possible for all insured persons, their dependents, and non-insured people whose income does not exceed £250 per annum, to have their eyes examined by an ophthalmic medical practitioner at his private consulting-room and to obtain a good, well-fitting spectacle frame or eye-glasses and best-quality lenses of any power; the total cost for consultation and glasses being 18s. . . . articles sold under the scheme are standardised as a safeguard to the public. A member of an Approved Society or of the Hospital Savings Association may be able to secure from one or other of these organisations a grant towards the cost of the examination and necessary glasses.

A GENERAL MEDICAL SERVICE

The uncertain and unequal distribution of additional benefits is an outstanding reason for abolition of additional benefits in single Approved Societies, and its replacement by unified administration. It is true that the assumed democratic organisation of these societies would thus be decreased in scope. But, as already indicated, this democracy for most insured persons is now a phantom of reality, the management nearly always being even less democratic than that of a large limited liability company with shareholders anywhere. If for the purpose of these benefits, and still better for all purposes, a territorial basis of organisation could be substituted, the machinery of records would be simplified, the expense of administration would be reduced, and much dissatisfaction among the insured would disappear.

An alternative has been proposed, that of unifying the medical benefit under the National Insurance Act with the medical services of public assistance and of public health authorities. This would give a gratuitous State Service of domiciliary medical attendance for those who are destitute, along with a contributory domiciliary service for the insured, and for many who cannot be classed as insured or destitute. It would still need to be supplemented by institutional and consultation services for special purposes, for insured and non-insured alike.

Events may grow in this direction. There are evident advantages in co-ordination and unification of medical work. But would medical certification and proper control of certified monetary benefit be more satisfactory in these circumstances? Probably it would be, if the medical practitioner in the altered circumstances became less dependent on the foibles of his patients, as he would be by every increase of his official work. But any development in this direction must necessarily be slow. The course of experience will show whether it would be entirely wise or not. Meanwhile great reforms are practicable with present arrangements.

In conclusion the views of the Royal Commission on National Health Insurance, 1926, on this intricate problem may be quoted:—

We are of opinion that the difficulties of a composite support to a completed medical service from insurance funds as well as from grants and rates would be so considerable alike in their financial, administrative, and social aspects that some more practical solution must be sought. In particular, we feel sure that the wider the scope of these services, the more difficult will it be to retain the insurance principle. The ultimate solution will lie, we think, in the direction of divorcing the medical service entirely from the insurance system and recognising it along with all the other public health activities as a service to be supported from the general public funds.

Need for Further Medical Benefits

Apart from the restricted and unequal extensions of medical benefit provided by those Approved Societies which possess available surplus funds—and not completely supplied even by these exceptional societies—medical benefits under the N.I.A. are incomplete in certain serious respects.

1. There is no provision for treatment in hospital or, alternatively, treatment at home, for serious operations or other conditions requiring expert medical service.

2. Apart from the limited consultations possible with regional medical officers, who may be described as generalised specialists, there is no provision under the Act for consultation as to diagnosis in obscure cases of disease, or for treatment of eye, ear, throat, gynæcological or other cases needing special diagnosis and treatment. This omission is harmless and even desirable for any cases of tuberculosis and venereal disease which come under the care of an insurance doctor, as in these instances national provision is made for consultations and special treatment when needed for the insured along with the rest of the population.

3. There is no provision for pathological and physical aids (X-ray examinations, etc.) in the diagnosis of disease and in guidance as to its treatment. This subject is discussed on page 212. In 1914 national funds had been set aside for providing these facilities for insured and non-insured alike, apart from the insurance organisation, but the war inter-

vened.[1] For some diseases already national provision is made, and insurance provision in these instances would be redundant.

4. There is usually no provision for nursing the sick. Both in respect to hospital provision and to nursing, insured persons, like others of limited means outside the insurance scheme, depend on voluntary and official hospitals, and on the Queen's Nurses and County Nursing Associations which are fairly general throughout the country. Payments are made for nursing services in many cases, but a large part of this help is gratuitous. It is supported by voluntary gifts and in some instances by subsidies from local authorities.

The fact that in the above and some allied respects the medical benefit under the N.I.A. is defective or wanting is not a valid argument against sickness insurance so far as it functions. The possibilities of an insurance service, to the expense of which national taxation supplies only a quota, must depend on economic conditions. A wider and, indeed, a complete service could be provided if funds were available, and if it were justifiable thus to treat exceptionally a limited third of the population, in part at least out of funds to which the entire community contributes. In respect of hospital accommodation and of expert consultations at hospitals, a large proportion of the insured are now making partial provision under a voluntary system of insurance (see p. 69). Compulsory contributions to an insurance scheme are necessarily conditioned by the economic state of the country. The Report of the Royal Commission (1926) emphasises this point in the remark, "it is small consolation to a bankrupt to be told that his doctor's bills have been the main cause of his disaster".[2] But this is a rather super-

---

[1] At the same time funds were allotted for providing specialist help for insured persons, but this also fell through on account of the war.

[2] Employers' organisations submitted to the Royal Commission (1926) that "there is a definite limit to the amount of money which any country can afford to spend in the providing of social services," and they were confident that this "limit had in Great Britain already been largely exceeded". They gave a table of which the following is the gist. In Great Britain the cost of five social services—poor law, workmen's compensation, old-age pen-

ficial view. It is not clear that great economies might not be effected in the administration of medical benefit in its present scope: and the rapid increase throughout the country of the voluntary insurance mentioned on page 69 is significant of desire for more complete protection.

EVIDENCE IN FAVOUR OF EXTENDED MEDICAL BENEFIT

The most eloquent testimony to the need for extended medical benefit is given by the dramatically rapid extent to which people in Great Britain are insuring the provision of hospital and consultative services for themselves and their families on a voluntary basis.

The B.M.A. support the idea that "The medical provision . . . (of the N.I.A.) should be as far as possible complete". They would also make some of the various medical services provided by the public health and education authorities an integral part of an Insurance Scheme, including the whole family of the insured person while increasing the service in the directions indicated in paragraphs 1–4 on pages 142–3. Obviously this would imply extending the medical benefits to all dependents of the insured, thus bringing from 1/2 to 2/3 of the total population within a contract system of medical treatment.

For financial reasons the Royal Commission limited themselves to recommending money allowances to dependents equal to those given in unemployment insurance.

The National Conference of Friendly Societies, which represents 4,000,000 State insured members and a total

sions, health insurance, and unemployment insurance—per head of total population is 78s. 6d. (about $20), and the figures given below show the expenditure in other countries corresponding to this sum taken as 100:—

Great Britain	..	..	..	..	..	100
Germany	..	..	..	..	..	48
France	..	..	..	..	..	17
Czecho-Slovakia	..	..	..	..	..	14
Belgium	..	..	..	..	..	7
Italy ..	..	..	..	..	..	4

Although I quote these figures from the evidence given to the Royal Commission, they are scarcely comparable for the last four on the list, except as indicating varying degrees of social insurance. France and Italy have scarcely initiated health insurance.

voluntary membership of 7,400,000, have pointed out that the medical services of public health, education, and poor-law authorities overlap with the insurance medical service, and very shrewdly say that merely to extend medical benefit on its present basis to dependents of insured persons would intensify this overlapping of services, would be extremely costly, and yet would leave outside the scheme many impoverished families .They add that this extension would in effect mean that a large number of insurance prac-titioners would be working full-time, on a basis which was devised for part-time work. This is true, and there would be an almost irresistible tendency to the appointment of whole-time salaried doctors for the work. The friendly society opinion already quoted receives some tentative support in the *Report of the Royal Commission on Sickness Insurance*, which states :—

Whether a contribution to medical provision for dependents is to be made from insurance funds or not, the fact remains that medical service for dependents is too large a problem to be considered apart from medical service for the whole working-class and, perhaps, middle-class population.

The members of the same Commission, who signed a Minority Report, are more definite, and make the recom-mendations which are quoted on page 138.

There is strong reason for the view that all public medical services including insurance should be unified in one organisation for the prevention and cure of disease, but not that other medical services should be merged into that of insurance. The first-named mode of unification appears to be the ultimate goal. Whether it will work for good or not will depend on the extent to which preventive medicine is brought into action.

This subject will be more fully discussed in my con-cluding volume, in which an attempt will be made to draw general conclusions from the general survey of facts.

CHAPTER VI

MEDICAL SERVICES FOR MOTHERS AND CHILDREN

THE PRACTICE OF OBSTETRICS IN ENGLAND[1]

THE history of British practice of midwifery in past centuries shows that parturient women have more usually been cared for by women than by surgeons or physicians. Commonly these women have been neighbours with some past personal or other experience. Often a particular woman has obtained local celebrity for her obstetric skill; and until recent years such midwives and the less skilful "handy women" of limited experience have cared for most of the wives of wage-earners and the poor in their hour of need. In 1827 the President of the Royal College of Physicians said that "midwifery was an act foreign to the habits of a gentleman of enlarged academic education". During the eighteenth century there had been much controversy between the midwives and the obstetricians as to their relative functions, each group fighting for supremacy. The obstetricians, of whom Dr. Smellie was the protagonist, were dubbed "he-midwives" by their rivals. The conflict undoubtedly led to some increase of efficiency in both groups.

Gradually the unnecessary suffering and deaths of women in childbirth attracted attention, and, in particular, the Obstetrical Society of London, from the time of its inauguration in 1858, agitated persistently in favour of improved obstetric teaching and training both for medical students and for midwives.

A first-fruit of this agitation was the appointment in 1883 of a representative of obstetric medical work on the General Medical Council, and the training of medical students was improved. In 1872 the Obstetrical Society started an

[1] The arrangements in Scotland differ in some minor details from those of England.

Examination Board for Midwives, and when the official roll under the Midwives Act was started, 7,465 midwives then in practice who had passed this examination were ready to take their place on the roll.

There was a long struggle, fought by obstetricians and a minority of other medical practitioners, backed by an increasing volume of public opinion, before the Midwives Act of 1902 became law. The fight was against a medical majority who considered that the training and official authorisation of a new order of certificated midwives would be detrimental to their interests. It may be accepted that they also considered that the practice of midwifery by midwives would increase the risk to mothers. What was not appreciated was that midwifery was already being practised by unqualified, ignorant women, over whom the community had no control, and that there was no reasonable hope of forbidding this practice, unless possibly by the introduction of a gigantic system of obstetric attendance by doctors subsidised by the State. This being outside the range of practical action, the choice lay between tolerance of an existent serious evil, and the training of midwives with gradual elimination of the "handy woman".

A committee of the London Obstetrical Society in an inquiry made by them in 1869 found that from 50 to 90 per cent. of the total births were attended by midwives, a proportion not dissimilar from the present proportion, with the important difference that most midwives are now qualified for their work, and this work is carefully supervised.

The Midwives' Institute, an association of midwives, co-operated with the Obstetrical Society in the struggle for legislation.

In 1902 the Midwives Act was passed through Parliament —"An Act to secure the better training of midwives and to regulate their practice". This Act forbade any woman to use the title of midwife after April 1, 1905, unless certified to do so under the Act.

After April 1, 1910, it was enacted that "no woman shall habitually and for gain attend women in childbirth otherwise than under the direction of a qualified medical practitioner unless she is certified under this Act".[1]

Existing midwives who held a midwifery certificate, or who without this produced satisfactory evidence that they "had been for at least one year in *bona-fide* practice as a midwife", were allowed to be certified as midwives.

A Central Midwives Board was formed for England and Wales whose duties comprised—

the regulation of the issuing of certificates and the conditions of admission to the roll of midwives;

the regulation of the course of training, etc., for midwives;

the making of rules for the regulation, supervision, and restriction of the practice of midwives; and

the publication of an annual official roll of midwives.

The rules made by the C.M.B. require to be approved by the Minister of Health. The councils of counties and county boroughs were appointed local supervising authorities:—

to supervise the work of the midwives within their area;

to investigate charges of malpractice, negligence, or misconduct; and

to suspend midwives from practice in certain conditions, and to report this to the Central Midwives Board.

Every midwife is required to report her intention to practise in an area to its local supervising authority.

In connection with the above incomplete summary of the Midwives Act, it should be noted that many untrained women already in practice were necessarily put on the Roll of Midwives when it was first published. The number of trained women then entered on the roll was 9,787, and of untrained women 12,521.

[1] By the Midwives Act, 1926, this condition was made more stringent, and an unqualified woman is now forbidden to attend women in confinement, except under the direct supervision of a medical practitioner, unless the Court is satisfied that the case was one of sudden or urgent necessity. Thus the question of remuneration is eliminated.

On March 31, 1918, the roll contained the names of 42,949 women, of whom 24,076 had passed the statutory examination of the Central Midwives Board and 9,472 had been admitted by prior certification. This left 9,401, or 21·9 per cent. of the total, on the roll who were untrained except by practice. In 1925 this proportion had declined to 4·4 per cent.

The number practising midwifery or giving notice each year, as required by law, of their intention to practise, differs greatly from the number qualified to practise. In 1918 the number practising was 11,449, of whom 39 per cent. were untrained. In 1927 the corresponding number was 16,610.[1]

This discrepancy in numbers between qualified and practising midwives arises in part from the unattractiveness of midwifery as a calling, and in part from the fact that the midwifery certificate has been commonly taken without any intention to practise as a midwife, but as a step towards appointment as a health visitor (public health nurse).

Nevertheless, the majority of births in England are attended by midwives—in 1927 over 61 per cent. of all births. Of the midwives attending these births, 90·5 per cent. were trained, while 96·6 per cent. of the total midwives on the Midwives' Roll were trained.

An amending Midwives Act was enacted in 1918. This gave the Central Midwives Board power to make rules for suspending a midwife from practice for a stated period, instead of striking her name off the roll. The same Act empowered local supervising authorities to aid in training midwives, and to make grants for this purpose. Midwives are required to call in a registered medical practitioner in the emergencies outlined on page 151, and in such cases the supervising authority is required to be responsible for paying the practitioner's fee in accordance with an official scale. The scale of payment at the time of the passing of the Act was fixed by the Local Government Board, and was sub-

---

[1] This number exceeds the number actually practising, as many midwives practise in more than one area.

sequently modified in December 1922 by the Ministry of Health. It is as follows :—

	£	s.	d.

1. Fee for all attendances of a doctor at parturition (i.e. from the commencement of labour until the child is born) whether operative assistance or not is involved, including all subsequent visits during the first ten days, inclusive of the day of birth 2 2 0

2. Fee for attendance of a second doctor to give an anæsthetic, whether on account of abortion or miscarriage, at parturition or subsequently .. 1 1 0

3. Fee for suturing the perineum, for the removal of adherent or retained placenta, for exploration of the uterus for the treatment of post-partum hæmorrhage, or for any operative emergency arising directly from parturition, including all subsequent necessary visits during the first ten days, inclusive of the day of birth 1 1 0
   This fee not to be payable when the fee under (1) is payable.

4. Fee for attendance at or in connection with an abortion or miscarriage, including all subsequent visits during the ten days from and including the first visit 1 1 0

5. Fee for visits to mother and/or child not included under (1) to (4):
   Day (9 a.m. to 8 p.m.) 5 0
   Night (8 p.m. to 9 a.m.) 10 0

6. The usual mileage fee of the district to be paid for all attendances under (1) to (5) of this scale.

7. Fee for attendance on mother and/or child at the doctor's residence or surgery 2 6

No fee shall be payable by the local supervising authority :—

1. Where the doctor has agreed to attend the patient under arrangement made by or on behalf of the patient, or by any club, medical institute, or other association of which the patient or her husband is a member, or when the doctor is under obligation to give the treatment to the patient under the National Health Insurance Acts, 1911 to 1922.

2. Where the doctor receives or agrees to receive a fee from the patient or her representative.

3. In respect of any services performed by the doctor on any date later than the 10th day from the date of his first attendance unless he has reported to the local supervising authority that he considers, for reasons stated by him, that his further attendance is necessary, or in respect of any services performed by the doctor after the expiry of four weeks from the day of birth.

All claims must be submitted within two months of the event. The emergencies for which a midwife is required to send for a doctor are given in the following official list :—

Conditions in which Medical Help Must be Sent For

In all cases of illness of the patient or child, or of any abnormality occurring during pregnancy, labour, or lying-in, a midwife must forthwith call in to her assistance a registered medical practitioner, using for this purpose the form of sending for medical help (see Rule 23 [*a*]), properly filled up and signed by her.

In calling in medical assistance under this rule the midwife shall send for the registered medical practitioner desired by the patient, or, if the patient cannot be consulted, by the responsible representative of her family.

The foregoing rule shall particularly apply :—

1. In all cases in which a woman during pregnancy, labour, or lying-in appears to be dying or dead.

Pregnancy

2. In the case of a pregnant woman when there is any abnormality or complication, such as :—

Deformity or stunted growth.
Loss of blood.
Abortion or threatened abortion.
Excessive sickness.
Puffiness of hands or face.
Fits of convulsions.
Dangerous varicose veins.
Purulent discharge.
Sores of the genitals.

Labour

3. In the case of a woman in labour at or near term when there is any abnormality or complication, such as :—

Fits or convulsions.
A purulent discharge.

Sores of the genitals.

A malpresentation.

Presentation other than the uncomplicated head or breech.

Where no presentation can be made out.

Where there is excessive bleeding.

Where two hours after the birth of the child the placenta has not been completely expelled.

In cases of rupture of the perineal body, or of other injuries of the soft parts.

Lying-in

4. In the case of a lying-in woman when there is any abnormality or complication, such as :—

Fits or convulsions.

Abdominal swelling and tenderness.

Offensive lochia, if persistent.

Rigor with raised temperature.

Rise of temperature to 100·4° F. for 24 hours, or its recurrence within that period.

Unusual swelling of the breasts, with local tenderness or pain.

Secondary post-partum hæmorrhage.

White leg.

The Child

5. In the case of the child when there is any abnormality or complication, such as :—

Injuries received during birth.

Any malformation or deformity endangering the child's life.

Dangerous feebleness in a premature or full-term child.

Inflammation of, or discharge from, the eyes, however slight.

Serious skin eruptions, especially those marked by the formation of watery blisters.

Inflammation about, or hæmorrhage from, the naval.

Note.—The foregoing lists are not exhaustive, and do not include all cases in which medical help should be summoned. According to Rule E20, "any abnormality" requires medical help. The instances in Rule E21 refer to some of the most striking and important abnormalities.

Note.—In cases where the eyes are affected the duties of the midwife are :—

1. To call to her assistance a registered medical practitioner, using for this purpose the form for medical help.

2. To send notice to the local supervising authority that medical help has been sought.

The local supervising authority is empowered to recover the doctor's fee from the patient or her husband. The extent to which this is done may be seen in the local instances (pp. 264, 317, 347, 361, 398, etc.).

A candidate before sitting for a certificate in midwifery is now required to have undergone a course of training in midwifery extending over a period of not less than 12 months. In the case of a nurse who has been certified by the General Nursing Council for England and Wales as fully trained, the period of midwifery training is reduced to six months. The certificate must show that the candidate has received instruction in the supervision of not less than 20 pregnant women; that she has witnessed 10 labours, and, in addition, has personally attended and delivered women in 20 further labours. Of the last-named 20, at least 5 must be attended in their own homes, and 5 within an institution where there is training approved by the Central Midwives Board. The candidate must also have nursed 20 mothers and their infants in the days following labour: and she must have attended at least 30 lectures on the subject of her examination given by recognised medical lecturers.

The details briefly outlined above indicate the intimacy of the relation between the work of doctors and midwives.

The training and practice of midwives will be discussed in a concluding volume, as will also that of medical students.

CHAPTER VII

MATERNITY SERVICES, INCLUDING ANTENATAL SERVICES

IN Chapter VI the present position of the practice of mid-wifery by midwives, as determined by national law and regulations, has been outlined.

The enactment of the Midwives Act, 1902, of subsequent additions to and emendations of this Act, the formation of the Central Midwives Board, its disciplinary action and the regulations issued by it for the guidance of local supervising authorities, and the control of the methods of practice of individual midwives by these authorities, have placed mid-wifery as practised by midwives on a firm basis from which it will not be displaced.

The control of the work of midwives is in the hands of county and county borough councils acting as local supervising authorities (p. 149). Each local supervising authority is required—

To exercise general supervision over all midwives practising within its area; to investigate charges of malpractice, negligence, or misconduct, and, should a prima facie case be established, to report the same to the Central Midwives Board; to suspend any midwife from practice, if such suspension appears necessary in order to prevent the spread of infection; to report at once to the Board the name of any midwife convicted of an offence; during the month of January in each year to supply the Board with the names and addresses of all midwives who, during the preceding year, have notified their intention to practise within its area; to keep a current copy of the Roll of Midwives, such roll to be accessible at all reasonable times for public inspection, and to report at once to the Board the death of any midwife, or any change in the name or address of any midwife, so that the necessary alteration may be made in the roll.

Midwifery inspectors are appointed by these authorities to visit midwives, inspect their records and outfits, give them friendly advice, warn them in respect of irregularities in their practice, and to investigate complaints of malpractice, or cases in which a discharge from the infant's eyes has been reported. They may also inquire respecting cases in which puerperal pyrexia has been reported, but such inquiries are preferably made by a medical inspector: and it is becoming the practice to an increasing extent to appoint a medical woman as chief inspector of midwives, with assistants, who must possess the certificate of the Midwives Board.

For our purpose it is unnecessary to describe this organisation further, except in so far as it impinges on the work of the private practitioner of medicine. It is evident that there is a close and intimate relationship between the work of doctors and midwives, in private practice and in the work of maternity hospitals and homes and at antenatal clinics.

Further details as to local midwifery services are given in other chapters. In rural areas the midwifery service is carried out mainly by the district nurse-midwives who are employed by district nursing associations. Most of these associations are affiliated to corresponding county nursing associations.

In some districts the combined work of district nursing and midwifery is associated with work as a health visitor and school nurse. Thirty-seven of the 62 county councils make contributions to county nursing associations for the provision of trained midwives in certain areas of these counties, where otherwise the supply of midwives would be inadequate for their needs.

Sending for Medical Help

Midwives are required to send for a medical practitioner chosen by the patient, on the occurrence of such emergencies as are enumerated on page 151. The extent to which they send for medical aid varies greatly.

On page 150 is given the official scale of payment of doctors for each of the chief emergencies. The fee of two guineas (about $8·40) is not regarded as adequate by many doctors, and it certainly is not in some instances as much as would have been obtained if the doctor has been engaged apart from a midwife for the confinement.

Local authorities can recover the medical fee guaranteed to a doctor thus called in from the patient if she is able to pay. As will be seen in the local reports, the amount thus recovered varies greatly.

There has been much increase in the sending for medical assistance since the fee was guaranteed by the local authority; and in some areas suspicion has been entertained that midwives acted in collusion with special doctors to secure demands for their attendance. This is probably exceptional.

Under powers given by a further amending Midwives Act, 1926, a local supervising authority, with the consent of the Ministry of Health, can make arrangements whereby an expectant mother, by the prior payment of an agreed sum, insures against the liability for the payment of a doctor's fee if he is needed. Some local authorities have acted on this scheme.

This has been done in various towns, the usual sum charged for this insurance being 5s. Thus in Birmingham (population 976,000) the number insuring in 1928 was 3,068 (18 per cent. of total births), and medical help was required in 1,196, i.e. over a third of the total cases. Among uninsured women attended by midwives (7,587 cases), the doctor was sent for in about 25 per cent. of the cases. Insurance fees came to £767, doctors' fees for these cases were £1,945. Among the non-insured who required medical aid, the majority paid the doctor themselves. Only 567 were left to be paid for by the City Council, at a cost of £746, of which £444 was recovered from the patients at a cost for recovery of £228.

In Portsmouth (population 257,000), with a similar system, the net cost to the local authority in 1929 was £603, as compared with £541 before the scheme began. The net result was that the local authority paid 48 per cent. of the doctors' fees. Among the insured women a doctor was sent for in 38·5 per cent., and among the uninsured in only 24·2 per cent. of the cases.

It has been found that insurance on these lines leads to a medical practitioner being sent for to a greater extent, sometimes unnecessarily; and some local authorities counteract this possibility by limiting this form of insurance to cases where there has been antenatal examination of the mother, either at the antenatal centre or to cases in which a certificate is received from a private medical practitioner that the case is normal. An insurance scheme on the above lines must relieve expectant mothers of much anxiety.

MATERNITY HOSPITALS AND HOMES

The provision of hospitals for the delivery of women who could not be safely treated at home was included in 1914 in the earliest Government grants for maternity and child welfare work. The provision was intended for women suffering from some morbid condition requiring careful watching or special surgical skill, and for women living in circumstances which made confinement at home precarious. Gradually the use of these officially provided hospitals and homes has extended, and many local authorities, as well as voluntary hospitals, admit women who prefer institutional treatment, and who are willing to pay part or the whole of the cost of this.

According to the *Ministry of Health's Annual Report*, 1928-29, there are 2,480 such beds in 152 institutions, provided in nearly equal numbers by local authorities and by voluntary agencies, which are recognised for the purpose of Government grants. These figures do not comprise the entire institutional accommodation for parturition; there is additional provision in poor-law infirmaries and in a large number of private institutions.

Now that poor-law infirmaries have become hospitals of public health authorities their use for parturition will probably greatly increase. Scales of charges are arranged according to family income. Already some 15,000 births (i.e. about 7 in each institutional bed) probably occur in the above 152 institutions in a year, which is equal to about 2 per cent. of the total births in England and Wales.

The extent to which beds are being provided for maternity cases in several areas can be seen in the local reports which follow.

The B.M.A. have expressed their view on maternity provision in institutions in the following resolution passed in 1926:—

Where the local authority makes provision for the institutional treatment of maternity cases this should be mainly or primarily for serious cases of antenatal complications, for cases requiring major obstetric operations, for cases where isolation and treatment of septic infection are specially indicated, and other cases where the home conditions are unsuitable or dangerous for confinements.

This proposed limitation of municipal activity has not been accepted by local authorities; and there is occurring in England, especially in towns—though to a less extent apparently than for the urban population of the United States—increasing arrangement for institutional care during parturition and in the lying-in period. As will be seen in subsequent chapters, charges are made for such cases on a scale arranged according to the family income. Above a certain income-limit, the whole cost of treatment may be charged; but in a high proportion of the total cases some portion of the cost is borne at the public expense.

ADMINISTRATION OF MATERNITY HOMES

Although with modern precautionary measures childbirth in an institution is safer than in the home under present conditions of domiciliary medical and nursing care, this often is not so.

The administrative arrangements at the municipal maternity hospitals and homes vary. As a rule, midwives are in charge of uncomplicated cases, a doctor being sent for if an emergency arises. A special doctor attached to the institution, or a number of private practitioners on a rota, or the patient's doctor of choice may be called in. In a large institution the staff usually is self-contained, and experience has shown that maximum safety from complications is then secured. In smaller institutions—and many municipal homes have only a few beds—the patient may arrange to have her own private doctor, paying him separately from her payment to the institution. In others there is a small rota of local doctors who attend in turn when the midwife calls for them. This may work well if each doctor is experienced and skilful and is a patient obstetrician; but in some instances calamity has resulted from undue haste, from deficient experience, or from neglect of strict antiseptic precautions.

ANTENATAL CONSULTATION CENTRES

A frequent cause of mortality as the result of pregnancy and childbirth is lack of medical diagnosis of abnormal conditions, as, for instance, albuminuria, cardiac disease, or disproportion between pelvic measurements and the size of the fœtal head. It must be remembered that although antenatal causes of death of mother or infant are very serious, even more important is the intranatal mortality, due in large measure to unsatisfactory midwifery. To combat morbid antenatal conditions rapid increase in provision for antenatal consultations has been, perhaps, the most important result of the maternity and child welfare schemes initiated with and helped by Government grants since 1914. It is recognised that these centres must be staffed by medical men or women with special experience, though there is no reason why every practitioner should not be competent for the work. As shown by the experience narrated on page 177, a specially trained nurse-midwife may undertake much of the work, subject to the reference of any patient presenting morbid signs to the doctor.

Under the rules of the Central Midwives Board it is the duty of each midwife to examine her patient as early as possible in pregnancy and record the result. The following is a copy of the record required to be kept by her:—

No...........   ANTENATAL RECORD

Name...Age.......................
Address...

Date of Booking...................................Temp...............Pulse.....................
Date of Expected Confinement...
Date of Last Period...........................Regular...............Irregular...............

PREVIOUS HISTORY

Previous Pregnancies...
    „   Labours...
    „   Miscarriages..
    „   Stillbirths.   Probable Cause.....................................
    „   Puerperia..

PRESENT PREGNANCY.   GENERAL HEALTH

Anæmia..............................	Heartburn..............................
Bowels................................	Œdema-Swelling....................
Breasts................................	Sickness................................
Cough.................................	Teeth....................................
Deformity...........................	Vaginal Discharge.................
Lameness............................	Varicose Veins......................
Headache............................	Other....................................

ABDOMINAL MEASUREMENTS AND EXAMINATIONS

Date	Interspinous	Intercristal	External Conjugate
	Height of Fundus	Position	Fœtal Heart Sounds Heard

Head pushes into Pelvis
Head engages in Pelvis

If she finds any abnormality she refers the patient to a private doctor, sending the following card:—

ANTENATAL CARE

Dr._____   *Date*_____

Address_____

I have advised Mrs._____

of_____to see you.

I shall be obliged if you will let me have your opinion
and advice on this case. The patient $\dfrac{\text{wishes}}{\text{does not wish}}$ to insure.

Signed_____

Address_____

Or the patient is sent to a consultation centre, and the
doctor of the centre is expected to fill up the following
form and return it to the midwife:—

ANTENATAL CLINIC

WELFARE CENTRE_____

Name_____   Register No._____

Address_____

I have seen the above-named patient, and the conditions found
and recommendations are given below.

1. MEASUREMENTS AND EXAMINATION:—

    Interspinous_____   Intercristal_____

    External Conjugate_____   Height of Fundus_____

    Position_____   Fœtal Heart Sounds_____

2. URINE:_____

_____

3. GENERAL HEALTH:_____

_____

4. RECOMMENDATIONS:_____

_____

To:_____

    Signed_____

I should be glad to see your patient again on_____

The issue of these forms presupposes—and this obviously is necessary if midwives are to practise midwifery—that midwives have wide discretion in the supervision of expectant mothers. It is clear, furthermore, that—as they attend a majority of total births—antenatal supervision and its extent must depend very largely on them. Even if they were to carry out most of the antenatal work now known to be desirable, and carried it out under strict medical rules (as in the instance given on page 177), it could not be stated truthfully that they would be encroaching on medical practice as it now exists.

Medical obstetric work in the past has usually consisted in booking a confinement, and expecting not to hear of the patient from the monthly nurse until parturition has made considerable progress. Antenatal supervision has been a natural result of the efforts made by official and voluntary bodies to lower the heavy puerperal mortality which still persists; and happily the medical profession generally is now alive to its serious importance. The real difficulty for them is to obtain from their prospective patients remuneration which will be on an adequate scale for the care which is needed.

Many midwives are still incompetent for this work; others do it intelligently and well. But it is obviously important that the rules laid down by the C.M.B. (pp. 151 and 152) should be rigidly adopted, and that there should be skilled antenatal supervision in every pregnancy.

In 1928–29 (*Annual Report C.M.O. Min. of Health*) the number of antenatal clinics in England and Wales approved by the Ministry was 887, of which 522 had separate sessions, and 365 sessions were held on the same day as infant consultations. Of the total, 521 were municipal and the rest voluntary.

It is set out in a recent official circular that the medical officer of the clinic, whether whole or part-time, should be trained and experienced both in obstetrics and antenatal work, and should preferably have held a resident appointment in a maternity hospital, with experience at its antenatal clinic.

In another recent circular, however (Memo. 156/M, M.C.W., Dec. 1930), the Ministry have given their assent to the county or county borough authority "making arrangements with private medical practitioners whereby the latter will undertake the routine antenatal examination of uninsured women who have engaged midwives for the confinement". No limitation is announced in this assent as to special experience on the part of the doctor thus employed, though presumably the local authority could make distinctions. To do so would mean much friction. The proposed arrangement is intended "to meet the needs of those uninsured women who are reluctant to visit a centre for the purpose of antenatal examination", and in rural districts for those women who live beyond a reasonable distance from an available centre.

It is too early to comment on the doubtful advisability of this particular proposal.

This is a convenient point to note the proposals made by the B.M.A. for a NATIONAL MATERNITY SCHEME, published in *Supplem. Brit. Med. Journ.*, June 29, 1929, as "a contribution to the improvement of the present unsatisfactory position of the puerperal morbidity and mortality rates of this country". On the assumption that early notification of pregnancy can be obtained, the scheme proposes that:—

(1) Every pregnant woman should be examined at least once by the practitioner chosen by her, not later than the 36th week of pregnancy, and on further occasions if he thinks this necessary, and that it should be the duty of the midwife chosen by the patient for her confinement to persuade her to this effect.

(2) Every woman is to be encouraged to have at least one postnatal medical examination.

(3) A doctor should be made available whenever his attendance is requested by the midwife. (This is already an accomplished fact for all serious complications) (p. 156).

(4) A further consultant shall be available for certain serious conditions.

It is suggested that the scheme shall be applicable to

persons of the economic status of insured persons, and on this basis it is estimated that 500,000 of the 654,172 births in England and Wales in 1927 would come under the scope of the scheme, and that its cost annually would be £2,100,000. Certain savings on present services may possibly be set against this.

The B.M.A. also emphasise the need for improvement in the training of doctors for maternity work.

The B.M.A. estimate that some 3 per cent. of the total births would require institutional treatment for medical reasons.

I need not discuss the financing of the scheme which is still only on paper. It is doubtful if any early action will be taken in the direction adumbrated, as a pre-condition is legislation for the unification of the present public services (insurance and public health) into a service with somewhat wider scope. The subject is further discussed in my concluding volume.

The B.M.A.'s scheme is important as showing the desire of the organised medical practitioners of the country to take an active part in what is needed to prevent unnecessary suffering and mortality in childbirth, and as indicating their acceptance of the principle that the midwife commonly is adequate to normal confinements.

Before any national scheme of maternity care can be instituted, radical changes will be required in the maternity benefit under the National Insurance Act. The conditions of this benefit are set out below.

THE MATERNITY BENEFIT UNDER THE N.I.A.

Under the National (Health) Insurance Act the wife of an insured man receives on the birth of her child the sum of £2, and if she is also an insured employed person (married or not) she receives the same amount. The grant of £2 or £4 is paid to the mother by the Approved Society of which she or the husband is a member. There is no control on the part of the society or the public health authority over the expenditure of this sum. Most of it goes to pay the midwife's or doctor's fee.

The benefit in this form was a mistake from its initiation. It would have been preferable to supply skilled service instead of a money benefit, by making such attendance part of the medical benefit, or by arranging for it in connection with the maternity service of local authorities.

The matter, as already seen, is complicated by the provision by public health authorities of a considerable amount of skilled help for women in pregnancy and confinement (p. 184). The partial midwifery help thus provided is usually given by midwives or in lying-in homes or hospitals (p. 157): added to which is the public health guarantee of the fee of the doctor called in by a midwife in an emergency.

Evidently it would be to the public advantage if the two services of insurance and public health could be combined, at least in respect of midwifery, and made available for both insured and non-insured below a stated level of income. There would be little difficulty in arranging this on a national basis, were it not for the vested interest of the Approved Societies which at present administer the maternity benefit. Were this done it would be possible, so far, at least, as a majority of the total births in Great Britain are concerned,[1] to arrange for antenatal consultations, and thus avoid the development of many conditions producing excessive puerperal mortality.

The British Medical Association have recommended unification of these services. In their view provision in connection with maternity and child welfare should be made "an integral part of the Insurance Scheme or brought into proper relation thereto". In view of the more comprehensive sphere of action of these authorities, the alternative plan of placing the administration of maternity help for all needing it in the hands of public health authorities is indicated.

[1] The Government Actuary has estimated that 80 per cent. of all births occur in the families of insured persons, and that of the remaining 20 per cent. one-fifth occur in a corresponding social stratum.

GENERAL REVIEW

The relation between doctors and midwives varies greatly in different parts of the country, as may be seen from the samples of local experience given in later pages. It is clear that there always has been this sharing of midwifery work between doctors and midwives; and it is doubtful whether, if we allow for the unrecorded work of unqualified women in the past, there has been as much supersession of doctors by midwives in recent years as is commonly stated. But there has been some transfer, midwives now attending parturient women for an inclusive fee of two guineas (about $8), who formerly would have paid two to three guineas to a medical practitioner.

Many doctors in a past generation have utilised the services of unqualified midwives, as also of unqualified medical assistants. Both of these are now illegal. It must be remembered also that midwifery had no place in the recognised medical curriculum before the Medical Act, 1886, and that midwifery practice was disliked by many doctors, although it was regarded as the necessary portal to family practice. With the introduction of insurance medical work its value in this direction has decreased.

Even now the training of medical students for midwifery practice is unsatisfactory. It is too short and not so practical as it should be. The difficulty of extension of training lies in the student's crowded curriculum. But if this is not done, medical midwifery will tend to become a specialism, and normal midwifery will go more and more to a midwife better trained than at present.

Teachers of obstetrics appear to be unanimous as to the need for more protracted training of medical students, for less facile "signing up" of students (whether medical or midwives) for attendance on a given number of confinements, and for the provision of specialist obstetric consultants to be available in every large area, in addition to the present provision for medical aid. There is an increasing volume of medical testimony, especially on the part of obstetric specialists, that the midwife is the proper person to conduct normal labours. This obviously tends towards the divorce of the general practitioner from obstetric practice, and his supersession as a consultant in difficult cases by an obstetric specialist. The increasing formation of allied groups of doctors all engaged in general medical practice, but each member of the group making himself specially responsible for difficult cases in one branch of practice, may help to avoid this contingency. Post-graduate courses of instruction for both doctors and midwives also will help; and these are being made available in some centres. If difficult cases of midwifery are to be satisfactorily treated, the doctor treating them must be as well equipped in his work as is the operating surgeon who has had ample hospital experience.

Subject to the needed reforms indicated above, it is likely that in England midwives and doctors will continue to share midwifery work and such emoluments as attach to it, and it is unlikely that midwives will entirely supersede doctors even for ordinary normal confinements.

Even if this happens, it is evident that doctors will continue to be required for the exact medical diagnosis needed in some parts of antenatal work, and for the serious complications of pregnancy and parturition, and post-partum.

The State has recognised this need in subsidising antenatal clinics, and in making it obligatory on local authorities (county and county borough councils) to pay the fee of the doctor called in by a midwife in an emergency. It is true that the authority may recover this fee from the patient; but the calling in of a doctor is ensured.

If midwives still further supersede doctors in obstetric practice, how will doctors acquire the skill and experience demanded to enable them to give midwives the help needed in the serious complications of parturition? This question has often been raised but not satisfactorily answered. Foreign experience (see Volumes I and II, *International Studies*) seems to show that this risk has been exaggerated.

The midwife in a complicated case can send for any doctor in the vicinity who is named by the patient, and the doctor coming to help may be unskilful or inexperienced. The best aid that might be obtained is not guaranteed. Possibly obstetrics will become more and more a speciality in medical practice. It is so already to some extent. In order to secure the most highly efficient service, this may be the ultimate development.

The indications in this direction are strengthened by the recent decision of the Ministry of Health to require the notification of "puerperal pyrexia", i.e. of each case of a temperature of 100·8° F. or more during the puerperium. Already it is officially recommended that a consultant should be available in each area to advise with the doctor in attendance on such a case. This consultant may be nominated by the practitioners in the area. It may be, hereafter, that the same consultant will be employed chiefly or exclusively for all cases in which a midwife sends for medical aid.

The policy of the B.M.A. on consultative work for diagnosis of the cause of puerperal pyrexia occurring in a family doctor's practice is set out in the following resolution passed by its Representative Body in 1927.

It is desirable, owing to the fact that puerperal pyrexia may be due to causes other than obstetric, that a panel of consultants, which may be instituted under the Regulations, should include competent physicians, surgeons, and pathologists in addition to consulting obstetricians; further, that some standard of competence should be adopted, such as membership of the staff of a local general or obstetric hospital, or the possession of special qualifications or experience by private practitioners.

The system is still in process of development, and doubtless medical officers of health in advising local authorities as to the appointment of consultants will have in view the many causes of pyrexia after parturition.

Excessive Puerperal Mortality

Medical and public journals in recent years have contained many contributions discussing the high mortality still caused by the complications of pregnancy and parturition. It only enters into this report in so far as it bears on the relative work of doctors and midwives.

A word of warning must be given as to the complete comparability of international statistics of maternal mortality. The following among other possibilities of error arise in instituting comparisons.

1. In some countries and in special areas the intentional induction of abortion and premature birth for non-medical reasons is much commoner than in others. This must affect the amount of puerperal sepsis, though probably not to an extent to vitiate broad comparisons.

2. Even with the same international rules of statistical comparison it is not certain that there is uniformity of practice in regarding a given death as having been due to pregnancy or childbirth. It is likely that this is a serious source of error.

3. There is the natural wish of the certifying practitioner in certain cases to oblige his patients' relatives by avoiding mention of parturition in a death certificate.

4. First-births are commonly twice as dangerous for the mother as the subsequent three or four births. Evidently, therefore, an arithmetical correction is called for in comparing countries or districts with high and low birth-rates respectively.

Making full allowance for these factors, there remain remarkable real differences in experience of puerperal mortality, for explanation of which one is driven to conclude that skilled and conscientious work as compared with work not manifesting these characteristics forms the chief explanation.

In support of this conclusion, I give in the next chapter an account of the experience of a particular lying-in hospital in an extremely poor part of London (home as well as institutional treatment), and I now give an extract from the appendix to the B.M.A.'s Report on a National Maternity Scheme, which further illustrates the same point:—

I. *That the normal case can be safely treated at home.*

1. In 1927, in the practice of the Queen Victoria Jubilee Nursing Institute Midwives in England and Wales, there were 53,502 deliveries, with only six deaths from sepsis in normal births. The overwhelming majority of these cases were attended in their own homes by midwives.

2. During the last ten years the General Lying-in Hospital, York Road, London, has attended in their homes 16,518 cases with three deaths, only one of which was due to sepsis—that is, a mortality of 0·18 per 1,000.

3. In the outdoor practice of the Edinburgh Maternity Hospital during four years, 5,000 cases were delivered, with two deaths only from sepsis.

4. In Glasgow, a city with an abnormally high maternal death-rate, 6,974 cases were attended by the Maternity Hospital in the homes of the women during 1926 and 1927, with four deaths, the causes of which are not stated in the report.

5. In Liverpool 1,547 patients were attended in their homes by the Liverpool Maternity Hospital without a death.

II. *That maternal mortality and morbidity can be very greatly reduced when proper antenatal care and supervison during confinement are provided in all cases, together with institutional accommodation for cases of complicated labour.*

The East End Hospital, in whose practice these principles are observed, had in ten years a total of 21,875 unselected cases (that is including both normal and abnormal, and both domiciliary and institutional cases) with 14 deaths—that is, a mortality of 0·64 per 1,000. This is a mortality equal to less than one-seventh of that obtaining over the country as a whole. The General Lying-in Hospital had 26,198 similarly unselected cases with 42 deaths—that is, a mortality of 1·6 per 1,000. This is a mortality equal to less than one-third of that obtaining over the community generally.

It may be assumed that proper antenatal care and supervision during confinement would lead to a reduction in maternal morbidity in a ratio similar to that which can be confidently expected to occur in the death-rate.

III. *That maternal morbidity can be greatly reduced with proper postnatal care and treatment.*

This is not capable of being supported by statistics, but it is well known that much chronic ill-health in women springs from the damage caused by child-bearing. It is commonly recognised that from 40 to 60 per cent. of gynæcological disease is caused in this way, and that much suffering and permanent ill-health can be prevented by the early detection and treatment of such conditions as displacements of the pelvic organs, infection, etc.

In giving the above extract I must warn against the assumption that the above-quoted puerperal death-rates are strictly comparable with puerperal death-rates as given in the Registrar-General's reports and in local statistical reports by health officers. The latter include mortality from abortions and miscarriages, and many such cases are not included in the above institutional statistics. But when full allowance is made, the above experiences are much more favourable than aggregate experience in private medical practice.

CHAPTER VIII

AN ILLUSTRATION OF EXCEPTION-
ALLY LOW MATERNAL MORTALITY

THE East-End Maternity Hospital, Commercial Road, London, E.1, is an institution in which an exceptionally low rate of maternal mortality in parturition had been experienced. In June 1929 I visited this institution and examined its records. The results of this examination, with some observations, are embodied in the following pages.

This institution was founded in 1884, and then consisted of seven beds at a house in Shadwell. Since that time it has steadily grown in size, the available beds increasing to 56. In 1927–28 there were 2,517 confinements in it, with three deaths. During its history the maternal mortality per 1,000 births among the patients confined in the hospital or at home under the care of its staff was as shown in tables on page 173.

Thus during the entire experience of the hospital, deaths of mothers have occurred at the rate of 2·1 per 1,000 infants born in the hospital, and at the rate of 0·74 per 1,000 infants born in the home practice of the hospital, or 1·35 per 1,000 infants born in its entire experience.

As this rate of mortality is only about one-third that of the metropolis as a whole, its record must be examined somewhat critically.

If there were marked superiority in the work of the hospital, one would at first blush expect this to manifest itself in its intern experience; but in this department the death-rate is more than double that experienced in the home work of the hospital. If one limits the comparison to the period 1914–28, the same superiority of home over hospital experience is shown (1·45 as against 0·51). In both instances the difference probably represents not inherently safer parturition at home as compared with parturition in hospital under reformed midwifery conditions, but only that a larger proportion of difficult cases become in-patients at the hospital, as well as a larger proportion of cases in which home conditions are unfavourable to successful lying-in.

But is the total experience of the hospital, intern and

A. Hospital Patients

Period	Number of Mothers Admitted	Number of Deaths	Deaths per 1,000 Births
1884–89	427	1	2·34
1890–97	1,629	12	7·37
1898–02	1,278	2	1·57
1903–07	1,966	6	3·05
1908–13	3,223	6	2·13
1914–20	4,970	10	2·01
1921–26	6,373	7	1·10
1927–28	2,517	3	1·19
1884–1928	22,383	47	2·10

B. Patients Attended at Home

Period	Number of Mothers Attended	Number of Deaths	Deaths per 1,000 Births
1884–89	—	—	—
1890–97	1,548	3	1·94
1898–02	1,530	5	3·27
1903–07	2,384	1	0·42
1908–13	5,597	1	0·18
1914–20	7,490	8	1·07
1921–26	7,027	2	0·29
1927–28	1,608	—	—
1890–1928	27,184	20	0·74

extern (1·35 deaths per 1,000 births), comparable with the puerperal death-rate for London as a whole, which for the single year 1928 was 3·09 per 1,000 births?

The metropolitan figures comprise deaths due to complications in all stages of pregnancy, including abortion, whereas those for the East End Hospital refer particularly to births after the seventh or eighth month of pregnancy. How much does this affect the comparison?

There are no available English statistics as to deaths due to pregnancy, classified according to its stage; but it is stated officially that the number of deaths occurring in the first seven months of and recorded as due to pregnancy weighs lightly in the total result.

In 1911–20 in England and Wales, 3,235 deaths were returned as due to "accidents of pregnancy" out of 32,971 from all accidents of pregnancy and childbirth. A mental allowance is necessary, therefore, for the fact that the total national and the metropolitan experiences are handicapped when these are compared with the experience of the East London Hospital. It is probable, however, that only a relatively small change would be effected (say one-tenth) if allowance were made for the unstated complications of earlier pregnancy in the hospital experience.

The rate of mortality (under 1 per 1,000 births) of the extern experience makes it highly probable that there has been much elimination of cases likely to be abnormal. Whether these all have been drafted into this charity or not cannot be stated. This point is in doubt. Emergency cases from outside are excluded as far as possible, in view of the possible introduction of infection. Thus cases of failed forceps are rarely admitted. They may go to the London or St. Bartholomew's Hospital, or elsewhere. I am unable to state to what extent allowance for these possibilities of incomparability would alter the figures, but I do not believe they would more than partially explain the superior experience of this institution.

Of the births in the hospital, 310 in 1927 and 384 in 1928 were of inhabitants of Poplar, and many Poplar women are attended from the hospital in their own homes. In the four years 1925–28 the total Poplar births were 14,026, and the puerperal deaths were 42, equal to a rate of 2·95 per 1,000 births. It appears probable that in Poplar, as in the rest of London, serious causes of excessive puerperal mortality exist and continue, which are avoidable, and which, in the experience of the East End Maternity Hospital, are largely avoided.

The conclusion that real saving of maternal life—and with it lessened suffering short of a fatal result—is being experienced in the work of this institution is confirmed by its experience of still-births and of deaths of infants within a fortnight after live-birth.

DEATHS OF INFANTS IN THE HOSPITAL PRACTICE OF THE EAST END MATERNITY HOSPITAL DURING 1925–28 INCLUSIVE

	In the Hospital	In the Patients' Homes	England and Wales
Births	4,889	2,643	—
Still-births	144	69	—
Deaths during the first fortnight after live-birth	71	28	—
Still-births per 100 births	2·95	2·62	3·30 (1926)
Deaths in first fortnight after birth per 1,000 births	14·5	10·7	26·5 (1927)

Thus the favourable maternal mortality is associated with a low proportion of still-births, and with a remarkably low death-rate among living infants while under the care of the charity. Here, again, certain possibilities of incomparability cannot be entirely eliminated. The charity is limited to married women, and there may possibly be exceptionally little syphilis among its patients. The question of proportion of *primipara* also arises. In 1928 primiparous births were 43 per cent. of the total births, which does not support the view that multiparous births are more frequent in this charity than elsewhere.

The number of attendances at the antenatal clinic averaged 3⅓ for every mother. One-fifth of these attendances were made to the medical officer's clinic.

In the same year the total original breech presentations were 104, cephalic version being successfully performed in 48, and attempted unsuccessfully in 17 cases.
In 12 other such cases the condition was not discovered
before birth, and in 27 for various reasons version was
not attempted.

In 3·2 per cent. of the total cases forceps were applied.
The proportion of forceps cases in extern cases was 1·65
and in intern cases 4·31 per 100 patients.

The preceding analysis of the mortality experience of this
institution, and a comparison of its figures with those for
the whole country, for London, and for one of the two
metropolitan boroughs in which the work of the institution
lies, makes it difficult to avoid the conclusion that—allowing
for all causes of accidental variation—the favourable experience of the East End Maternity Hospital was in large
measure the result of work of a more efficient character
than that in the general community. If so, the practice of
this institution deserves careful study.

Some special features of this practice emerge in the
following description of the working of the charity.

There is continued oversight and care for the mother
throughout pregnancy from the moment she registers for
midwifery attendance; also in parturition; and for her infant
and herself for a fortnight afterwards.

The women attended are all married. They are all poor,
and I am informed that even when the pecuniary maternity
benefit under the National Insurance Act is forthcoming,
the managers of the hospital seldom feel justified in claiming
any part of it. For multiparæ 10s. is paid for maintenance
in hospital during two weeks, and 21s. for primiparæ. The
total amount received from patients was £1,291 in 1928,
the total expenditure for the year being £7,640.

Patients book for maternity attendance usually in the
sixth or seventh month of pregnancy. Out of over 2,000
patients in 1928, only about a dozen had failed to book.
Very few emergency cases are admitted.

This implies that the first condition of successful midwifery is secured in most of the cases attended by this institution, namely

ANTENATAL CARE

Each primiparous expectant mother is expected to attend, and does attend, an antenatal consultation at the hospital. This attendance is in effect a condition of subsequent maternity attendance. A fortnightly consultation is held at which all primiparæ and other pregnant women with an unfavourable history in previous pregnancies are required to attend. Other multiparæ are seen and examined three times during pregnancy.

These fortnightly consultations are held four times each week, and a fifth weekly consultation is also held by Dr. W. H. F. Oxley, the honorary visiting officer of the institution, to whose skill and constant care the institution owes much. The first-named consultations are held by the assistant matron, specially skilled in this work, which she has carried out for many years. Any patient found by her to have even a trace of albuminuria, or to present a malpresentation of the fœtal head, or any other abnormality, is always referred to the medical clinic. The principle claimed for this scheme is that a skilled nurse with many years' experience of midwifery and antenatal work can be trusted to pick out the patients who should consult with the medical officer. There is the closest co-operation between the assistant matron and the doctor; and in the circumstances of this institution the economical system here adopted works admirably.

A serological blood test for syphilis is not made as a routine; it is only made when symptoms or the history of the patient indicate its desirability. All patients with syphilis are referred to the special venereal disease clinic at St. Bartholomew's Hospital, where they can have treatment without delay or waiting. Such cases are few in number in the experience of the lying-in hospital. They are attended for parturition by this institution and come into the general statistics.

In discussing the carrying on of the antenatal clinic in

ordinary cases without medical aid, the very competent assistant matron was confident that this arrangement in experienced hands worked well. She urged that for the doctor to see the patient once or twice or even three times during pregnancy gave a false and misleading sense of security, and that the nurse should know enough to ensure immediate reference to a doctor whenever required.

In the lying-in hospital five midwives and one relieving sister are employed. In the district work two sisters and eight midwives are employed, who live in the hospital.

The discovery of wrong presentations is an important part of the antenatal work. The midwives are trained to recognise these, and version for breech presentations is usually carried out in the thirtieth week of pregnancy. This has been done for the last fifteen years, and it partially accounts (by preventing "breech" births) for the low infant mortality in the experience of the institution. The midwife is encouraged to perform these versions under the doctor's guidance. If she does not succeed at the first attempt, it is then done by the doctor.

As pregnancy approaches its term, determination of the position of the fœtal head, and of its size in relation to that of the pelvis, becomes an important part of the skilled midwife's work, as determining the line of procedure to be adopted.

The urine is tested in every case fortnightly from the time of booking, which is usually early in the seventh month. Any case with the slightest albuminuria is referred to Dr. Oxley. One of the midwives or midwife-pupils then visits the patient weekly, and reports whether the albumen has disappeared under dietetic treatment. If not, the patient is usually admitted to hospital, and if the albuminuria then continues, labour is commonly induced, as otherwise chronic nephritis may follow.

As for other complications, the main indication is to prevent their occurrence. Eclampsia occurs chiefly in patients who have not come under supervision. In the experience of this charity the last death from this cause occurred in 1919, since when 20,000 patients have been attended. During the last four years only one slight case of eclampsia has occurred among 8,000 patients, and this patient had neglected to come for antenatal examination for three weeks.

A few of the midwives are able to make blood-pressure tests; but as high pressure is rare apart from albuminuria, the test is rarely needed except as a prognostic guide.

The detection of vaginal discharge is an important part of antenatal work. This is treated at the hospital, the patient sometimes being admitted for this condition.

Dental caries, if considerable, is treated, patients being referred to other centres for this.

The methods of dealing with other complications of pregnancy and parturition need not be detailed.

GENERAL OBSERVATIONS

The preceding details give only a partial possible explanation of the favourable experience of the Maternity Hospital. But there can be no question as to the importance of the rigidly required and cheerfully accepted antenatal supervision, practised as in this charity. For:—

1. It is the beginning of the system of supervision and preventive action characterising the entire work of the institution.

2. The doctor and matron alike are confident that the consistently good results are due to three factors, all operating as the result of the remarkable spirit of service and devotion characterising the staff.

(a) The patient is quickly made to realise that a deep interest is being taken in her welfare.

(b) The patient almost without exception obeys in every detail the instruction given to her.

(c) These instructions are reduced to their utmost possible simplicity.

Not too much is asked from the nurse or the patient. An impossible asepticism is not aimed at, but the utmost cleanliness of hands, mackintosh, etc., is required. Lysol and other antiseptics, which in adequately strong solution will be uncomfortable for the nurse's hands, are eschewed, and mercuric chloride solution is always used after previous soap and water. There is no prohibition of vaginal examinations.

About 7 per cent. of the cases confined at home are seen also by the doctor, who is called in by the midwife. It will be borne in mind that the home-attended cases have been partially "weeded" of patients likely to need medical aid.

While reserving a discussion of the general problem of excessive puerperal mortality in the light of this local experience, and experience in various countries, a few observations may be made.

Much puerperal mortality must be ascribed to the ignorance and unwitting neglect of the mother herself. The entire machinery of the East End Maternity Hospital is calculated to overcome this ignorance and neglect. Sympathetic co-operation of a high order between doctor, midwives, and patients is secured and maintained.

The dangers of malpresentation, of contracted pelvis, of antecedent disease are reduced to a low level. The care given in parturition secures relative immunity from sepsis, which is perhaps most frequently due to trauma.

It appears probable that much of the excessive puerperal mortality in private medical practice is due to delay in institutional treatment when this is found by the doctor to be indicated. This is not merely a question of actual deficiency of institutional beds. If the patient is sent by the private doctor to an institution (e.g. for severe albuminuria or for narrow pelvis, etc.), the doctor loses his prospective fee for the case. Perhaps as important as this is the fact that he loses prestige in his practice by sending a patient to a hospital. These human factors need to be weighed and provided for in securing safer parturition.

This subject is discussed more fully in my concluding volume.

CHAPTER IX

CHILD WELFARE SERVICES

THE history of public provision for ensuring the safety of childbearing and of the infant cannot be given in detail here. During the last 50 years both these objects have occupied the attention of social workers, obstetricians, and medical officers of health. Earlier attempts were directed especially to the regulation of the practice of midwives and to the prevention of infectious diseases, in particular to the reduction of the devastating mortality from summer or epidemic diarrhœa. The extent to which this last-named object has been attained in England can be judged from the following diagram (Fig. 3). Diarrhœa is now becoming a relatively rare disease; and the mortality from respiratory and other infections also shows a remarkably great decline. In 1896–1900 diarrhœa caused one-fifth, and 1926–27 only one-tenth, of the total infant mortality.

Measures for the protection of mother and child were being promoted by public health authorities and voluntary agencies for a number of years before the Great War; for the infant these gradually extended beyond efforts to prevent measles, whooping-cough, and diarrhœa, and were directed increasingly to an improved standard of health as well as to the prevention of disease. The introduction of medical inspection of school children in 1907 in a few years showed the terrible amount of disease with which young children when they reached school age were already handicapped, and thus gave valuable impetus to increased activity in preventive measures at earlier ages.

For years before the prompt notification of births to the M.O.H. became obligatory, the addresses of infants were obtained in many areas from the registrars of births, and visits were made to their mothers, and especially in the months of June and July to the mothers of infants who it was known were being artificially fed.

Diarrhœal prevalence had much influence in the historical development of infant welfare work. In a few towns municipal milk depots were opened for the supply to poorer mothers of trustworthy cows' milk. In some early investiga-

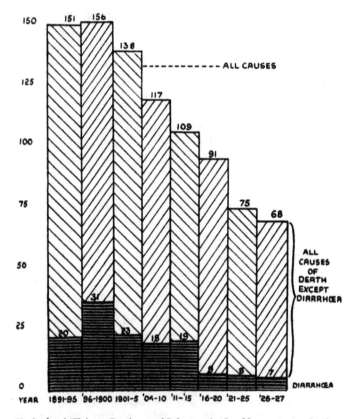

England and Wales.—Death-rate of Infants under One Year per 1,000 Births.

tions it was found that condensed milk was an even more dangerous source of food for infants than fresh cows' milk. The limited utility of milk depots became evident; and the need to avoid encouragement of artificial feeding led to the formation of schools for mothers, merging into the more comprehensive infant consultations, in which the problem of each infant was studied on its merits by a medical man or woman. The advice given at these consultations was largely hygienic, though it often became therapeutic; and as Budin, the distinguished founder of such consultations, said, "an infant consultation is worth precisely as much as the presiding physician".

Hygienic work for the children was rendered easier by two Acts of Parliament—the Children Act, 1908, and the Notification of Births Act, 1909. The first of these enabled legal action to be taken when children were neglected; and neglect and cruelty were interpreted as occurring when medical treatment had been neglected. Local authorities and the inspectors of voluntary societies, especially the National Society for the Prevention of Cruelty to Children (N.S.P.C.C.), were able effectively to warn neglectful parents, and in extreme cases to take legal action for their punishment.

In the provinces Huddersfield was a pioneer in obtaining early notification of births.

In 1909 the Notification of Births Act came into force throughout London, and was adopted rapidly in the rest of England. This Act provides that the parent, in addition to registering the birth of his child within six weeks of its birth, shall within 36 hours after the birth notify its occurrence to the M.O.H. of the district in which the birth occurred. This has made early as well as systematic home visiting of mothers and their infants practicable, and such visits are now almost universal. These visits, and the counsel given by competent and sympathetic visitors, form the most important part of child welfare work in England. The help thus given is made more valuable by encouraging the mother to bring her infant periodically to a stated infant welfare centre, where medical advice is available.

The visits of advice made after the birth of an infant at each parent's home gradually became more general, and their value was realised; practical measures of help were associated with these visits of advice, and in 1914, after several reports on Infant and Child Mortality and on Maternal Mortality from its Medical Department, the Local Government Board secured the consent of the Treasury to the giving of grants of money equal to the approved amount spent by each local authority or voluntary organisation on schemes for improving the health of mothers and their infants. The Board of Education already had been giving grants for schools for mothers under their general educational powers. Their work became subsequently merged into the infant consultations of public health authorities, the predominant note of which was the giving of individual counsel to the individual mother as to her own health and that of her infant, though collective instruction was also given to the mothers attending the infant consultation (Infant Welfare Centre).

The importance and wide scope of measures entitled to the 50–50 grants given by the Local Government Board on behalf of the Central Government can be seen from the following schedule, which may be regarded as the charter of child welfare work on which all subsequent English developments have been based. Notwithstanding more recent extensions and modifications, the schedule covers the main scope of medical and hygienic activities now in being :—

(Copy of official document)

MATERNITY AND CHILD WELFARE

A complete scheme would comprise the following elements, each of which will, in this connection, be organised in its direct bearing on infantile health.

   1. Arrangements for the local supervision of midwives.
   2. Arrangements for:—

Antenatal
1. An antenatal clinic for expectant mothers.
2. The home visiting of expectant mothers.
3. A maternity hospital or beds at a hospital, in which complicated cases of pregnancy can receive treatment.

3. Arrangements for:—

Natal
1. Such assistance as may be needed to ensure the mother having skilled and prompt attendance during confinement at home.
2. The confinement of sick women, including women having contracted pelvis or suffering from any other condition involving danger to the mother or infant, at a hospital.

4. Arrangements for:—

Postnatal
1. The treatment in a hospital of complications arising after parturition, whether in the mother or in infant.
2. The provision of systematic advice and treatment for infants at a baby clinic or infant dispensary.
3. The continuance of these clinics and dispensaries so as to be available for children up to the age when they are entered on a school register, i.e. the register of a public elementary school, nursery school, crèche, day nursery, school for mothers, or other school.
4. The systematic home visitation of infants and of children not on a school register as above defined.

LOCAL GOVERNMENT BOARD,
WHITEHALL, S.W.   *July* 1914

In the circular letter to which the above schedule of proposed work was appended, local authorities were urged to undertake work which would deal continuously with the whole period from before birth until the time when the child is entered upon a school register. It was definitely contemplated that "medical advice and, where necessary, treatment should be continuously and systematically available for expectant mothers and for children until they are entered on a school register, and that arrangements should be made for home visitation throughout this period".

Early notification of births was made universally compulsory in 1915, and the Act of that year empowered local authorities to exercise all their powers under the Public Health Acts "for the purpose of the care of expectant mothers, nursing mothers, and young children". In drawing the attention of local authorities to these powers the Local Government Board deprecated false economy during the war. They wrote:—

At a time like the present the urgent need for taking all possible steps to secure the health of mothers and to diminish antenatal and postnatal infant mortality is obvious, and the Board are confident that they can rely upon local authorities making the fullest use of the powers conferred on them.

Work proceeded with redoubled activity during the war, on the broad lines set out in the preceding schedule, both local authorities and voluntary organisations taking an active part in it.

In 1918 a further law was enacted, still further emphasising the importance of the work. This was the Maternity and Child Welfare Act, 1918. The Act imposed statutory duties on every local authority undertaking maternity and child welfare work. They were required to form a special maternity and child welfare committee. Two-thirds of its members were to be members of the council, and the remaining third, or part of it, might be introduced from without from among persons specially qualified by training or experience in subjects relating to health and maternity, of whom at least two must be women. Their duties were to "make arrangements for attending to the health of expectant and nursing mothers, and of children up to 5 years of age not being educated in schools recognised by the Board of Education". It is set out in the Act that its provisions "do not authorise the establishment by any local authority of a general domiciliary service by medical practitioners". The medical officer of health of each borough within an administrative county was required to send a weekly list of births locally notified to the county council.

In a covering circular to local authorities dated August 9, 1918, the Local Government Board re-emphasised its view that child welfare work was second only in importance to direct war work, and drew attention to the fact that the sanction of the Treasury had been secured to a considerable extension of the scope of the 50–50 grants. The following additional services were included:—

Hospital treatment for children up to 5 years of age.
Lying-in homes.
Home helps.
The provision of food for expectant and nursing mothers and for children under 5 years of age.
Crèches and day nurseries.
Convalescent homes.
Homes for the children of widowed and deserted mothers, and for illegitimate children.
Experimental work for the health of expectant and nursing mothers and of infants and children under 5 years of age.

In 1919 the Local Government Board was merged into the Ministry of Health, and, as will be seen below, infant and maternity work has continued progressively to increase.

The rapid growth of this work may be illustrated by the grants of money from the Central Government, by the increasing number of health visitors employed, and of special child welfare centres.

In 1914–15, the first year of 50–50 grants, the amount of money distributed by the Central Government was £11,488. It rapidly increased, notwithstanding the Great War.

In 1915–16 the amount was £41,466.
In 1916–17 the amount was £67,961.
In 1917–18 the amount was £122,285.
In 1918–19 the amount was £218,190.

. . . .

In 1921–22 the amount was £1,113,922.
In 1923–24 the amount was £754,961.
In 1925–26 the amount was £850,173.
In 1927–28 the amount was £983,031.
In 1928–29 the amount was £1,010,705.

A large part of the early post-bellum increase of grants was for the supply of milk. In 1920 for the country as a whole the supply of food and milk formed 17 per cent., in 1921, 25 per cent., and in 1922, 20 per cent. of the total expenditure of local authorities on maternity and child welfare. Since then the Ministry of Health has restricted this provision; but owing to prevalent unemployment, the amount remains large, even though it has been suggested by the Ministry that "applications should be considered only in those cases in which the medical officer of health or the medical officer of a centre certifies that the health of the mother or child would suffer unless a supply of milk or food is provided by the local authority". (*Annual Report, Ministry of Health*, 1927–28).

Of the total amount in 1927–28, a little over one-seventh consisted of grants made to voluntary societies. The percentage distribution of these large sums, and the equal sums contributed in each administrative area were devoted, is seen in the following table (*Ninth Annual Report, Ministry of Health*, 1927–28) giving the total net expenditure as 100:—

	Per Cent.
Medical officers	9·9
Health visitors	24·8
Midwifery	4·4
Fees paid to doctors called in by midwives	2·9
Nurses	0·9
Centres	11·1
Day nurseries	1·9
Maternity homes and hospitals, infants' hospitals and arrangements for treating puerperal fever and ophthalmia neonatorum	16·0
Milk and food	20·9
Orthopædic treatment	0·8
Home helps	0·3
Miscellaneous	6·1
	100·0

HEALTH VISITORS, that is, public health nurses with special knowledge of child hygiene, have been employed by public health authorities for many years. In Manchester they were working in 1900, the women employed being engaged chiefly in securing more cleanly domestic conditions. With the adoption of early notification of births, they became concerned in all areas with infantile hygiene. At first partly or fully trained nurses were employed for this work, preference being given to women who were also qualified as midwives. Then a special course of training in child hygiene was demanded, and the requirements in this respect have now become greater, and health visitors generally are fully qualified nurses with six months' additional practical training in their special work.

In 1918 already a large staff of health visitors was being employed. The number of these and the corresponding number in 1928 are shown below:—

ENGLAND AND WALES

	1918	1928
Whole-time health visitors doing only maternity and child welfare work	751	948
Part-time health visitors undertaking also school work or tuberculosis visits	760	1,347
District nurses engaged as health visitors ..	1,044	1,461
Additional health visitors employed by voluntary societies	320	351
	2,875	4,107

In 1929 the number of infant welfare centres in England had become 2,522, of which 1,623 were conducted by local authorities, and 899 by voluntary agencies (*Ministry of Health's Report*, 1928–29).

As we are concerned chiefly with the relation of medical practitioners to these special services, it is unnecessary to give details as to official expenditure for home nursing of infectious cases, day nurseries, the supply of milk and food to necessitous mothers, and other chiefly non-medical activities. My observations will be chiefly limited to home visitation of young children by nurses and the medical and hygienic care given at child welfare centres (infant consultations). The increasing provision by public health authorities of beds in maternity hospitals is noted on page 157.

HOME VISITATION BY NURSES IN RELATION TO MEDICAL PRACTICE

This, I have already stated, in my view is the most important part of infant welfare work in Great Britain. It is most efficient when the visits are preceded and supplemented by regular attendance at a child welfare centre for weighing, for hygienic advice, and for consultation with its medical officer at the first visit, and afterwards whenever the baby is not thriving. The home visits are made by a fully trained nurse who has had supplementary training in the hygiene of infancy and childhood. Usually the family doctor is not in attendance when she visits; but whether so or not, the judicious health visitor ascertains any dietetic or other instructions he may have given, in order to avoid clashing of advice. This is the rule under which she acts, and it is seldom contravened. The occasional instances in which the mother informs the doctor of divergent advice given by the health visitor, most often are instances of misquotation, and are at once rectified if the doctor communicates with the medical officer of health. In the main the health visitor is a valuable auxiliary to the family medical adviser. It must be noted that in a high proportion of the total families visited, the mother would lack the needed advice as to the management of her infant but for the health visitor's visits. Even fairly well-to-do families are very apt to neglect to seek medical advice, unless there is actual illness which appears to be serious; the health visitor's advice not only prevents much illness, but also accelerates the seeking of medical advice when needed.

As health-visiting now functions, it does not encroach on medical practice, *as this has existed in the past*, but increases the demand for it, by conducing to early medical attendance in illness, and by creating a demand for hygienic medical guidance.

Infant Welfare Centres in Relation to Private Medical Practice

The last remark in most districts is true for the hygienic and medical work of infant welfare centres. Where this is not so, it is contrary to the policy which has guided the giving of governmental grants from 1914 onwards. The work done in these centres, in the main, was not being done for the children of the social status who attend these centres, prior to their opening. On the contrary, lowered health was allowed to drift into ill-health, and this into actual disease in vast numbers of cases.

I give here an admirable summarised statement of work as carried out at a good centre :—

The babies are brought when they are about three weeks old; the family history is taken; they are weighed each time they come; and any collateral information bearing on each case is obtained. All babies are seen by the medical officer and carefully examined at their first visit, and a strict record is kept of all particulars; their diet is discussed, special stress being laid on the great importance of breast-feeding. The mother is supplied, if necessary, with printed instructions how to promote or increase the supply of milk, and advised as to the number and duration of feeds; further advice is given on clothing, bathing, ventilation, exercise, and all desirable hygienic necessities. If breast-feeding is not satisfactory, the mother comes to the centre for three or more "test feeds"—namely, weighing the baby before and after each feed; should the supply be insufficient an amount of modified cow's milk is ordered to be given immediately after each breast-feed, so that the total amount will produce 45 to 50 calories per pound weight per day. If breast-feeding is impossible, instructions are supplied to the mother how to feed the baby on modified cow's milk.

The mother brings the baby to the centre once a week; if all is not going well she sees the medical officer. This goes on at lengthening intervals during the first year. From the first to the fifth year the child is brought to the centre once a month; if any evidence of illness or disease is apparent the case is referred to the private medical attendant or to a hospital. For minor ailments simple remedies are prescribed. We frequently meet with cases of malnutrition, marasmus, and sometimes cœliac disease, where dietetic treatment is sufficient.—Dr. J. H. HAINES, East Islington Welfare Centre, London, *Brit. Med. Journal*, January 11, 1930.

It is evident that although the function of the centre is mainly hygienic, this embraces a vast range of subjects. In infancy, furthermore, the boundaries between ease and malaise, between health and sickness, are ill-defined and often traversed, and the medical officer of the centre finds herself obliged to prescribe for digestive derangements, to order cod-liver oil, etc. If there is bronchitis or other acute illness, or any risk of the onset of this, the mother is warned to call in a private doctor at once. (See under Brighton, p. 363.)

It is a good rule to give an intimation to this effect to every parent, in view of possible contingencies.

The organisation of these centres was considered in 1921 by the Medico-Sociological Committee of the British Medical Association, and their recommendations as approved by the annual meeting of the association in 1923 are noteworthy.

One paragraph of their report reads as follows:—

No medical treatment should be given at the centre as it is against the best interests of the centres to encourage women to go there for what they can *get* rather than what they *learn*.

If we except prescriptions given for temporary disorder, this is the general procedure at centres. Dr. Alfred Cox, the able medical secretary of the B.M.A., in a recent report (*Brit. Med. Journal*, November 3, 1928) based on a tour of inspection, has stated:—

In every area I visited it seemed to me that a genuine attempt was made (before giving anything except treatment for really minor ailments) to get the parent to consult the private doctor.

This is confirmed by the evidence collected in my own inquiries. (See the local reports which follow.)

Another paragraph may be quoted from Dr. Cox's report:—

The only drugs I saw given were an occasional grey powder, cod-liver oil and external remedies for the contagious skin disease, and, very occasionally, a simple cough mixture.

In short, it may confidently be asserted that as a rule both the hygienic advice and the treatment given at these centres deal with cases among the wage-earning classes which would never have found their way to a doctor's private consulting-room.

MEDICAL STAFFING OF INFANT WELFARE CENTRES

In most areas whole-time official doctors (usually women) do this work, and on this there has been much controversy. It is work which a general practitioner is competent to undertake, if willing to devote time to render himself proficient in this somewhat neglected branch of hygienic medicine. The report quoted above states :—

Medical education at present, though not ignoring the subject of infant welfare, cannot be said to devote sufficient attention to it. . . . (But) the experience of a suitable family doctor of some years' standing would be a very valuable asset in the work.

It is undoubtedly desirable to secure the sympathy and co-operation of the medical practitioners of the district, but the appointment of such practitioners to attend at centres has often been disadvantageous. For: (1) If there are several practitioners in the area, a rota is asked for, and this is generally and rightly condemned; or, in the alternative one practitioner may be giving advice at the centre to parents who usually employ another practitioner in illness. (2) The private practitioner not infrequently finds himself unable to keep his appointment at the centre. On this point the Representative Body of the British Medical Association have urged (1923):—

That private general practitioners or consultants accepting office under local authorities must realise that the duties of these offices require to be fulfilled strictly in accordance with the conditions of the appointments and in priority of all other engagements.

There seems to be little doubt that the policy of whole-time medical officers of infant welfare centres will persist for some years; but it is extremely important that these medical officers should consider themselves as acting in collaboration with the private practitioner, whenever the parent attending the centre has one. But on this point, see a further discussion in my concluding volume.

PAYING WELFARE CENTRES

Poverty in the home does not necessarily imply absence of skill in infant management, nor do riches always imply its possession; and appreciation of the value of the chiefly hygienic advice obtained at child welfare centres has led to sporadic attempts to secure similar advice for mothers who can afford to pay enough to make the centre self-supporting. For instance, in London a club has been started on these lines for mothers of the professional class who cannot afford repeatedly to call in a doctor for general supervision of their infants. It is made a condition that any mother wishing for this supervision must first inform her family doctor of her intention and obtain his co-operation. Cases of illness discovered at the club are referred back to him.

The Council of the British Medical Association tentatively approved of the movement illustrated above, but this approval was vetoed by the representative meeting of the B.M.A., which passed the following resolution:—

The Representative Body, while it fully appreciates the value of any educational work proposed to be undertaken at paying centres for middle-class mothers in the way of giving lectures on infant management, does not approve of these centres providing consultations and advice in respect of mothers and young children belonging to classes of the community who are quite able to consult their own family doctor.

The rules of the club appeared to safeguard the position of the family doctor, but if he is prepared to give the same continuous supervision and counsel on terms which are within the capacity of middle-class mothers the need for the club does not arise.

The problem here presented is part of the entire problem of the educational guidance of mothers and the hygienic supervision of the infant and the toddler. How many families can afford the frequent supervision which is needed, in supplementation of the weekly weighing, etc., which the intelligent mother can undertake? How many doctors have time to devote to this work for remuneration which would make it possible for most mothers to engage their services? It must be added that the training of doctors in the past has not been satisfactory in regard to infant dietetics, clothing, rest, exercise, ventilation, and general hygiene; and that in order to undertake this work—the same applies to the work of child welfare centres—they will need to be prepared to deal with minutiæ, which in other cases they leave to trained nurses, and they will need—if they are to secure many clients—to be prepared in a large number of cases to work on a financial basis which is very different from their ordinary scale of fees. Can this be organised by private medical practitioners on an insurance basis or otherwise? If so, it will be a source of gratification to all public health workers.

The work for the middle-class mother involves also home visits by a health visitor. She is needed not much less by this mother than by poorer mothers.

Ideally one may hope for the period when private medical practice will be so modified that every family even the poorest, will have their own doctor, when financial impediments to adequate access to the doctor will disappear, and when the family doctor will in the fullest sense be the hygienic as well as the medical adviser of the family. But when that comes, it will include consultation with specially skilled doctors in all cases requiring exceptional technical skill.

The movement to inaugurate infant welfare centres for middle-class mothers can only be retarded or prevented by family doctors devoting special attention to children, and by their forming family contracts, in lieu of payment by fees, which would encourage prompt consultations even for the slightly ailing or the well.

CHAPTER X

THE SCHOOL MEDICAL SERVICE

THE school medical service is an outgrowth of the system of elementary education which became national in 1870. With the making of school attendance compulsory in 1880 for all children aged 5–14, and still further with the abolition of fees for attendance in 1887, there gradually emerged the realisation that sickness was a chief cause of absence from school and of subsequent inefficiency in adult life. In 1902 a step towards bringing official educational work into relation with public health work was taken by transferring the duties of separately elected school boards to education committees of public health authorities. These committees are not directly elected by the people, but chosen from the elected members of county borough councils or county councils (and some smaller local authorities), additional members being co-opted to these committees from without. (See page 31 for constitution of education authorities.)

The detection of widespread serious physical defects and weakness in military recruits and in school children, and the need which arose in 1906 for the feeding of underfed school children during industrial depression, led to the passing in the last-named year of the Education (Provision of Meals) Act, and in 1907 of the Education (Administrative Provisions) Act, which imposed on education committees (local education authorities) the duty to provide for systematic medical inspection of all children, whether sick or well, immediately before, or at the time of, or as soon as possible after, their admission to a public elementary school, and on such other occasions as the Board of Education direct.

They were further empowered to make such arrangements as may be sanctioned by the Board of Education for attending to the health and physical condition of the children educated in public elementary schools.

This includes the power to provide treatment for those school children in need of it.

The legal position as regards treatment was profoundly modified by Section 2 (1) of the Education Act, 1918, which imposed on local education authorities the duty of treating such children in elementary schools as needed it.

It will be noted that the school medical service is not a general public health service, applicable to all children of school age, but "is rather an ancillary educational service which affects only the pupils in certain recognised educational institutions". For the children in elementary rate-aided schools it carries with it the duty not only of medical examination of the scholars in these schools, but also the duty of adopting measures to secure the treatment of any defects that are discovered.

By the Education Act, 1918, the duty of medical inspection, but without the correlative duty of treatment, was imposed on education committees having control of secondary and continuation schools supported chiefly out of rates and taxes.

In each administrative area the education committee entrusted with this medical work is a committee of the local authority like the Public Health Committee, but it has fuller delegated power than the latter. The work initiated under the above enactments has been a great factor in raising the national standard of health of the young. Centrally the new medical work was in the vigorous hands of the Board of Education, a separate department of the Government from the Local Government Board, which subsequently became the main element in the Ministry of Health.

It is unnecessary to discuss fully the drawbacks of this dichotomy of central supervision of hygienic and medical work for school children and for the rest of the community. At the beginning the division probably hastened the progress of school medicine. More recently the separation, to the extent to which it continues, is not entirely in the public interest. It should be added, however, that even though complete fusion of all educational and general health activities were to occur centrally as well as locally, there would still be needed a close liaison, amounting in certain particulars to partnership, between public health and education authorities. Confusion and extravagance of effort are inevitable so long as schemes for the medical supervision and treatment of school children remain separate from corresponding schemes for infants and toddlers. But such supervision and treatment are not the only need. While they form indispensable means for the prevention of disease and the enhancement of health, more general measures are needed for the same purpose, which belong to education authorities, such as the teaching of personal hygiene to every scholar, and the cultivation of mental as well as physical hygiene in their widest sense, including organised games and physical exercises. More and more as school hygiene advances, it will become less clinical and will resemble increasingly the medical service of infant welfare centres, which is chiefly hygienic. At the present day, in both school and pre-school public medicine, morbid conditions cry out for remedial treatment, and these—representing as they do a more urgent need than the hygienic personal supervision which should persistently be exercised—may sometimes undesirably limit this needed supervision. More general treatment of morbid tonsils, adenoids and teeth, and of crippling defects, whether caused by rickets, infantile paralysis, or tuberculosis, in the pre-school period will, ere long, make it possible for the school medical service to become more largely preventive in its work. This is already taking place in some areas. (See, for instance, pp. 349 and 415.)

The end in view is well expressed in Dr. Auden's school report for Birmingham (1929):—

The chief function of a medical department is not mere inspection and the treatment of defects, but rather to attempt to adjust each child to meet the demands of his future social relationships, and to improve the conditions of child life as generation succeeds generation.

Unless educators and hygienists join hands, only partial

success is possible. A statement made by me in *The Ministry of Health* (Putnams, 1925) may also be quoted: "As school medical inspection becomes increasingly preventive and less palliative and curative in its scope, the necessity for daily partnership between hygienic and scholastic workers in every area will increase."

MEDICAL TREATMENT OF SCHOLARS

Local education authorities have now had imposed on them the definite duty to provide or arrange for the treatment as well as to make medical inspection of the children attending schools under the local authority, and a large amount of valuable work has been done to secure treatment for school children found to need medical care.

Education committees are required to charge for treatment of school children, as can be seen from Section 81 of the Education Act, 1921, which reads as follows:—

1. Where a local education authority provide for the medical treatment of children or young persons attending any school or institution under the last preceding section, there shall be charged to the parent of every child or young person in respect of any treatment provided for that child or young person such an amount not exceeding the cost of treatment as may be determined by the local education authority, and, in the event of payment not being made by the parent, it shall be the duty of the authority, unless they are satisfied that the parent is unable by reason of circumstances other than his own default to pay the amount, to require the payment of that amount from that parent, and any such amount may be recovered summarily as a civil debt.

2. Nothing in this section shall be construed as imposing any obligation of a parent to submit his child to medical inspection or treatment under the last preceding section.

In fact assessments for payment for treatment of school children are made in a generous spirit, and in no case are they allowed to inhibit ready access to treatment. The conditions chiefly treated are those which in the absence of school clinics would be much neglected in the present circumstances of English life, especially in rural districts.

Information as to the scale of charges in various areas is given in the local chapters which follow. (See, for instance, Swindon, p. 350, Gloucestershire, p. 294, London, p. 417.) Some detail concerning the general working of school medical inspection and treatment is given in the chapters dealing with the work of local health and educational authorities, especially in the chapter relating to London, and only a brief sketch for the whole country need be given here. The annual reports on "The Health of the School Child" by the chief medical officer of the Board of Education, who holds the same position at the Ministry of Health, give an excellent picture of the varied health activities for the benefit of school children.

In 1928 nearly 5 million children were in average attendance at elementary schools in England and Wales, and 38·4 per cent. of these were medically examined in the course of routine work. Many other children were medically examined for special reasons, making the total proportion examined in a single year 57·2 per cent. of the number in average attendance.

It will be noted that school medical work is legally limited to the child attending school, and does not provide complete medical care for all children of school age. There is therefore very strong reason for unifying the medical work of public health and education authorities. A further urgent reason lies in the fact that a large proportion of children when they first attend school are suffering from defects and disease which ought to have had earlier treatment.

The limitation of school medical work to scholars at once implies that certain classes of illness and minor ailments come preponderantly within the range of work of school authorities.

The chief forms of medical treatment provided are for defective vision and squint, for enlarged tonsils and adenoids, for uncleanliness and verminous conditions, for dental disease, and for minor ailments, such as ringworm, impetigo, blepharitis, sores, etc.

The family practitioner is given an opportunity to treat wherever this can be arranged. Failing this a very large amount of treatment is carried out by local education authorities. The number of authorities who make provision for official treatment is given in the following table. The total number of education authorities is 317.

ENGLAND AND WALES
EDUCATION AUTHORITIES PROVIDING TREATMENT

For	Number of Authorities	Number of Clinics
Minor ailments	311	963
Dental defects	304	1,087
Defective vision	316	593
Supply of spectacles	310	—
Adenoids and tonsils	267	84
Ringworm by X-rays	176	46
Orthopædic treatment	183	191
Artificial light treatment	64	45

Further details of school clinics and of other arrangements for treatment of school children are given in the local reports which follow, especially for London (p. 413), for Cambridge (p. 271), and for Brighton (p. 374).

Much of the treatment of minor ailments is undertaken by fully qualified school nurses. These nurses in 1928 inspected over 14 million children for uncleanliness and verminous conditions, of whom over 700,000 required treatment in these respects. The success of cleansing work may be illustrated by the experience in the schools of Willesden, a borough on the borders of London. In 1914 of the total children inspected 20 per cent. had nitty or verminous scalps. In 1927 the proportion was only 4·9 per cent. In the same schools 79 per cent. of the medical and 97 per cent. of the dental defects were treated under official auspices, and 21 per cent. and 3 per cent. respectively by private practitioners.

In 1928 the medical and nursing staff employed in the school medical service of England and Wales was as follows:—

	School Medical Officers	Assistant School Medical Officers	Additional Practitioners Employed on Specialist Duties	School Nurses
Giving whole-time to School Services ..	13	254	—	1,298
Part-time, residue to Public Health Service	250	366	—	1,529
Part-time, part of residue to Public Health Service	40	61	—	—
Part-time, residue to private practice ..	14	295	—	78
—	—	—	1,593	—

The efficiency of school medical work can be partially measured by the extent to which treatment is secured for the children found on inspection to need it.

Gradually the proportion of cases diminishes in which parents neglect treatment, the need for which is discovered by school doctor or nurse; in a minority of cases the powers given by Section 12 of the Children Act have been found valuable. Under this section failure to secure treatment is construed to be causing "unnecessary suffering or injuries to the health" of the child, and the parent can be punished. Legal decisions to this effect have been secured in respect of children with severe adenoids and cleft palate.

THE PRE-SCHOOL CHILD

Reference has already been made to the many children who when admitted to an elementary school at the age of 4 or 5 are found to suffer already from caries, enlarged tonsils, and other defects. Some of these can be detected at an earlier age if the child is brought to a crèche or a nursery school. There should be no gap between the supervision exercised at child welfare centres and that by the school doctor. In some areas active efforts are being made to fill up this gap. Thus in Birmingham children under 5 who have been already seen by the health visitors are asked to attend a child welfare station and are there medically examined, in accordance with a medical schedule similar to that used for school medical inspection. In addition, remedial exercises clinics are being opened for pre-school cases of flat-foot, badly shaped chests, at which breathing exercises, etc., are given. (See Report for 1929 by Dr. G. A. Auden, School Medical Officer, Birmingham.) It is only by vastly extended efforts that children aged 2–5 years can cease to be "the great pool from which originate carriers of disease, crippling, and mental disorders". (J. Kerr.)

Some recent figures of experience in London emphasise the need for more vigorous effort to reach the pre-school child. Out of 1,000 entrants to London County Council schools 472 had decayed teeth, 185 morbid conditions of nose and throat, 17 had cardiac disease, 21 eye diseases (including squint but not defects in refraction), 11 had ear disease, 11·5 skin affections, and 3·5 some deformity. The need for overhaul before school attendance begins is further indicated by the fact that the examination of entrants may be postponed for some months after school attendance begins, or even longer than this.

In Edinburgh the toddlers' playgrounds, which are supervised by a health visitor, have been found valuable for the same purpose, and still more in securing a supervised open-air life to the child of the overworked mother.

Gradually the partial gap between the infant welfare centre and school medical inspection is being filled up; and when this is effected, school medical work will become more effective on its hygienic side, and less burdened on its clinical side.

A recent circular issued jointly by the Parliamentary chiefs of the Ministry of Health and the Board of Education (Circular 1054, December, 1929) is significant in this connection. It commences with the bold statement that "the

State made itself responsible for the health and education of all children from the age of five onwards", and then points out that hundreds of thousands of children for three or four years before going to school "have no help, direction, or succour from public sources, however much they may need it". Furthermore, "it is grossly uneconomic to allow the health and stamina of infants to deteriorate till 5 years old and then to spend large sums of money in trying to cure them between the ages of 5 and 15"; and it is recommended that, following on systematic health visitation and when any abnormal condition is found:—

Parents should be persuaded to have the child examined by their ordinary medical attendant, who would himself undertake any treatment which might be required, but it would be necessary for the authority to arrange for facilities for examination and treatment to be available for other children at a clinic or hospital. In many cases it may be possible to utilise school clinics for this purpose.

This recommendation of the Central Government has already been considerably anticipated in some towns, as in the instance of Birmingham already cited. The further example of Hyde, Cheshire, may be cited. The Medical Officer of Health sends to parents of children who, according to the birth register, were born three years earlier, the following letter:—

Dear Sir or Madam,—As a result of the school medical inspections, it has been found that when children commence to go to school, roughly three out of ten have already got medical defects or diseases which require treatment. A large number of the babies born in the borough are examined at the child welfare centre during their first year, but very few children are again medically examined (save in the case of serious illness) until they are of school age, and in view of the fact that so many are then found to have defects, often of long standing, it is felt that, in the interests of the children, parents should be given an opportunity to have their children examined, say, at two years of age. It is proposed, therefore, to have all the children of the district examined as they become two years old, if the parents are willing; and as our records show that your child is now of this age, I would be glad to know if you are agreeable to have him or her examined. Examinations will take place, by appointment, at the maternity and child welfare centre, and will be free of charge. In your own interests, and for the sake of your child's welfare, I would urge you to take advantage of the facilities offered. If you are willing to have your child examined, will you please return the enclosed postcard to me as soon as possible. (See *Medical Officer*, February 2, 1929.)

INADEQUACY OF SCHOOL MEDICAL WORK

It will be clear from the preceding paragraphs that school medical work, valuable as it is, only fills up gaps in medical aid otherwise not obtainable. Even in this particular it does less than could be done if public medical work for infants, for the toddler, and for the school child became a unified organisation. The National Union of Teachers, representing all the elementary school teachers in the country in a resolution passed January 5, 1929, have emphasised their conviction that "there is need for considerable improvement in the provision of medical treatment following medical inspection, and that the provision for minor ailments cannot be regarded as providing a satisfactory and comprehensive scheme of medical treatment". They express their gratification at the progress already made, but press for more complete action, especially in making provision for dental treatment.

The trend of the official circular quoted on page 203 and of the resolution of the N.U.T. quoted above is in the direction of largely increased therapeutic activities of education committees of public health authorities. The need for such work would greatly decrease if every pre-school child were satisfactorily overhauled and treated. It would not arise, furthermore, if family practitioners were able to organise hygienic and therapeutic treatment for all the wage-earning sections of the population, with the assistance of consultant services, whenever required.

This brings us to consider briefly the relation of the school medical service to voluntary hospitals, and the attitude of the British Medical Association, as representing private medical practitioners, to the school medical service.

SCHOOL MEDICAL TREATMENT AND VOLUNTARY HOSPITALS

The history of this relationship has important bearing on the relative responsibility of the State (i.e. of communal government) and of the family to secure medical treatment as needed. The present position is set out in some detail in the chapters which follow, the experience of London and of Brighton being especially enlightening. Let us outline the stages in the development of school medicine. Adequate medical treatment for the poor and their children has always been a difficult social problem; and vast masses of curable disease, owing to the difficulties of this problem, have remained untreated. In the past and now, voluntary hospitals—supported by the bequests and donations of the charitable—have partially filled this gap, and in them treatment has been undertaken which would otherwise have had to be secured at the expense of rates and taxes.

When the social and hygienic conditions of school children were realised, there came first, in 1906, the provision of meals for insufficiently nourished children. At first voluntary workers supplied the necessary funds; these later being supplemented from rates (p. 196). Then came the Act of 1909 making it obligatory on education authorities to provide for the medical inspection of children, to which was tacked on the authorisation quoted on page 196. It was stated in promoting this legislation that medical treatment was not primarily intended to be included; and local education authorities were advised to "encourage and assist . . . voluntary agencies and associate with themselves representatives of voluntary associations for the purpose". In a Circular (596) the Board of Education laid it down that:—

Before direct treatment of ailments is undertaken by a local education authority itself by means of a school clinic or otherwise, all reasonable advantage should be taken of the benefits of such institutions as hospitals and dispensaries.

It was further stated that treatment at a school clinic should only be given if treatment cannot be secured directly by the parents or through the agency of the poor-law or as above. In short, other available means of providing treatment were to be exhausted as far as possible before resorting to school clinics supported out of public funds. Very soon this attitude was modified; and the desirability or necessity of providing directly for a large portion of the defects found on medical inspection became clear. The process of transference from hospitals to school clinics was expedited by the hospitals themselves. The staffs of these institutions were often "snowed under" by the crowds of children needing treatment whose need had been revealed by medical inspection at school. Some of the hospitals were willing to treat these children in return for subscriptions from the local education authority or on a capitation arrangement with this authority. Even then the hospital, especially in great towns, was not always conveniently situated, and difficulties arose in securing prompt attention. The staff of many voluntary hospitals, furthermore, declined to give gratuitous services for the treatment of patients for whom the education authority had, by implication at least, made itself responsible. Such arrangements, however, persist in some areas to the present time.

In some areas groups of private practitioners have arranged special school clinics (see London, p. 416), the education authority remunerating the staff, which has been elected among the doctors themselves. The story of the struggle in Brighton is illuminating (p. 367).

In most areas it has been found necessary to establish official school clinics, to the most efficient of which have been attached beds for special cases needing post-operative stay in hospital. For dental diseases school clinics are now almost universal.

RELATION OF GENERAL MEDICAL PRACTICE TO SCHOOL
MEDICAL WORK

A vast amount of clinical work is being carried out for school children. A large part of it is being done by school nurses (small festering wounds, impetigo, dirty heads, etc.)

either at school or in minor treatment centres, more or less under the supervision of the school doctor.

Another large part of the school clinical work consists of the treatment of conditions which in the past were seldom undertaken by general practitioners.

A neglected no-man's land was occupied, exemplified by treatment of eye refraction cases and of ringworm by X-rays.

The orthopædic work of special school clinics and of the institutions in which this is undertaken is in a similar position. It includes remedial exercises and massage, the correction of deformities after poliomyelitis, chronic tuberculous joints, etc. Formerly some general medical practitioners operated on adenoids; but this operation is one implying exceptional skill; and most parents cannot afford a consultant's complete fee. Most of the dental work now being done at school clinics was previously almost completely neglected. Dental conditions have received much attention by school authorities; but even in this case, it is estimated that at present there is only, on the average, one whole-time dentist to every 11,000 elementary school children, whereas the number needed for adequate attention is at least one dentist for every 5,000 children.

From this incomplete enumeration it is clear that school medicine has opened out a new area of largely neglected treatment, and has only to a smaller extent encroached on treatment by private medical practitioners, which in the absence of school medicine they would have given. Furthermore, the general practice of sending letters signed by the school doctor to parents whose children need treatment has caused a very considerable increase of resort to the family practitioner, which otherwise would not have occurred. (See, for instance, pp. 327, 416, and 496.)

With these points in mind, we may note the attitude of the British Medical Association to school medicine. This is embodied in a general statement printed in the *Annual Handbook* of the Association for 1928:—

Briefly stated, the policy of the association as regards treatment of school children is to the effect: (1) that treatment by an education authority should be confined to those children whose parents cannot afford to pay privately for treatment, parents being recommended to secure treatment for their children from their family doctor; (2) that medical treatment and the treatment of refraction should be carried out by private practitioners; (3) that treatment of the children normally should not be carried out through voluntary hospitals, and that in cases where the work is so carried out, there must have been previous consultation with the hospital medical staff, who should be paid for this work; (4) that where treatment by private practitioners (whether general practitioners, specialists, or both) is adopted, it should be by means of a "Treatment" centre or clinic, or in sparsely-populated districts by "recognition" of places where the local practitioner(s) should carry out the necessary treatment; (5) that where practitioners in an area are desirous of carrying out treatment of school children found defective, they should through the Division (of the B.M.A.) make representation to the local educational authorities and place a scheme before the body; (6) divisions desirous of placing a scheme of treatment by local practitioners before the local education authorities will have the full support of the association, but for purposes of co-ordination such schemes should be submitted to the head office of the association prior to being forwarded to the education authorities; (7) that it is not part of the policy of the association to resist the adoption of some other scheme preferred by the education authority on the ground that it involves the employment of whole-time officers for the purpose of treating necessitous children; (8) that a scheme for treatment might be a combination of whole-time and private practitioners; (9) that there is no objection to treatment by provident dispensaries, public medical services, or other contract medical practice organisations, provided the remuneration of the practitioners is adequate, and that effect be given to the principle of free choice of doctor and of patient; (10) that any scheme for reference of children to the poor-law for treatment be opposed.

This is an omnibus statement which obviously implies that the local education authorities must decide for themselves the school medical policy most appropriate for local needs, though the association favours part-time doctors and clinics run by associated doctors. The local examples illustrate various types of school medical service,

and reference should be made to them. The consideration sadvanced on page 208 are being increasingly realised,
and friendliness between general practitioners and the
school medical service is becoming more general than
it has been.

In conclusion, there is nothing incompatible between the
growing provision for official medical supervision of
school children and the even more desirable periodical
examination by the family doctor of pre-school children,
as well as of scholars, where this can be organised. Possibilities in this direction will be discussed in a concluding
volume.

The Hiatus at Ages 14-16

Reference may be made here to the gap between leaving
school and the commencement of sickness insurance at the
age of 16. During these two years of life the partial medical
care on an official basis intermits, and serious defects may
develop. A pupil may leave school with good teeth, and
when he comes under medical care as an insured person his
teeth may be seriously carious. A scheme of periodical
examinations between the ages of 14 and 16 would do much
to raise the standard of adult health, assuming that action
followed inspection. In some large industrial works this is
being done.

It is not within the scope of this volume to describe the
English system of medical examination of boys and girls
when they begin work in a factory. Certifying surgeons
were first appointed under the Factory Act of 1844. The
Home Office (not the Ministry of Health) appoints in each
area a local practitioner to undertake this work. In some
areas there is a measure of collaboration between him and
the school medical officer, the records of the latter being
made available when the would-be factory worker is
examined by the certifying factory surgeon. In a few areas
the certifying factory surgeon is also the school medical
officer, and then unity of counsel and action is possible. But
the present position is unsatisfactory and calls for reform.

CHAPTER XI

SOME SPECIAL PUBLIC MEDICAL SERVICES

A. ACUTE INFECTIOUS DISEASES. PATHOLOGICAL SERVICES

WE have already seen that there are three chief medical services carried on entirely, or almost entirely, at the expense of the public rates and taxes—poor-law, public health, and the school medical service. These are now becoming almost completely unified locally into one great service; but meanwhile one must study the medical side of the important sub-divisions of public health work in their relation to private medical practice.

PROVISIONS FOR ACUTE INFECTIOUS DISEASES

Most of these are required to be notified to the local medical officer of health. A few diseases acquired in industrial work are required to be notified to the Chief Inspector of Factories, Home Office, London. These include anthrax, glanders, and other infections acquired in work; also lead and phosphorus and other industrial poisonings.

A fee of 2s. 6d. is paid to the certifying practitioner for every case notified from his private practice, or 1s. if the case has occurred in poor-law or hospital practice.

Cases of tuberculosis, pulmonary and non-pulmonary, are also required to be notified to the M.O.H. This is sometimes seriously neglected, the notification being sent only a short time before the patient's death, and preventive measures therefore being thwarted and delayed. With increasing co-operation between the private practitioner and the official tuberculosis officers this will be remedied.

In England every sanitary authority is empowered to

provide a hospital for the isolation of the infectious sick, and in Scotland this duty is obligatory. This duty becomes obligatory in England under the Local Government Act, 1930. It devolves on county and county borough councils, and many of the smaller isolation hospitals will doubtless disappear. Motor ambulances render it possible to provide more satisfactory treatment in larger institutions serving wider areas.

For many years patients suffering from an infectious disease, whether smallpox, enteric fever, diphtheria, scarlet fever, or other disease were required to contribute to the cost of their maintenance personally or through their parents or other guardians. The attempt to recover these sums—seldom more than a fraction of the total cost—caused much friction and was often ineffective: furthermore, when the contingency of such payment became known, parents often refused to allow the patient to be removed to hospital, thus possibly endangering the whole family and other families. During the last quarter of a century these payments have almost disappeared; though sometimes patients will pay for special accommodation in a private ward. It is now held that the patient thus isolated gives what is almost a *quid pro quo* in protecting the public through his volitional isolation. Though the results of hospital isolation of scarlet fever have not entirely fulfilled expectations in reducing the prevalence of this disease, there has been great social gain in this provision, and much medical gain for the individual patient; and the practice of gratuitous hospital treatment of these and other infectious diseases is now so firmly established that any attempt to diminish it or to charge for it would be strongly resisted by the general public.

In regard to infectious diseases, therefore, *there is* in Great Britain *gratuitous hospital treatment of all patients, of whatever social class*, whenever the private practitioner, acting in conjunction with the M.O.H., considers that this is advisable.

Disinfection of bedding and of premises is also carried out almost universally at the public expense.

Vaccination against Smallpox

The provisions for the compulsory enforcement of vaccination have been made before 1930 by the various boards of guardians. There is an official public vaccinator in every district, whose duty it is, in the case of every child who has reached the age of four months, to call at any house in the district served by him on receipt of the requisite notice from the vaccination officer, and offer to vaccinate the child with glycerinated calf-lymph. He has also fixed hours at his office for gratuitous vaccination of adults.

The public vaccinator is supplied with vaccine lymph manufactured in the governmental lymph establishment; private practitioners obtain their supply from commercial sources. It will be seen that *for vaccination also there is a universal gratuitous service* for all wishing to accept it, although many patients prefer that the family doctor should undertake this work for them. Certificates of successful vaccination are accepted from private medical practitioners, but there are no arrangements for paying them for vaccinating their private patients at the public expense, nor are they supplied with vaccine lymph by the Government.

In England and Wales, in 1927, the proportion of infants certified to have been successfully vaccinated either gratuitously by these public vaccinators or by the family doctor by private arrangement was 44·9 per cent. of the total births, while in 40·7 per cent. of the infants whose births had been recorded a declaration of conscientious objection to vaccination had been received from the parents. Such a declaration is accepted as exempting from the obligation to vaccination. The remaining 14·6 per cent. are partly accounted for by postponements of vaccination on medical grounds, by lost addresses, etc. Under the Local Government Act, 1929, the duty of enforcing vaccination devolves on the councils of counties and county boroughs; but it is unlikely that this will mean much greater assiduity in enforcing the law. Vaccination, to an increasing extent, is becoming a panic measure when cases of smallpox are reported; and it forms, of course, an indispensable precaution for all engaged in investigating and treating cases of smallpox, whether doctors, sanitary officials, disinfectors, wardmaids, or nurses. Their immunity against attack forms an outstanding and unchanging proof of the efficacy of vaccination in preventing attack by smallpox.

PUBLIC PATHOLOGICAL SERVICE

As part of the control of communicable diseases, there has grown up the practice of supplying laboratory aids to diagnosis.

The M.O.H. is expected to consult with any private physician having doubt as to the character of a suspected infectious disease; and this is done on a large scale, especially when smallpox is suspected. This service is gratuitous. In many areas the M.O.H. or his deputy also undertakes the abstraction of cerebro-spinal fluid in suspected poliomyelitis or meningococcal fever.

In addition, public health authorities arrange for the gratuitous examination of pathological smears from sore throats, of sputum, urine, etc., for tuberculosis, and of blood, fæces, etc., for the Eberth bacillus.

In 1912, in my Report as Principal Medical Officer of the Local Government Board, I summarised the work then being done by local authorities under this head. In the counties of England and Wales in 1911 specimens examined averaged 1·9 per 1,000 of population (chiefly tubercle, diphtheria, and typhoid), and in the county boroughs they averaged 9·1 per 1,000. These examinations were made either at municipal or county official laboratories, or at university or other laboratories with which the local authority contracted for the work. In London the ratio was 3·3 per 1,000 of population. In a few centres milk was examined for tubercle bacilli. There has been great extension in each kind of examination since the above return was first made, though more recent figures are unavailable.

The same report described the much more extensive pathological work being done in voluntary hospitals, and

extension of similar work by public authorities was advised.
It was added:—

Pathological work forms an important means of ascertaining the
distribution and character of disease in a district, and thus
enabling rational preventive measures to be taken. The total
pathological work carried on in hospitals and elsewhere is work
which local and central health authorities may legitimately carry
on or subsidise from public funds.

In my Report for 1913 I published fuller details showing
that: *The number of specimens examined per 1,000 of population on behalf of public health authorities in England and Wales
was:*—

Widal test	0·21
Swabs for diphtheria	4·13
Sputa, etc., for tubercle bacilli	1·89
All others	1·48
TOTAL	7·71

In the same year proposals were put forward and included
in the Government's Budget providing for a large extension
of pathological facilities at the public expense, for instance
for examination of suspected morbid growths, cancer, etc.
The Great War prevented the adoption of these proposals,
and this gap, so far as concerns provision at the public
expense, remains almost unfilled.

The chief additional advance has been the universal
provision of facilities for examination of pathological
material from suspected cases of venereal disease. In 1917
the Local Government Board (now the Ministry of Health)
organised *inter alia* the provision of laboratories throughout
the country for the examination of material from patients
suspected to have V.D.

In my official memorandum written at that time stress
was laid on the utilisation of the pathologist for consultation
and for the taking as well as for the examination of specimens. I added: "If a pathologist is looked upon as only a
person undertaking certain technical processes, and is
required merely to give a positive or a negative answer to

a definite question, his special knowledge is partially wasted."

For this reason the Board insisted on each pathologist under the venereal disease scheme being a physician "able to apply the knowledge obtained by medical training to problems arising in connection with specimens taken from patients, etc." In 1928 there were 77 approved laboratories in England and Wales which had been doing this work for a series of years, and the number of specimens examined in these V.D. laboratories (*Report, Chief M.O. to the Ministry of Health*) increased from 33,889 in 1917 and 71,943 in 1918 to 225,352 in 1924 and 313,428 in 1928. Of this last number—

1,993 were microscopic examinations for spirochætes,
125,914 were microscopic examinations for gonococci,
185,521 were Wassermann tests.

The numbers for 1928 are exclusive of 60,842 specimens examined at treatment centres for spirochætes or gonococci.

These examinations are all made at the public expense, and any qualified medical practitioner can make use of this provision without charge. Thus there has grown up provision at the communal expense of such pathological aids to the prompt recognition of disease as experience has shown to be desirable. There is an increasing practice of extending these aids to diagnosis beyond communicable diseases to cancer, to tests of assimilation and elimination, etc. As will be seen later, the use of X-rays at the public expense is steadily increasing.

From the above sketch it will be seen that private practice for pathologists has already been greatly restricted by the activities of public authorities added to the encroachments produced by the work of pathologists attached to large voluntary hospitals. If the proposals of the Government in 1914 had fructified, this private practice would have been even more encroached upon. Such a transfer is to be deprecated, unless it fulfils the condition that the practitioner should have the advantage of personal consultation with the pathologist. In Aberdeen consultations on these lines are provided by the local authority, and in a few areas in England the scope of pathological examinations at the public expense has already become very wide. This process, if it extends, will mean the steady diminution of private pathological practice. There is no provision in the National Insurance Act for this work; and attempts to promote it would probably end in national provision not limited to the insured population. The provision would then be comparable to that for education, and for many branches of public health work.

This subject has engaged the attention of the Consulting Pathologists Group of the British Medical Association, who have reported on the "unfair competition of laboratories established by public health authorities". They have received the support of the Representative Body of the B.M.A. (Supplement, *British Medical Journal*, August 4, 1928), who resolved as follows :—

That the work of laboratories established by public health authorities should, in the opinion of the Representative Body, neither provide for pathological examinations nor furnish reports on individual cases, except (1) in cases which directly involve questions of public health, or (2) where provision is made for such reports by statutory right, or (3) when the patient is stated by the practitioner to be unable to pay a fee; provided that in parts of the country where facilities for pathological examinations and reports are not afforded either by private practitioners (pathologists) or by the service of the local hospital, the local public health laboratory may properly make examinations and furnish reports as these are required by practitioners for patients who are in a position to pay the usual professional fees.

The first item (1) necessitates definition. Does not the early diagnosis of the nature of suspected cancerous tissue, or of the character and extent of a patient's anæmia, directly involve questions of public health? The supposed distinction between "public" and "personal" can scarcely be maintained in view of the present scope of public health administration.

CHAPTER XII

SOME SPECIAL PUBLIC MEDICAL SERVICES

B. Tuberculosis Medical Services

As we are concerned chiefly with the relation of private medical practitioners to official medical action against tuberculosis, it is unnecessary to discuss sanitary measures for securing a tubercle-free milk supply. The main problems, indeed the only problems so far as concerns pulmonary tuberculosis, are the control of the spread of infection from the human patient to other persons, and the control of the circumstances which favour the development of the tuberculous seed when implanted in human tissues.

In this control scientific aid in ensuring personal hygiene and in guiding the treatment of the individual patient is indispensable. Both personal hygiene and treatment are hygienic in that they promote the health of the patient and diminish the risk of infecting others; and it is futile to attempt to separate them in any scheme of satisfactory action. Hence the solution of housing difficulties, the maintenance of meticulous cleanliness, the provision of abundant fresh air and sunshine, and of adequate nutrition, form part of the needed medical provision, as much as the actual clinical care of the patient.

Tuberculosis in all its forms is a notifiable disease, and it is thus practicable to investigate each notified case so far as concerns (1) the patient's own comfort, care, and hygiene; while at the same time (2) all unfavourable environmental circumstances can be discovered and so far as practicable removed; and (3) the earliest evidence of similar disease in members of the patient's circle can be detected.

Such measures may include not only the correction of personal habits conducing to infection, but also in certain cases the provision of additional bedroom accommodation, or additional food for an impoverished family.

Official action on some of the lines indicated above had been taken in Britain long before 1911, when major attempts to control tuberculosis by direct action were begun on a national scale. The additional impetus given in that year originated in the enactment of the National Insurance Act. In this Act a special "Sanatorium Benefit" was included, for the provision of sanatorium treatment for tuberculous insured persons.

In the same year the annual National Budget allotted £1,500,000 as a grant towards the cost of erecting sanatoria in Great Britain, which, with further money supplied by local public health authorities, led to a rapid increase in residental institutions (hospitals and sanatoria) for consumptives. In 1911, in addition to the large provision of hospital beds for destitute consumptives made by boards of guardians, public health authorities in England and Wales had about 1,300 beds for the institutional treatment of tuberculosis, and there were 4,200 further beds in private sanatoria and voluntary institutions. In 1917 the total available beds (again outside the poor-law) numbered 12,441, of which about one-half had been provided by local authorities.

In 1929 the available accommodation in different categories was as follows (*Annual Report, Ministry of Health*, 1928–29, p. 41):—

Local authorities had 155 sanatoria for pulmonary tuberculosis (P.T.), and in 44 isolation hospitals similar accommodation was provided. The total beds in the above institutions numbered 13,811. Voluntary bodies provided 68 institutions, with 5,114 beds, for P.T.; while in 162 general hospitals a number of additional beds were provided.

In addition, there were 65 institutions for non-pulmonary tuberculosis, with 1,001 beds, provided by local authorities, and 2,620 beds provided by voluntary bodies. The total beds numbered 23,260.

In 1912 schemes for local control of tuberculosis were inaugurated. These included the appointment of a medical *Tuberculosis Officer* (T.O.), who is required to have had special experience in the diagnosis and treatment of tuberculosis. Regulations recently issued by the Minister of Health (February 1930) crystallise the requirements which a T.O. must fulfil as follows :—

Any person appointed by the council of a county, county borough, or metropolitan borough, or by a joint committee of any such councils, to be a tuberculosis officer or medical superintendent shall be a registered medical practitioner who, prior to the 1st April, 1930, has held the appointment of tuberculosis officer or medical superintendent with the approval of the Minister, or, who, subsequent to qualification, (1) has had at least three years' experience in the practice of his profession; (2) has spent in general clinical work a period of not less than eighteen months, of which not less than six months have been spent in a hospital as resident officer in charge of beds occupied by general medical or surgical cases; and (3) has received special training, for a period of not less than six months, in the diagnosis and treatment of tuberculosis.

The T.O. is a whole-time official in the department of the M.O.H., and he is expected to undertake or to initiate all action needed on the receipt of notifications of cases from medical practitioners, to arrange the home visits of public health (tuberculosis) nurses, to supervise with them the home circumstances of each patient and the taking of all necessary domiciliary precautions, to arrange for home nursing when required, and to decide in consultation with the notifying practitioner whether subsequent treatment shall be domiciliary or institutional. He is also expected to cultivate consultations with private practitioners as to cases of doubtful diagnosis, and to arrange for X-ray photographs when desirable. Commonly examination of contacts is done by the T.O., with the consent of the practitioner.

In 1928 there were 382 approved tuberculosis officers in England and Wales carrying out the special official anti-tuberculosis work, and in particular conducting clinical and preventive work in 473 dispensaries throughout the country.

In each locality a *Tuberculosis Dispensary* is established, at which patients sent by doctors are examined; also contacts. Patients may attend independently; in which case the usual practice is to write a letter to the patient's doctor, if he has one, stating what has been found in the patient, and to make suggestions.

As a rule ordinary treatment is not undertaken by the T.O. at the dispensary, but only such special forms of treatment as the giving of tuberculin, refills in the treatment of pneumothorax, artificial light therapy, etc.

There has been much misunderstanding of the function of the dispensary. It forms the special bureau of the Public Health Department, in which all the anti-tuberculosis work of the public health authority is concentrated, including the making of arrangements for the provision of institutional treatment. The work centring in it is more preventive than clinical. It is an organisation rather than a building; in it all the preventive work at the homes of the patients and in institutions finds its nodal point.

The most common weakness of the T.O.'s work has been the predominance of clinical medicine. The T.O. must be a good diagnostician, able to command the respect and esteem of the practitioners of the district in which he works; but his supremely important work is preventive.

Another weakness of his work in very large communities, not so easily remedied as the above, consists in the divorce between his work and that of the residential institutions for the treatment of tuberculosis. The secrets of increased success in tuberculosis work lie (*a*) in always putting prevention in its first place, and (*b*) in ensuring that the T.O. can keep touch with tuberculous patients at every stage of their illness. Especially is it necessary for him to be able to watch patients in "observation beds".

The large industrial county of Lancashire may be instanced as having secured this. Dr. Lissant Cox records (*Medical Officer*, October 27, 1928) that 83 per cent. of all cases come to the consultant T.O. before notification by the patient's doctor for an opinion as to diagnosis. This shows excellent co-operation with the family doctor. The administrative county of Lancashire, with its large industrial population, has been able to organise a graded tuberculosis service, with T.O.s who see the patients also at the sanatoria. The T.O.s have beds at local hospitals for advanced cases, which greatly enhances the value of their work. In London (p. 432) one of the great difficulties in tuberculosis administration is constituted by this divorce between institutional and domiciliary and dispensary supervision.

The *home-visiting* of tuberculous patients forms an essential part of a tuberculosis scheme. This is carried out at frequent intervals by whole-time tuberculosis nurses, or—

by district nurses subsidised by the local authority, or
by nurses who also spend a part of their time in visiting infants and their mothers, or as school nurses.

These three different arrangements for home visiting can be regarded as appropriate for areas having differing distributions 'of population. In rural areas the second or third arrangement may be preferable (see pp. 278 and 298, also 316).

The *Institutional Treatment* of tuberculous patients comprises sanatoria and hospitals, and in a few instances colonies at which convalescent patients continue to reside and do suitable work. The last named are excellent in selected cases, but obviously only a portion of the total cases are suitable for colony, i.e. special village, life.

It is unnecessary that I should stress, as I have done elsewhere, the supreme importance of providing adequate hospital beds for advanced and bed-ridden consumptives, who in the most helpless stage of their illness are most liable if untrained to give infection in massive doses to their relatives and nurses. It is important to make this provision as attractive as is practicable, if protracted domestic infection is to be reduced to a minimum.

As early as 1912 more than one-half of the deaths from pulmonary tuberculosis in London and about one-third of the total in the whole of England and Wales occurred in poor-law and other hospitals in circumstances which usually for many months had minimised risk of infection; and since then the proportion of institutional treatment has increased.

In 1928–29 local authorities in England and Wales spent £3,209,544 on tuberculosis schemes, of which 19 per cent. was for dispensary services and 81 per cent. for residential institutions.

At every point the working of a tuberculosis scheme impinges on that of a private practitioner.

(a) *As to Notifications.*—There is considerable delay in notification on the part of many practitioners. In 1928 out of 77,881 total new cases coming to the knowledge of health authorities, in 5·5 per cent. information was only received after the death of the patient. This occasional failure to co-operate can be reduced by the cultivation by the T.O. of cordial relationships with medical practitioners, and by his steady effort to give the practitioner expert assistance. From an annual return made by the Ministry of Health it is possible to compare this and other indices of efficient work in 159 areas in England and Wales, including 78 county boroughs.

The proportion between number of new cases of tuberculosis and deaths from tuberculosis gives an indication of the completeness of notification of sickness. I confine my comparisons to county boroughs, taking extreme instances :—

Bolton	..	..	..	..	143	
Birmingham	..	..	..	..	184	
Bootle	..	..	..	..	242	cases were notified
Gateshead	..	..	..	..	275	to 100 deaths.
Doncaster	..	..	..	..	353	
Sheffield	..	..	..	..	431	

(b) *As to Use of Free Facilities for Examination of Sputum.*— Stating the number of such examinations of sputum per 100 new cases and contacts examined we find the following illustrations :—

Birmingham	..	..	..	..	228	
Bradford	..	..	..	..	213	per 100 new cases
Blackburn	..	..	..	..	65	and contacts examined.
Wallasey	..	..	..	..	38	

The differences are not likely to be explicable by variations in personal examination of sputum by individual practitioners, apart from the municipal laboratory, or by very great variations in diagnostic competence in the practitioners of the towns enumerated. One is compelled to conclude that, in addition, there are great variations in the earnestness of practitioners to secure an accurate diagnosis.

(*c*) *As to Degree of Co-operation between T.O. and the General Practitioner.*—This may be measured by the proportion which consultations between these two bear to every 100 deaths from tuberculosis.

There are wide variations :—

Coventry	..	..	..	..	74
Warrington	..	..	..	..	105
West Ham	..	..	..	..	141
Derby	..	..	..	..	355
Sheffield	..	..	..	..	783
Leeds	..	..	..	..	867

consultations per 100 deaths.

Making large allowance for different methods of administration and of enumeration, the above figures display great variations in the standard of medical practice.

Similar differences are found in the proportion of contacts who are examined, in the utilisation of X-ray examinations for diagnosis, in the extent to which home visits are made by the T.O. and by health visitors, and in the extent of social care and after-care given to the patients.

The medical practitioner is not the only offender in regard to delayed notifications of tuberculosis. The frequent unwillingness of patients to come for treatment at an early stage is another cause of delay. But there is a decreasing though still large number of practitioners who fail to examine their patients carefully, and who may attend them for weeks or even months for winter cough or other vague conditions, when it would be practicable for them alone, or with the help of the official provisions indicated above, to make a prompt and accurate diagnosis.

RELATION OF THE TUBERCULOSIS PROBLEM TO SICKNESS INSURANCE

As already stated, the National Insurance Act when enacted included a "Sanatorium Benefit", and local authorities were expected on payment to provide treatment for tuberculous insured patients. Strenuous representations were made on behalf of the Local Government Board and local health authorities to the effect that it was unwise in a national scheme intended for the prevention and treatment of tuberculosis to treat insured persons preferentially or separately. Local authorities were then given capital sums for erection of sanatoria, and half the total cost of approved expenditure on tuberculosis schemes for the entire population was promised from national funds. This resulted in 1921 in the cessation of the sanatorium benefit of the N.I.A.

Panel doctors still had their duty to attend insured consumptives when treated at home, and were required to make periodical returns concerning such patients to the tuberculosis officer of the local authority; but institutional treatment was to be supplied by local authorities. In certain instances local authorities are authorised to certify for the provision of extra nourishment when, in the opinion of the T.O., this is necessary for the proper treatment of the case.

About one-third of the total tuberculous population is insured, and domiciliary attendance for them is assured. The panel doctor can have no financial objection to their attendance at the tuberculosis dispensary whenever this is desirable, nor does he suffer financially if the patient is admitted to a residential institution. For the rest of the population official tuberculosis arrangements might conceivably tend to interfere with private medical practice; but the general consensus of opinion is that medical practitioners have no grievance against tuberculosis officers in respect of the official arrangements for the control and prevention of tuberculosis. The chief occasional exception to this rule is when an over-zealous health visitor gives hygienic counsel that should have been anticipated by the family doctor.

THE PRIVATE PRACTITIONER AND TUBERCULOSIS

I quote a paragraph from an address by myself, published in the *Lancet*, October 30, 1926, which sums up this part of my subject:—

For insurance and non-insurance patients alike there is needed closer co-operation between consultants and general practitioners, first for the use of available special services, but also for similar and extended provision for others now excluded from these services. The days for single-handed practice have gone by. We all have to admit our need for help from brother practitioners who have skill in a special department of medicine. The appreciation of this need and action upon it does not diminish the importance of the general practitioner, who in the interest of his patient is the assessor and executor of the special knowledge which the expert contributes as a guide in the treatment of the patient.

In no disease more than in tuberculosis is the hygienic work of the private practitioner so important. Is this fact universally appreciated? Do we lay adequate stress on the importance of teaching the patient to cough with his mouth screened, as well as on suitable disposal of sputum? Do we impress upon the patient, and do we adequately realise ourselves that 14 to 15 per cent. of the total deaths registered from tuberculosis occur at ages under 15 years; that juvenile tuberculosis is concerned also in many deaths registered, for instance, as broncho-pneumonia; and that it is highly probable that infection of human origin in childhood bears a large share in producing adult mortality from pulmonary tuberculosis? Above all, do we realise that this mortality in childhood and youth, as well as in adult life, results not merely from circumstances of life favouring effective infection, but is due to repeated and excessive doses of infective material received from adults who are in our professional charge, and to whom we may not even have revealed the nature of their disease? There can be no reasonable doubt that if a simple hygienic code of conduct were rigidly followed by every consumptive patient a much more rapid decline of tuberculosis, especially among children, would follow. For the partial character of the success already secured, not only the medical attendant, but also public health authorities who are slack in their administrative and educational work against tuberculosis, and patients and their relatives who fail to adopt the—often inadequately impressed—precautionary measures which are needed, must share the heavy burden of responsibility.

NON-PULMONARY TUBERCULOSIS

The obligation to report non-pulmonary has been less strictly fulfilled than the corresponding duty to notify pulmonary tuberculosis; although it has been found that non-pulmonary disease in children often gives the clue to unrecognised pulmonary tuberculosis in adults. In recent years a rapid development of official schemes for the treatment of cripples, whether from tuberculosis or other diseases, has occurred. General practitioners have welcomed these schemes as providing skilled treatment for a class of patients very difficult to deal with in their homes. The provision of such schemes, as in the corresponding experience for pulmonary tuberculosis, has led to increased readiness and completeness of notification of cases.

CHAPTER XIII

SOME SPECIAL PUBLIC MEDICAL SERVICES

C. MEDICAL SERVICE FOR THE CONTROL OF VENEREAL DISEASES

IN public health administration two diseases or groups of diseases, namely, tuberculosis and venereal diseases (gonorrhœa and syphilis) in many countries have been made the subject of special measures of control, including treatment of these diseases at the public expense. The justification for this lies in their devastating prevalence, in the fact that they are chief causes of mortality, and especially of premature mortality, and that apart from their lethal effect, they are responsible for a vast amount of illness and of inadequacy for life's work in workers and their dependents, and especially at the ages when the worker should be at the height of his working capacity.

Although very dissimilar in origin, the two groups of diseases have this in common, that treatment and disinfection form an essential part of any effective campaign against them; and this, with the considerations mentioned above, amply justifies the special effort of public health authorities to control them.

Venereal diseases originate in anti-social conduct. Their main source is sexual promiscuity, commonly the promiscuity of commercialised vice, though during and since the Great War, the occasional prostitute, who has other sources of income, has been found to be even more dangerous.

In England earlier public attempts at the control of venereal diseases were directed to the disinfection of prostitutes and their segregation while contagious. In a few military towns prostitutes were subjected to sanitary supervision, including physical examination, followed by hospital treatment and disinfection when necessary. These attempts at control were never very successful. They only reached a fraction of those concerned, and even in these the control was largely futile; while men—except soldiers and sailors partially—were left uncontrolled. The attempt to give by these medical means an artificial security to promiscuous fornication did not succeed.

In 1913 a Royal Commission on Venereal Diseases was appointed to investigate the subject; and in February 1916 this Commission, of which the writer was a member, made the following, among other, recommendations (summarised):—

1. A service for the diagnosis of V.D. by laboratory methods should be organised by the large public health authorities, to form part of more general provision of laboratory facilities having for their object the prevention, diagnosis, and treatment of diseases in general.

2. The best modern treatment of venereal diseases should be rendered readily available for the whole community, and the arrangements should be such "that the persons affected by these diseases will have no hesitation in taking advantage of the facilities for treatment which are afforded".

3. The organisation of these means of treatment should be in the hands of the large public health authorities.

4. As the first step in the preparation of their schemes by local authorities, the voluntary general hospitals in each area should be approached for the institutional treatment of V.D.

5. At any institution in a local authority's scheme (this includes the treatment of out-patients as well as of in-patients), treatment should be free to all. "There should be no refusal to treat a patient who is unwilling to go to his own doctor."

6. A person applying for treatment at any centre should have no residential restriction imposed on him.

7. Evening clinics convenient to working classes should be arranged.

8. Local authorities should be empowered to supply

salvarsan or its substitutes gratuitously to medical practitioners, subject to proper safeguards.

9. National Funds should subsidise the expenditure incurred by local authorities as above and for educational work on the same subject, to the extent of 75 per cent. of the total expenditure, 25 per cent. being paid by the local authorities themselves.

10. The advertisement of remedies for venereal diseases should be prohibited.

These recommendations were almost immediately put into force by the Local Government Board. It was made obligatory on the councils of counties and county boroughs to make arrangements, subject to the approval of the Local Government Board:—

(1) To enable any medical practitioners to obtain, at the cost of the council, scientific reports on material from persons suspected to be suffering from venereal disease; and

(2) To submit to the Board a scheme for the treatment at and in hospitals or institutions of persons suffering from venereal disease, and for supplying medical practitioners with salvarsan or its substitutes.

Facilities for the diagnosis and treatment of venereal disease were rapidly provided throughout the country. The circumstances of the war gave impetus to the movement to this end, and led also to the organisation of valuable educational work, both civilian and military.

Among other statements the Royal Commission had emphasised the mischievous part played by unqualified medical practice in the perpetuation of these diseases in the following words:—

We have no hesitation in stating that the effects of unqualified practice in regard to venereal diseases are disastrous, and that in our opinion the continued existence of unqualified practice constitutes one of the chief hindrances to the eradication of those diseases.

To stop this evil the Venereal Disease Act, 1917, was passed by Parliament forbidding such practice, and making advertisements or recommendations to the public of any supposed remedy for V.D. a punishable offence.

From this brief summary it will be seen that against V.D. the British Government has enacted two great and far-reaching principles which have not been adopted for any other single disease:—

(1.) That no one is permitted to treat V.D. except a qualified medical practitioner; and

(2.) That everyone, rich or poor, can claim gratuitous treatment for V.D. at officially organised clinics in every county and town in the country.

This does not imply that the medical officer of the clinic may not suggest in a given case that the patient should see a private doctor; but treatment, and, in fact, continued treatment, may not legitimately be refused.

In addition, (3) the supply of laboratory diagnostic facilities for every patient[1] gives every private practitioner the same gratuitous help as is afforded for diphtheria, enteric fever, and some other acute infectious diseases:

And (4) salvarsan or one of its substitutes is supplied gratuitously for his private patients to any medical practitioner who is familiar with the procedure in intravenous injections.

ATTITUDE OF THE MEDICAL PROFESSION

When the Government's order was issued in 1916 making it obligatory on local authorities throughout the country to provide, as set out above, for the treatment of V.D., the country was engaged in the Great War, and the unanimous acceptance of the proposals owed much to the general realisation of the immediate need for national efficiency. The medical profession shared this desire to help to the utmost, as is clearly brought out in the following extracts from the official journal of the B.M.A.:—

The Council of the B.M.A., reporting on the Report of the Royal Commission on V.D., expressed their appreciation of

[1] This includes free supply of outfits and payment of expenses of postage incurred by the practitioner.

the courtesy of the President of the Local Government Board, who had given them access to drafts of the proposed regulations for the control of V.D. and the memorandum of the Medical Officer of the L.G.B. on the organisation of medical measures against V.D. which it was proposed to send to county and county borough councils.

In replying they indicated to the Board that in their opinion it was essential that the local medical profession should be asked to nominate representatives to serve upon any committee having control of the arrangements under the local scheme. They then recommended that the Representative Body of the B.M.A. should approve the Commission's Report.

They followed this up by definite recommendations endorsing the main recommendations of the Royal Commission, of which the following are the most important:—

(a) That provision should be made for facilities for the diagnosis and treatment of V.D. by laboratory methods.

(b) That "measures should be taken to render the best modern treatment of V.D. readily available for the whole community, and that the arrangements should be such that persons affected by these diseases will have no hesitation in taking advantage of the facilities for treatment that are afforded."

(c) That treatment at any institution included in a local authority's scheme should be free for all. There should be no refusal to treat a patient who is unwilling to go to his own doctor.

The Council of the B.M.A. recognised that this last resolution, which accorded with the Royal Commission's recommendations, was "a new departure of a most important kind". They added the following comment, subsequently endorsed by the Representative Meeting of the B.M.A., which is a striking illustration of the victory of national considerations over the immediate monetary interests of medical practitioners.

The policy of the Association in connection with treatment at hospitals has always been that persons who are able to pay for their own treatment should not be treated at charitable institutions except in emergency, but should be referred to a private practitioner. In endorsing the recommendation of the Royal Commission the Council recognises the exceptional nature of venereal disease; the reluctance of patients affected by them to go to their private medical attendant; the risk that they may go to unqualified persons for treatment with disastrous results to themselves and to others; and the importance to the community of adopting all possible measures for inducing sufferers from venereal disease to seek early and adequate treatment. On these grounds the Council is of opinion that the recommendations of the Royal Commission should be accepted and approved by the Association.

In a letter dated August 29, 1916, the Local Government Board recommended to the local councils responsible for the administration of anti-venereal measures the need for securing cordial co-operation of the medical profession.

The free supply of salvarsan or its approved substitutes was, as we have seen, a further provision of the new schemes. Each practitioner wishing for such a supply in his private practice was to receive it without charge. In order to avoid the risk of its unskilled use, the practitioner wishing for a private supply was asked to produce evidence that he had adequate experience of the administration of these drugs by intravenous injection, or that he could produce evidence of having hospital experience in their administration.

It will be seen that the principle of diagnosis, and, if needed, of treatment, at the public expense of all applicants who believed themselves to be suffering from V.D. was accepted by the medical profession as a whole; and this attitude has been consistently maintained to the present time, and is now fully accepted.

Seldom is any complaint heard from private doctors that they are being deprived of patients. A philosophical view of this diversion of patients is perhaps encouraged by the fact that a third of the population are medically insured, for whom payment is on a *per capita* basis, and that public treatment of V.D. relieves the insurance doctor from a task which is often repugnant to him. Reference to local reports shows that many doctors dislike these cases and are glad to send them on to the clinics. Other doctors have frankly informed me that the modern treatment of V.D. is a problem for the expert, and that the general practitioner as a rule should not undertake it. The prolonged treatment needed is often not worth while for the practitioner. There still remains much private medical attendance on these diseases, and free laboratory diagnosis, free arsenobenzol preparations, and free consultation with the expert at the V.D. clinic helping to make private treatment efficient, were contemplated and aided from the initiation of official schemes.

V.D. Clinics have usually been instituted in a special department of general hospitals, the intention being thus to aid in rendering recourse to treatment easy, without identification of the particular illness. There is the further point, that consultation with other departments of medicine is thus made easy.

A considerable number of special *ad hoc* clinics have also been opened and have proved successful.

It is unnecessary to discuss the general organisations of V.D. clinics. The medical officer is salaried. He may be a member of the general hospital staff or not. He may be engaged for this work on a whole-time or part-time basis.

In England and Wales there are 188 V.D. clinics. Their number has been almost stationary since 1920. The rapid development of the system is indicated by the fact that in the first year, 1917, there were already 117 clinics.

The following figures for 1928 (*Annual Report, Ministry of Health*, p. 51) show the number of new cases coming under treatment in that year:—

Number of new cases of syphilis	21,126
Number of new cases of gonorrhœa	39,033
Number of new cases of soft chancre	965
Number of other cases found not to be suffering from V.D.	26,899
	88,023
Total Number of attendances at the Treatment Centres	2,310,322

In 1928, out of 49,961 cases which ceased attendance during the year,—

17,864 were discharged after completion of treatment and observation;

14,125 ceased to attend after completion of one or more courses of treatment, but before final tests as to cure;

17,972 ceased attendance at an earlier stage.

The general course of events is more clearly shown in the following diagram, in which the number under each heading in 1918 is given as = 100.

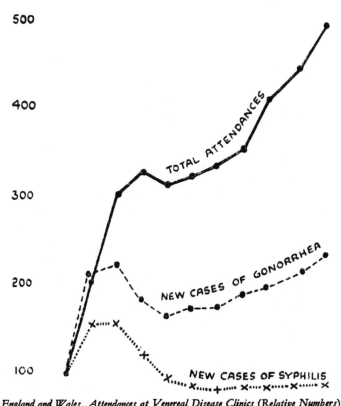

England and Wales. Attendances at Venereal Disease Clinics (Relative Numbers).

It will be noted that the number of new cases of syphilis has declined. This is concordant with the national mortality figures.

There has been some increase in gonorrhœa cases, which may mean that an increased proportion of the total cases are coming for treatment. A very satisfactory feature of the diagram is the remarkable increase of attendances as related to number of patients. Evidently patients are continuing treatment more satisfactorily with each succeeding year, and the number of chronically infective cases must, as a result of this, be reduced.

There has been remarkable reduction in the national death-rate from the group of diseases which can be regarded as giving a good index of the prevalence of syphilis. The increasing distance from the circumstances of war has meant reduction of infection; but I have no doubt that the reduction of infection secured by treatment at the clinics has borne a very important part in bringing about the favourable change. Increase in the registered death-rate from syphilitic diseases is shown in 1927-28. This, in part at least, is ascribable to the new forms of medical certification of death used in those years. These forms now encourage fuller statement of the more remote causes of death.

The main points of administrative action are embodied in the preceding outline. It is unnecessary to detail special arrangements made to secure the examination of material from still-born fœtus, for examination for spirochætes, and for the treatment of pregnant women and of young children at child welfare centres found to be suffering from syphilis. The importance of determining when syphilis or gonorrhœa is present in the expectant mother has not yet received the attention it needs. Much social work is being done to help to secure satisfactory treatment for infected women in unsatisfactory lodgings. The treatment of seamen is becoming a matter of international co-operation.

Syphilis is not a compulsorily notifiable disease, though by some this is regarded as desirable. In Bradford a limited measure making notification of syphilis in young children compulsory is being tried. Notification as a means for securing compulsory continuance of abandoned treatment is strongly advocated by some. Apart from the difficulties

associated with any attempt at treatment against the will
of the patient, it is doubtful whether more success would
follow threat of compulsion than the tactful counsel of a
medical officer who has enlisted the confidence of his
patient.

Ophthalmia neonatorum is compulsorily notifiable both
by doctors and midwives, and blindness due to it is greatly
decreasing. A large majority of these cases is caused by the
gonococcus.

Educational measures have a close bearing on the value of
V.D. medical work. The most valuable counsel is that given
by a trusted medical adviser; and the decrease of V.D.
depends largely on his impressing on his patients the right
attitude to this social problem.

Valuable educational work is done by the British Social
Hygiene Council; commonly public authorities employ this
Council or its local branches in educational work having
special bearing on the prevention of V.D., and the Ministry
of Health, in a recent circular, has expressed the hope that
local authorities will contribute at the rate of 5s. per 1,000 of
population to its work. The advertisement of facilities for
treatment by local authorities is an important item in the
work of local authorities. The following cutting from a
Birmingham newspaper illustrates the means taken to insure
that everyone shall know of the facilities provided for
treatment :—

VENEREAL DISEASES

The WORCESTERSHIRE COUNTY COUNCIL have arrangements with HOSPITALS in WORCESTERSHIRE—BIRMINGHAM,
KIDDERMINSTER, DUDLEY, and STOURBRIDGE—whereby
ADVICE and TREATMENT can be obtained FREE OF COST
by all WORCESTERSHIRE PERSONS SUFFERING, or supposed
to be suffering, from VENEREAL DISEASES (Syphilis and
Gonorrhœa).

Further information and a pamphlet as to times when
patients can attend may be obtained from the County
Medical Officer, 29, Foregate Street, Worcester.

All correspondence will be treated as confidential, and
replies will be sent in plain envelopes.

The rapid progress of anti-venereal medical work has been stimulated by the fact that only one-fourth of its cost comes out of local rates. Under the Local Government Act, 1929, this ceases, and new methods of adjustment between contributions from local and national funds are substituted, which it is hoped will not lead to curtailment of the present anti-venereal work.

(An admirable account of the British system of control of V.D. in Great Britain is given by Colonel L. W. Harrison, D.S.O., in the *Journal of Social Hygiene* for April 1929. It contains fuller details of the working of V.D. clinics than can be given in this chapter.)

CHAPTER XIV

D. NURSES' WORK IN SICKNESS AND HEALTH

WE are concerned in this chapter with the relation of the practising physician to the nurse's work. The success of medical practice depends very largely on efficient nursing; furthermore, the successful application of preventive medicine on its personal side depends largely on such work as is now being done by health visitors (public health nurses) to a happily increasing extent in most countries.

This at once introduces the dual aspect of the nurse's work: she is a nurse for the sick, and a supervisor to see that medico-hygienic precautions and practice are adopted in sickness and as a means of preventing sickness.

The hygienic value of the nurse's domestic attendance on the sick is very great. Hygienic advice as to ventilation, personal cleanliness, and cleanliness of the sick-room, and as to diet, is much more highly appreciated during illness than at other times; and such advice has the further advantage that the nurse herself demonstrates in her work the needed ritual of health.

Partly for this reason in many communities the district sick nurse undertakes also the hygienic visitation in tuberculosis and in infant and pre-school health work; and in other chapters will be found examples of this combination (see, for instance, pp. 278 and 298). There is something to be said for and something against this combination of clinical and hygienic functions.

In sparsely populated areas the combination works well, and the duties of village midwife are occasionally super-added, though there is risk that clinical work, especially for acute cases, may at times encroach too much on hygienic work. In the early days of health-visiting, in new communities, the offer of sick nursing has opened doors for hygienic work which would otherwise remain closed (see Vol. II, *International Studies*, p. 103, for instance).

When a nurse is employed by a public health authority to visit the mothers of infants of tender age, or to pay hygienic visits to tuberculous patients, occasional friction has arisen, her reputed advice having been said to conflict with that previously given by the family doctor. When this occurs, it nearly always has meant inaccurate quotation by the mother of the nurse's remarks, and a telephone message of the doctor to the M.O.H. would at once prevent further misunderstanding. The public health nurse is always instructed to support advice already given by the family doctor if there is one. The head of the family commonly is not willing to pay for visits by the doctor as often as are required if the upbringing of infants is to be hygienic and safe; and he is a wise doctor who asks for a health visitor to call at intervals to supplement his advice and to secure adherence to the course of life he has laid down.

But in the more usual circumstances the family either has no regular doctor, or the remuneration needed to secure his services cannot be afforded; thus if a member of the family has tuberculosis, or the mother has recently given birth to a child, or a toddler is slowly convalescing after measles or whooping-cough, or a parent needs directions as to the treatment, for instance, of pediculosis or impetigo in a scholar, or as to future admission to a hospital, and in many other instances the health visitor's work is invaluable, and cannot be intermitted without serious injury to the communal health. The methods and details of her work can be seen in the appropriate sections of subsequent local chapters.

SICK NURSING

We need not concern ourselves directly with institutional nursing, as this is now well organised, and in most hospitals is adequate to needs, though not in regard to social service (p. 244). Nursing of cases of sickness at home is still inadequately organised, although the last half-century has seen vast improvements in this respect. Fully-trained nurses are now registered in an official Roll by the General Nursing Council for England and Wales, which was formed under the Nurses' Registration Act, 1919. This Council consists of 25 members, of whom 9 are appointed by Government Departments and 16 are registered nurses. They remain in office for five years.

A nurse, in order to secure a place on the Roll, must have had three years' training in a general hospital, or part of the time in a children's hospital, a hospital for women, or a hospital for infectious diseases, and must have undergone a three years' course of instruction. Such fully-trained nurses hold all the chief appointments in nursing; but in villages a nurse who has had only a year's training is sometimes employed for district work.

DISTRICT NURSING

In order that the sick poor may be satisfactorily nursed in their homes, district nursing has gradually been organised in nearly every considerable village as well as in every town in the country. Such district nursing was first organised in Liverpool in 1859, and it was there first demonstrated that not only could valuable help be given in the restoration of the sick, but that with this help could be associated even more important assistance in lifting the family towards independence and moral health.

In a few years other towns followed Liverpool's example. In 1874 the Metropolitan Nursing Association was founded; and Queen Victoria, in 1887, gave £70,000, the Women's Jubilee offering, in memory of her fifty years' reign, to promote district nursing. The Queen's gift was devoted to training nurses fully equipped for district work—these to be supplied to affiliated nursing associations; to the supervision of this work; and to establish a central training-home in London. Since then central training-schools have also been established in Cardiff, Edinburgh, and Dublin.

Up to 1889 nursing associations were almost limited to towns, especially large towns. In 1888 the first rural nursing association was started in the West of England, Hampshire following in 1891, and Lincolnshire in 1894. The general object of county nursing associations is to do for each county what the Queen's Institute is doing more generally for the whole country. They encourage the formation of local nursing associations, raise funds for training nurses and midwives, and supervise their work. The work of county nursing associations in undertaking work for county health authorities in midwifery and nursing can be referred to on pages 278 and 298. In order that the local nurse-midwives might be competent to undertake health-visiting and school nursing, as well as midwifery and sick nursing, special courses of instruction were arranged for them. At the end of 1926 there were 57 county associations and 2,676 village nurses employed by local associations affiliated to them (Dr. Shadwell, *The Times*, September 28, 1926).

Most of the existing nursing associations became affiliated with this central organisation, and only a few county associations now remain unaffiliated to the Queen's Institute of District Nursing.

In 1897, the occasion of Queen Victoria's Diamond Jubilee, a further sum of £48,000 was handed over to the Queen's Institute, and on the death of Queen Victoria a further memorial fund of £84,000 was contributed for the same purpose.

QUEEN'S NURSES

Two grades of nurses are employed in the work of district nursing associations. Queen's Nurses have all had three years' training in a recognised hospital, and, in addition, six months' special training in district work tested by an examination. Many also are qualified as midwives. The training in district nursing is given at about one of about 84 homes in England and Wales by the local superintendents of nurses.

VILLAGE NURSES

Village Nurses are not hospital-trained. They have a year's district training and often have also qualified as midwives. Their work is excellent, although they would not be competent to undertake the nursing of an operation case or to do some of the more skilled work of a fully-trained nurse. It must be recognised, however, that women are needed who, while not fully trained, are able to undertake the nursing of many patients, who otherwise would be nursed by wives or mothers in the family of the sick. Economic circumstances call for a class of nurse who, while conscientiously carrying out medical instructions and adequate for many illnesses, are not fully equipped in every respect. To employ a fully-trained nurse in minor illnesses is an extravagance in the use of financial resources, and is not always justified, though the work of auxiliary nurses will always need supervision by fully-qualified superintending nurses.

The question as to how far nurses may undertake minor medical work not infrequently arises, especially in work following medical inspection of school children. In the aggregate, school nurses undertake a vast amount of treatment of minor conditions, such as chilblains, cut fingers, impetigo, pediculosis, and no serious objection is raised to this. The work is authorised by the school doctor and is partially, but often very slightly, supervised by him.

In addition, school nurses give valuable help in massage and other forms of mechanical treatment for deformities. In the school dentist's work specially trained nurses have been utilised for scaling teeth, and even in a few districts for extractions of temporary teeth or for stopping these. The general weight of professional opinion is against this, but given personal supervision by a qualified dentist, there is much to be said for the regulated use of specially trained nurses for this work, as there is for their employment under strict regulations in the administration of anæsthetics (p. 49).

In infant welfare centres and in the home visiting of infants nurses are invaluable. These nurses are now required to have had six months' training in their work in addition to their full qualification in nursing.

As will be seen by reference to pages 279 and 323, health officers differ greatly in their view as to the advisability of allowing district nurses to undertake health visiting. Against the combination it is urged that, although the medical knowledge of a nurse is needed, she should have the social outlook of the M.O.H., rather than the clinical outlook of the family doctor. It is urged also that the bed-side nurse's attitude is necessarily one of obedience to the doctor, but for her work in health visiting she requires the spirit of initiative; and that the bed-side nurse has little knowledge of healthy infants and young children, of general health conditions, or of the social circumstances of wage-earners. These points may easily be pressed too far; and in rural work, at least, much can be urged in favour of combining several varieties of nursing—bed-side nursing, the work of a school nurse, of a tuberculosis public health nurse, and of a health visitor—in one person.

Industrial Nurses

Industrial nurses are now largely employed in factories and other large establishments, and their utility has been abundantly proved. They act under the general direction of the special doctor employed by the industry in question. Such arrangements have been less frequently adopted in England than in the United States.

Hospital Almoners

Hospital Almoners have duties which link up the home and hospital work of nurses in clinical, preventive, and social respects. Their work is very fully described by a pioneer in it, Dr. Richard Cabot, and can only be briefly summarised here. He points out (*Proceedings, International Conference of Social Work*, Paris, 1929) that the first appointment of "Lady Almoner" was in 1895 at the Royal Free Hospital, London, though previously some hospitals had inquiry offices to prevent the "abuse of hospital charity". Her first duty was to investigate the financial circumstances of patients, and to transfer such patients as were suitable for treatment in poor-law institutions. In the United States, Baltimore and Boston had similar officers, and the admirable work of almoners at the Massachusetts General Hospital is well known.

Their work has been widened and made more social, as Dr. Cabot points out, by the more general appreciation of the facts that each sickness has its "human" and social as well as its medical aspect; and that much can be done in the family by bringing social agencies and public health activities into play. Anti-tuberculosis work has been pre-eminently successful in breaking down the wall of partition between the medical and the non-medical treatment of disease.

By means of the almoners it has become possible to supply the medical and surgical staff of the hospital with important information as to the patient's home conditions, and thus expedite or delay his discharge, or lead to the taking of specific precautions. Co-operation with public assistance and other social agencies has been secured, and convalescent treatment frequently arranged. Continuance of domestic nursing and treatment has been secured by correspondence with the local nursing association; and the utilisation of the hospital out-patients' departments has been facilitated. All this has been in addition to arranging the contribution, if any, which the patient will pay for his treatment in hospital.

The almoner cannot report to the private doctor, beyond announcing the fact that his patient has been sent home. Such an announcement does not diminish the desirability of a definite medical report from the hospital to the doctor who was responsible for the patient's admission.

Evidently the almoner's time for home visits is limited, and there usually are no such visits. It ought to be possible to secure from the M.O.H. a statement of the patient's home circumstances ascertained by a health visitor and to arrange for the hospital doctor to possess this information, to guide both in treatment and in time and method of discharge from the hospital. In Toronto there is a service of hospital social workers who are in close touch with the field nurses of the public health service.

The chief object both of health visitors and of hospital almoners or social workers is identical. It is to rehabilitate the families visited by means of available medical and social measures; and I have no doubt that in future developments of health visiting, visits to the homes of patients sent into hospitals for all kinds of sickness, and to the same patients after their discharge from hospital will form a much larger proportion of total hygienic work than it does at present.

NURSING OF THE SICK IN LONDON

The special conditions of sick nursing in London are here described somewhat fully; but the main features apply in large measure also to experience in provincial towns.

Although metropolitan arrangements for sick nursing are complicated, a vast amount of beneficent work is being accomplished which, while it does not completely meet all public needs, probably approximates as near to this as in any large community in the world.

In every part of London we find nurses employed by nursing organisations for the supply of skilled nurses and other nurses in independent practice. These nurse the well-to-do. They are fully trained, having had a three years' training in various hospitals and nursing-schools, and having obtained a certificate of efficiency.

But nursing by these efficient and well-paid nurses is only within the reach of the well-to-do; and, even for many who are much above the weekly wage-earning class, payment for a nurse's services may imply a heavy financial burden. For wage-earners this is an impossible burden; and for most of them skilled nursing is only possible through the help of the voluntary nursing associations now to be described.

Neighbours help in sickness to a remarkable extent: but neither neighbourly kindness, nor even the devotion of wife or mother, will compensate for the lack of skilled nursing in acute illness. Efficiency is necessary as well as devotion, and, happily, efficiency can be and is associated with the devotion of the nurse who regards her calling as a sacred mission.

That for the ordinary wage-earner, and a large proportion of the poorer salaried population, individual provision for nursing in sickness is impracticable is generally recognised: and it is somewhat strange that hitherto little has been done in England to make this provision by insurance methods. Under the National Insurance Act medical aid is provided, but nursing benefit is only exceptionally given as a special benefit. In some child welfare centres, especially in the East End of London, small organisations have been formed on insurance lines for supplying home-helps during the lying-in period. Home-helps are selected women of a similar social status to that of the mother, who carry on the household work while the mother is disabled (p. 187).

At present there are, according to the *Directory* issued by the voluntary Central Council for District Nursing in London, 31 district nursing associations in London, supplying different parts of the metropolis, whose areas— in part owing to the efforts of the Central Council—are now fairly well delimited, thus avoiding overlapping of effort.

The definition of fully-trained district nurses usually accepted is that of the Hospital Sunday Fund, which describes them as including—

> Nurses who have received three years' hospital training and six months' district training.

Outside these local nursing associations a number of parishes in London have trained nurses who are not attached to any association. There are, furthermore, many nurses working in ecclesiastical parishes, or attached to religious organisations, who have no definite boundaries for their work. A considerable further number of nurses work in connection with Medical Missions.

In London—unlike the practice in many parts of Britain— district nurses do not act as midwives, except in Hampstead. Midwives in London practise independently. The only exception to this is the work done by midwives in maternity institutions and in the extern maternity departments of general hospitals and of lying-in hospitals.

The voluntary nursing associations provide domiciliary nursing assistance in nearly every part of London. In their distribution needs are only approximately met. There is need for further developments, and it is probable that growth on an insurance basis would be most satisfactory. The data given below were collected by Miss Richardson, the secretary of the Central Council for District Nursing in London, and analysed by myself with the help of Miss Richardson. This was in April 1925, but the data may be taken as approximately representing the present position.

In the following statement of proportions of district nurses to population for the different metropolitan boroughs, it should be remembered that some of the extensive differences would be mitigated, if one could allow for the fact that nurses' work may not follow borough boundaries.

At the date given above there were 247 district nurses attached to the 31 nursing associations in London, including the nursing superintendents of these associations. These work out at 1 nurse to 18,120 population for the metropolis. In the City of London there was 1 to 6,854, but the circumstances of this chiefly non-residential part of the metropolis are exceptional. In other central boroughs of London the proportion was also relatively high. Thus it was—

> 1 nurse to 8,368 population in Holborn, and
> 1 nurse to 10,856 population in Finsbury.

Among less central and more clearly residential quarters the nearest to the above were:—

> 1 nurse to 10,887 population in Lewisham,
> 1 nurse to 11,161 population in Greenwich,
> 1 nurse to 11,945 population in Bermondsey.

At the other end of the scale there was:—

> 1 nurse to 27,561 population in Islington,
> 1 nurse to 29,309 population in Bethnal Green,
> 1 nurse to 31,588 population in Fulham,
> 1 nurse to 33,550 population in Battersea.

Making all allowances for overlapping of the district nursing service in different boroughs, and assuming, as may safely be done, that no borough is over-served, it is evident that notwithstanding the extent of this invaluable voluntary service, it is inadequate to the needs of the metropolis.

It may be assumed that the need for district nurses is greatest in the most densely populated areas; but when the relation between size and social character of dwellings and number of nurses in a given borough was tested, I was unable to find any connection showing that the supply of nurses is greater as the need for them increases.

At the time when the above investigation was made, I quoted some figures supplied by Miss Beard as to the Boston (Mass.) Instructive District Nursing Association. This great association had one nurse to every 6,562 of population, and judging by the estimate that 40 per cent. of the population are likely to be sick at some time or other during a normal year, the nurses of the Boston Association reached only 5 per cent. of its sick population in such a year.

If it be assumed, after allowing for the portion of the need met by private nurses, by hospital nurses, and by nurses not affiliated to the Central Council for District Nursing in London, that at least one district nurse should be available for 8,000 persons, then the work of the federated associations in London needs to be largely supplemented. The total need for the metropolis on this assumption would be 560 district nurses, instead of the 248 nurses provided in 1925.

As a rule, the nursing associations are supported by :—

(a) the gifts of the charitable, in subscriptions and donations;
(b) by small payments made by patients according to their means;
(c) for special services (see p. 252) by the London County Council and the Borough Councils of London;
(d) by grants from the Metropolitan Hospital Sunday and Saturday Funds.

About one-fourth of London is served by the *Ranyard Nurses*. The history of this association dates back to the years just before 1868, when Agnes Jones joined Mrs. Ranyard in the project of training a corps of nurses to live and work among the poor. Agnes Jones was the pioneer in workhouse nursing reform at Liverpool, where she died in 1868. The Ranyard Society was a religious organisation in two branches, a Bible Mission and a Nursing Society. The latter grew rapidly and was eventually separated in actual working from the Mission, though still linked to it. Gradually the nurses were hospital-trained: and the Ranyard Nurses, with two or three other societies, gradually spread their work over London. In 1868 5,000 visits were paid to 99 persons: in 1874 the number had become 111,601 visits to 4,392 persons. Their work and that of other district nurses stand in the front rank as a means of social ameliora- tion. The Ranyard Nurses work under the direction of private doctors, who are supplied with postcards for summoning the nurse, and with papers for giving her directions. No case is undertaken unless a doctor is in attendance. Each nurse, who must already be fully qualified, is trained locally for district work under an experienced superintendent before she undertakes independent district work.

In 1928 there were 90 Ranyard Nurses at work, and during the year they attended 10,924 cases and made 255,707 visits to these. In addition, 3,613 visits were made by sisters or superintendents. During that year £126 was received from patients. Working for the L.C.C. at their minor ailment centres and dispensaries the Ranyard Nurses made 250,560 attendances and paid 2,732 home visits to patients attending these school centres.

Among the chief nursing associations in London are those given in the table on p. 251 (an incomplete list).

Most of these associations are affiliated to the Queen Victoria's Jubilee Institute for Nurses.

The main duty of their nurses is to nurse the sick poor in their homes, payment for this coming from voluntary sub- scriptions to the association and to a small extent from patients' small contributions.

A very important branch of home nursing carried out by these associations is that of patients discharged from metropolitan hospitals who still require nursing attention; or of patients who, were it not for the fact that home nursing is available, would have needed indoor hospital treatment. Hospital almoners refer cases to the nurses of the appropriate District Nursing Association, and it has been estimated

	In the Year	
	Cases	Visits
Brixton District Nursing Association ..	5,599	90,378
Camberwell District Nursing Association	1,310	19,295
Chelsea and Belgrave District Nursing Association	1,544	20,026
East London Nursing Society	13,437	175,973
Hammersmith District Nursing Association	1,392	13,894
Kensington District Nursing Association	2,150	40,156
Metropolitan District Nursing Association	2,994	50,204
North London Nursing Association for the Sick Poor	4,140	63,987
Paddington District Nursing Association	3,000	41,349
Ranyard Nurses	11,165	255,979
Shoreditch District Nursing Association	2,025	29,946
South London District Nursing Association	4,065	60,852

that approximately one-fourth of the work of district nurses is concerned with patients sent out from hospitals and with out-patients at these hospitals. But for the relief thus given, the strain on voluntary hospital beds would be even greater than it now is.

The rules governing the work of all voluntary nursing associations in London are somewhat similar. They act under the direction of the medical attendant of each patient, and without the aid of these nurses private medical attendance would lose a large part of its utility.

But their work is not limited to life in a sick household, in which the family and the medical attendant have to face the problem of illness. It extends as already seen (2) to hospital patients, out-patients, and former in-patients; (3) they are utilised in large measure by the boards of guardians (now public assistance committees) for the sick poor, who are authorised to contribute to the funds of nursing associations; and (4) they are being largely employed in the medical service of the L.C.C. and of the metropolitan borough councils.

The powers of borough councils to undertake the home nursing of cases of sickness are not general. They do not extend to the general nursing of the sick, but are limited, as officially stated by the Ministry of Health, to the items set out below:—

1. The provision of nursing assistance for the purposes of Section 67 of the Public Health Acts Amendment Act, 1907, where in force;
2. For the purposes of the Public Health (pneumonia, malaria, dysentery, etc.) Regulations, 1919;
3. For patients suffering from influenza, measles, german measles, encephalitis lethargica in need of nursing assistance; and
4. For expectant and nursing mothers, for cases of puerperal fever, for cases of ophthalmia neonatorum, and also for cases of measles, whooping-cough, epidemic diarrhœa, and poliomyelitis in young children.

In setting out these limitations, the Ministry of Health have recommended that a district nursing association should be established in sanitary areas on voluntary lines to undertake general nursing. The local authorities can, if they desire to do so, subscribe to the funds of the association in respect of services rendered to the class of case set out above.

The nursing of new-born infants suffering from ophthalmia necessitates energetic measures undertaken with skilled knowledge: and the Central Council for District Nursing in

London has been instrumental in arranging for district nurses in London to obtain special instruction in this work. All candidates for district nursing from the Queen's Institute of District Nursing and from the Ranyard Nurses arrange for a special course of two weeks' training in special ophthalmic hospitals: and other smaller associations have been urged to adopt the same procedure.

In the treatment of patients under the National (Health) Insurance Act district nurses are largely utilised, a definite agreement commonly being made between the greater insurance societies and the nursing associations. Most approved insurance societies pay at the rate of 1s. 4d. a visit. Under special arrangements the Prudential Society pays 1s. a visit. It is probable that this does not completely cover the share of the cost of the nurse which ought to be borne by the insurance society; but the call on charity is reduced by these payments.

In addition to the invaluable domiciliary nursing outlined above, there is the vast army of nurses engaged in like work in hospitals and other residential institutions. And there is, furthermore, the work of health visitors, of tuberculosis nurses, of school nurses, and others who are concerned chiefly or solely with personal hygiene. These may be looked at as engaged in the van of the army of Preventive Medicine: but the nurses who attend to the sick are also equally indispensable in the warfare against disease. The two together represent in a special manner the modern outlook on disease and its prevention.

SUMMARY

From the above necessarily incomplete sketch of nursing in England as related to medical practice—clinical and preventive—it will be seen that voluntary effort has been very markedly successful in supplying a large part of the skilled nursing which is a necessary element in a satisfactory medical service. There are too few nurses available in some areas; but there is, I think, no part of the country in which a nurse cannot be obtained for an urgent case of illness without any cost to the patient. I am not referring to the provision of nurses by public assistance committees, but to possibilities apart from this.

This result is a remarkable instance of success in organised systematic voluntary work, supported by contributions of the charitable, and to a small extent by payments of beneficiaries.

The result is noteworthy, furthermore, as demonstrating the practical recognition of the fact that the nursing of a large section of the total population is beyond their means, and must be provided by efforts of the well-to-do.

For those thus benefited there is growing up, through the working of sickness insurance and otherwise, the practice of nursing provision on an insurance basis. This pooling of funds provided by the regular contributions of both healthy and sick for a common purpose is the best method of ensuring adequate nursing for wage-earners; unless one falls back on a general nursing service paid for by general taxes, to which these wage-earners would necessarily contribute their share. This is the practice in regard to elementary education. The insurance method is more likely to prevail in the provision of home nursing.

NOTE.—Since this chapter was written the Medical Department of the London County Council has published a recent survey of district nursing in London (P. S. King, 1931); and the Report of the *Lancet* Commission on Nursing, dealing with the shortage of candidates for nursing the sick (*Lancet*, August 15, 1931), should also be consulted.

PART II

SOME LOCAL MEDICAL SERVICES IN ENGLAND

CHAPTER XV

CAMBRIDGE, TOWN AND COUNTY[1]

I HAVE selected the medical and hygienic activities of the university town of Cambridge and the administrative county in which it is included for separate description for several reasons :—

1. Both in the university town and in the entire surrounding county there is evidence of the leavening of the ideals of men, and still more of women, of university rank, including the wives of professors and heads of colleges.

2. The town has not completely independent administration, but it has made a success of those branches of public health and medical work in which it is filially related to the County Council.

3. Both in town and county there is evidence of active co-operation between official and voluntary (unpaid) agencies for health and welfare; and this has been coincident with a frank acceptance of the necessary supremacy of the official organisation, which supplies a large share of the "sinews of warfare". Much elasticity of action is left to the voluntary workers. Enthusiasm happily characterises these workers, but it would be erroneous to assume that enthusiasm is their monopoly.

4. Not least important, the town and county of Cambridge each has a public dental service for the juvenile population which, perhaps, is the only one in England which can claim to be approximately adequate for every child and scholar needing dental attention.

In the description of the various medical activities which follows, the arrangements for Cambridge itself and for the county cannot in all respects be separately stated. This arises out of the governmental arrangements of the two.

[1] Date of investigation, April 1929.

As in other areas, we are concerned with four aspects of public work, viz. that carried on by:—

Public Health Authorities	⎰ Borough Council ⎱ Urban District Councils Rural District Councils County Council
Poor Law Authorities	Boards of Guardians
Education Authorities	Committees (almost autonomous) of Borough Council and County Council

Insurance Committee of the County.

Since April 1930 the boards of guardians have been superseded by the Cambridgeshire County Council.

There are two local elementary education authorities in the geographical county, one for the town (borough) of Cambridge, one for the rest of the administrative county. Many of the following pages will be concerned with their medical work.

Public health work, including its medical part, is carried on:—

1. By the County Council, so far as tuberculosis and venereal disease are concerned; also the control and maintenance of asylums for the insane and feeble-minded, the welfare of the blind, of children with mental deficiency, and of maternity and child welfare in rural districts.

2. By the Borough Council of Cambridge, which for most of its public health work acts separately from the County Council.

3. By other small local authorities within the administrative county.

In Cambridgeshire these small authorities are all for rural districts, six in number, of which the aggregate population in 1921 was 70,338. Census population, Cambridge (1931) 66,803.

The population of the municipal borough of Cambridge

in the same year was 59,264. The total population of the administrative county was 129,602.

The rural district councils are concerned chiefly with elementary sanitation and the control of infectious disease, each district having its own part-time M.O.H., except in one instance where a whole-time M.O.H. acts for two districts in Cambridgeshire, and for several in the adjoining counties of Essex and West Suffolk. In Cambridge Borough a highly developed public health service is in existence; and the borough in Dr. A. J. Laird, and the county in Dr. F. Robinson, have the good fortune to possess chiefs of their public health work who are outstanding in reputation in the public health world.

The Borough Council presents a special feature. Under its charters it is governed by a council which consists of forty-five councillors directly elected, and fifteen aldermen elected by the councillors; but it has also eight members (six councillors and two aldermen) representing the University. Its mayor is elected annually, councillors triennially, and aldermen every six years.

The County Council has forty-eight councillors and sixteen aldermen similarly elected. In both Borough and County Councils, the Council can co-opt on to its Maternity and Child Welfare Committee, its Midwives Committee, its Committee for Mental Defectives, and its Education Committee men and women from outside the Council to take part in their work.

The responsibility for the medical care of the population of Cambridgeshire, as elsewhere, is shared in the main between the following :—

1. General and special medical practitioners engaged in private practice.
2. Since 1930 the Public Assistance Committee of the County Council.
3. The public health authorities (Town Council, County Council, and smaller Sanitary Authorities).
4. The education authorities (Education Committees of the Town Council and the County Council).
5. The Local Insurance Committee arrange for domiciliary attendance of insured persons by "panel" doctors.

The conditions of insurance medical practice are common to Cambridgeshire and the entire country. On these, see Chapter V. Insured persons are mainly associated in various friendly societies and other insurance societies, which, if they possess surplus funds, sometimes pay for specialist medical services. Out of these surplus funds dental help is given in Cambridgeshire; and some small payments are made from insurance society funds to the County Nursing Association for the services of nurses. In addition, special payments are made for ophthalmic treatment and for obtaining spectacles. Some of the insurance societies in the county subscribe to the Addenbrooke's Hospital, and their members are then relieved from certain small charges made to ordinary patients; and a few societies are able out of their surplus funds to send members to convalescent homes. The friendly societies have arranged collections and parades at which considerable sums for Addenbrooke's Hospital, Cambridge, have been collected.

Hospital Provision

Cambridge Borough.—The borough poor-house combines the functions of poor-house and infirmary. Its inmates are chiefly old and infirm, patients suffering from chronic disabling or incurable disease, some lunatics and feeble-minded, and a small number of children.

During 1927, 10·9 per cent. of the total 748 deaths of Cambridge inhabitants occurred in the poor-house, while 25·9 per cent. of total deaths in Cambridge occurred in public institutions, of which 8·8 per cent. were in Addenbrooke's Hospital, and 6·2 per cent. in other institutions.

There are five poor-houses in the county. These at the census of 1921 had 429 inmates. Two of these serve also some areas outside the county. The county lunatic asylum at the last census had 586 inmates.

At the poor-houses scanty provision has, hitherto, been made for modern medical and surgical work. Under the new conditions, these institutions become a part of the public health service, and developments and improvements may be anticipated. Of voluntary hospitals, Addenbrooke's Hospital in Cambridge has 190 beds, and there are two smaller hospitals in the county, as well as eight registered nursing-homes with fifty-three beds.

Vaccination, as in other parts of the country, has up to 1930 been in the hands of the boards of guardians in the county, when undertaken at the public expense. In 1926, 39·2 per cent. of infants born in Cambridge borough were certified as having been successfully vaccinated, the majority remaining unvaccinated because of "conscientious objection". The rest of the county has a somewhat similar experience.

MIDWIFERY ARRANGEMENTS

Cambridge.—For two years no deaths due to puerperal conditions have occurred. In these years 1,827 births occurred. There are fifty-four midwives practising in the administrative county, of whom thirteen reside in Cambridge. The control of midwives devolves on the County Council as the local supervising authority for the administrative county; but in order to help the borough's scheme for maternity and child welfare work, the detailed administration of the Midwives Act has been delegated to the Town Council. The county's inspector visits the midwives in the borough and reports to Dr. Laird, the borough M.O.H., and the County Council intervenes when disciplinary action is needed in regard to any midwife. Fifty-five midwives practise in the county, including thirteen who practise chiefly in the borough. All of these have been fully trained for their work. The superintendent of midwives is competent and helpful, and encourages midwives to refer cases in which difficulty is anticipated to the gynæcologist of Addenbrooke's Hospital. Furthermore, midwives are encouraged to examine for albumen the urine of their prospective patients, and in fact do so.

Under the arrangement for the borough made with the County Council notifications of abnormal conditions at birth (which midwives are legally bound to send) are sent direct to Dr. Laird, the borough M.O.H., the county superintendent subsequently investigating and reporting. These visits average two annually to each midwife.

In 1920, 57 per cent. and in 1927, 71 per cent. of the total births in the borough were attended by midwives. Medical assistance is secured adequately in the confinements attended by midwives.

The County Council is under legal obligation to pay the fees of doctors called in by the midwives. The midwife can call in any practising doctor chosen by her or the patient. The fees of these doctors are paid in accordance with an official scale (p. 154).

Very few expectant mothers attend the welfare centres, described hereafter, but the trained midwives themselves have learned to give a certain amount of antenatal care when engaged in good time and to refer their patients to doctors if danger is presaged. Their antenatal visits are stated to average three per case.

In addition, two whole-time health visitors do a certain amount of antenatal visiting in the town of Cambridge. Much of this arises incidentally from their health-visiting of infants.

Visits by the health visitors, especially when continued beyond the first birthday, imply friendly contact with many expectant mothers, and thus much helpful advice and even assistance in obtaining medical help when needed is given.

Through the health visitors about one-eleventh of all expectant mothers were brought into touch with hygienic advice.

County.—As midwifery arrangements overlap for the county and town, we may complete our statement for the county at this point.

In 1927 three deaths from puerperal sepsis and three from "other accidents and diseases of pregnancy and parturition" occurred in the county. These deaths occurred in connection with 1,883 births, showing a maternal mortality much below that of the country as a whole.

During the same year 273 notifications were received by the County M.O.H. from midwives in accordance with the Midwives Act as to conditions calling for medical care.

There has been a progressive increase of cases in which the midwife sends for medical aid. In 1919 this proportion was 5·2 per cent., in 1926 it was 9·3 per cent., and in 1927 it became 12 per cent.

During 1927 the Town Council maintained 10 beds for puerperal patients in Addenbrooke's Hospital, and they have also arranged for the reception of complicated maternity cases or cases in which home conditions are unsatisfactory into the new block of the public assistance infirmary recently opened.

The County Council since 1913 have given scholarships to assist in the training of 37 nurse-midwives, and during 1927 they contributed maintenance grants to the total amount of £49 to three district nursing associations within the county, in respect of the services of the nurse-midwives in their employ. Through the activity of the County Nursing Association, aided by the financial support of the County Council, only 26 parishes, with a total population of 7,700, are left within the county without nurse-midwives. The total number of rural parishes is 129, with a population of 70,338 in 1921.

The above facts throw light on the low puerperal mortality in the town and county. Added to this is the advantage of Addenbrooke's Hospital and of the high standard of medical work in a university town.

PAYMENT OF DOCTORS' FEES

Where practicable the County Council obtains some portion of the doctor's fee from the patient (p. 280), the Surgical Aid Association assessing the amount claimed and collecting it for the town. This action of a voluntary organisation is a good example of collaboration of a voluntary with an official body (see also p. 277). In the county the health visitors collect the information required by the county M.O.H. to enable him to assess the charge, if any, to be made.

There is but little friction between doctors and midwives as to midwifery work either in town or county. A few doctors still prefer to retain all the midwifery cases in their area. In such cases the local midwife acts as a maternity nurse under medical direction. This arrangement is liable to the abuse that the midwife may be given responsibility which belongs to the doctor.

It has become a recognised practice for midwives —accepting lower fees than doctors—to attend the majority of confinements in the families of wage-earners; and the administrative control of midwives is now so complete that medical assistance when needed is seldom neglected. Furthermore, the legislation which has made it obligatory on the local supervising authority to be responsible for the payment of a doctor when a midwife has called him ensures that medical practitioners have an assured remuneration for this arduous work.

CHILD WELFARE WORK

This is undertaken by official and voluntary agencies, acting in close co-operation, both in the town and county.

Cambridge.—For this special work two whole-time health visitors (qualified nurses having special knowledge of midwifery and child hygiene) are employed in the borough of Cambridge. Their chief duty is the visitation of homes from which notification of a birth has been received.

Taking the average of the three years 1925–27, at least 83 per cent. of the mothers of all infants born in the borough were visited at their homes by the health visitors, and on an average the mother of each infant was visited three times during the infant's first year. Many visits were made also to children in the "toddler" stage, thus enabling preventive and curative action to be urged, which must diminish the need for medical treatment in school-life.

The County.—In the county home visitations are undertaken in part by the district nurse, when there is one, she acting also as school nurse; in other districts by two county health visitors.

In 1927, 7,589 visits were made by the county health visitors, and 18,549 visits by district nurses. Of the total visits 2,383 were to expectant mothers, and 14,984 to children aged 1–5.

By means of these visits 54·7 per cent. of expectant mothers in the county received supervision and advice, calculated on births in all social classes. The proportion in the working classes is higher than this.

The home-visiting of mothers and infants is an essentially important part of the work of the health visitors. It forms part of the complete policy which comprises occasional attendance at maternity and child welfare centres.

Cambridge Centres.—There are five of these centres in the borough, each of which has a weekly session. Each centre is conducted by a lady superintendent, who is a voluntary worker, assisted by one or more other voluntary workers, and by one of the two whole-time official health visitors of the borough. A doctor attends fortnightly (in three instances a lady doctor) to see special cases and to advise the lay-workers generally. The fee paid by the Town Council to the doctor for each session is one and a half guineas (about $7·50). The work consists chiefly of the giving of hygienic advice, the baby being weighed and a record of his progress being kept. Some minor medical aid is given; but this is small in amount, and no responsibility is taken for the continuous medical care of children attending the centres. As the sessions are only weekly the need for this rigid restriction is evident. Each sick child is referred to a private doctor, or failing this to a hospital; and parents are warned of the need for medical attendance in any emergency.

An additional mothers' welfare centre is held weekly, at which mother-craft guidance is given. The Cambridge centres have voluntary helpers who hold a high social position in the University or town, and who—many of them—have scientific knowledge of child hygiene and social problems.

County Centres.—There are seven maternity and child

welfare centres in the county outside the borough of Cambridge. None of these is directly administered by the County Council, but the Council gives financial help for their outfit and maintenance. The services of the district nurses who assist the voluntary workers at each centre are given in return for the general grants made for child welfare work to the nursing associations. The annual cost of each centre is about £25, including the fee of the doctor who attends at every alternate weekly session and 5s. per attendance for the district nurse, where a district nurse is employed who is not affiliated to the County Nursing Association's staff. Usually £10 is subscribed by the County Council towards the expense of each centre, while 50 per cent. of the remaining expenditure is paid by the Ministry of Health.

Milk is supplied if the doctor attached to the centre certifies it is necessary for an infant or for a mother who has been examined by him. There is a definite scale of charges, varying with weekly income per head from *nil* to the total net cost of the milk. In the borough when a charge is made for milk or for cod-liver oil and malt, it varies from cost price to half or quarter price according to circumstances. For rural districts the County Council spends about £240 in a year in supplying milk, receiving perhaps £15 from those able to pay in part. In the county the M.O.H. certifies all applicants for milk on the report of the health visitor or doctor.

The giving of food except through the special public assistance organisation is open to theoretical objection, and destitute families are in fact referred to this by the Council. In practice these objections scarcely emerge in the giving of milk. Recent researches have shown that even healthy and satisfactorily fed children improve rapidly on an additional ration of milk. Considering the economic position of a large proportion of the agricultural population in England the giving of milk at the child welfare centre justifies itself in the impetus which it gives towards improved general hygiene.

The population of Cambridgeshire outside Cambridge is chiefly engaged in agriculture. The number of agricultural labourers in each of the five rural districts of the county at the census of 1921 varied from 46 to 60 per cent. of the male population aged 12 years and over. The usual wage for an agricultural labourer is £1 10s. or less a week, a little more for carters and some others. A few additional pounds per annum are earned as harvest money. It is scarcely possible out of such weekly earnings to supply the additional milk required for sick or weakly children.

TUBERCULOSIS WORK

The tuberculosis death-rates in Cambridge and in the county approximate that of England and Wales as a whole, being under 1 per 1,000 of population.

Cambridge not being a county borough, the administrative control of tuberculosis, so far as it relates to diagnosis and treatment at the public expense, rests with the County Council.

The County Council provides supervision, but not treatment, except in residential institutions. This supervision is given in patients' homes, at a tuberculosis dispensary, and in sanatoria and hospitals.

One dispensary in Cambridge serves the whole county area, a whole-time tuberculosis officer conducting its work with the help of two whole-time tuberculosis nurses. Every case of tuberculosis diagnosed by a private medical practitioner is required to be notified to the M.O.H. These notifications are dealt with by the tuberculosis officer, the nurses making domiciliary inquiries and reporting to the tuberculosis officer. The tuberculosis officer also examines any suspected children referred to him by the school medical officers.

The total cases of tuberculosis examined or treated at the dispensary in the year 1927 were 2,244 old cases and 702 new cases. These patients are visited from time to time at home. In 1927 the tuberculosis medical officer made 2,283 such visits, the dispensary nurses 1,679, and the general nursing staff of the county 1,596 visits to notified tuberculous patients.

This amount of visitation means a very active supervision over the hygienic conditions of home treatment, and shows that the tuberculosis officer plays an important part in the domiciliary as well as in the dispensary part of the organisation. The tuberculosis officer, Dr. W. Paton Philip, is accepted by the medical profession throughout the county as an official gratuitous consultant for cases of suspected tuberculosis, and his services in this capacity are much appreciated. His use of radiographs in his consultative work greatly facilitates continued co-operation with private practitioners. During the year 1,151 X-ray examinations were made, a film being developed in 682 instances.

The details of domiciliary supervision need not be detailed. Open-air shelters are lent by the Council for both adults and children, and six new shelters, with bedding outfits, were purchased during the year, bringing the total acquired up to 159.

Dental treatment is provided at the dispensary when in the opinion of the tuberculosis officer this is necessary for successful treatment. Over half of the patients attending the dispensary are insured under the national scheme of sickness insurance, and in some of the Approved Societies to which they belong dental treatment is included. Altogether fifty-five tuberculous patients received dental treatment in 1927, including the provision of artificial dentures. Part payment is recovered from the patient where practicable.

Sanatorium treatment was provided for 278 patients, including 98 children, during 1927. Most of the adult cases are treated at the Papworth Tuberculosis Colony, which does not belong to the Council. Other patients are sent to institutions provided by various authorities.

The Cambridgeshire Tuberculosis After-Care Association is an important voluntary auxiliary in helping tuberculous adults. The County Council makes a grant of £100 annually to the association. Further funds come from friendly societies to supplement the earnings of tuberculous insured persons who are only able to work part-time. Some 30 patients were thus helped in 1927, and further assistance was given to other patients who had not been in a sanatorium. The tuberculosis officer has impressed on the voluntary workers of the association that the success of anti-tuberculosis work depends in large measure on adjustment of the working hours and conditions of ex-patients and on the remedying of faulty home conditions, and deprecates undue concentration on so-called sanatorium treatment. The After-Care Association comprises representatives of the County Council and of friendly societies in nearly equal numbers, and is advised by the tuberculosis officer.

Effective after-care of insured tuberculous patients is hampered because they cannot receive their financial benefit under the National Insurance Act if they are partially occupied for gain. There is needed an assessment of benefit according to the patient's certified condition. Meanwhile the association, by its special work, has greatly helped. Through it the earnings of insured tuberculous persons are supplemented by friendly societies, the general principle adopted being that for insured persons the contributions should equal the sickness benefit they would have received if they had continued to be certified as unfit for work.

VENEREAL DISEASE WORK

Addenbrooke's Hospital (Voluntary) in Cambridge forms the official centre for the treatment of venereal diseases for the town and the county. Males and females are dealt with at separate hours, and every effort is made to ensure privacy.

Any person is entitled to receive treatment free of charge, and can obtain particulars as to hours of attendance by application to the county or district medical officers of health. Afternoon and evening clinics are held weekly for both sexes, and six beds are reserved for in-patient treatment. Facilities are afforded for irrigation in gonorrhœa between clinic days.

At this clinic 108 patients were under treatment at the end of 1927. New patients during the year numbered 197. They made 1,830 attendances on clinic days and 3,663 on other days (chiefly irrigation cases), and the aggregate "in-patient days" was 946. Of the total 369 patients under treatment during the year, 120 left without completing treatment on the basis of the somewhat high official standard. Under the national venereal disease scheme free diagnosis and treatment are provided for all comers, of whatever social status. In addition, eight private medical practitioners were supplied gratuitously with arseno-benzol preparations for their private patients.

Pathological examinations of material (316 Wassermann tests and 315 bacteriological examinations in 1927) are made by a University pathologist. Any medical practitioner can send such specimens for gratuitous examination.

In addition, educational work directed to promote sexual morality and hygiene and to secure prompt treatment if infected is undertaken in lectures and films, the films being supplied by the British Social Hygiene Council. The expense is defrayed by the County Council under their general scheme.

SCHOOL MEDICAL WORK

Cambridge has a separate elementary education authority, formed by the Education Committee of the Town Council; while the Education Committee of the County Council acts for the rest of the county. For higher education the County Council is the sole authority.

Cambridge has 20 elementary schools, 40 departments, and 7,060 children on its school registers. In addition, there is an open-air school and a class for backward children, each providing for some 40 children. The school medical work is organized by Dr. Laird, the M.O.H., with Mabel Gurney, M.D., (whole-time) as chief assistant. There are two whole-time qualified dental officers, two whole-time school nurses, and two whole-time dental assistants (women); also clerical assistants. Children are examined medically soon after coming to school (entrants) and twice afterwards (intermediates and leavers). Many special as well as these routine examinations are made.

At each routine examination of children some 30 per cent. of all the scholars are examined; and it is satisfactory to note that three-fourths of the parents attend when their children are examined. Their attendance is very important from the standpoint of adult hygienic education.

One of the earliest gains from routine inspections and what follows on these has been the reduction of pediculosis. At the last inspection only 3·7 per cent. were found affected. Incidentally medical inspection reveals the unfortunate fact that only 29 per cent. of the children inspected in 1927 showed vaccination marks.

Head teachers and attendance officers assist in preventing epidemic and skin diseases by reporting them to the M.O.H.

The treatment of minor ailments found in medical inspection is undertaken at the borough's school clinic; 512 such cases were treated in 1927. In addition, 78 children were treated for defective vision, 34 children for diseases of the throat and nose, 2,876 children for dental disease, 1,018 children for uncleanliness.

A large proportion of these cases are treated on behalf of the Education Committee at the Addenbrooke's Hospital: thus the X-ray treatment of ringworm of the scalp (5 cases), removal of tonsils and adenoids (33 cases), treatment of otorrhœa (22 cases), and variety of other conditions, including curvature of the spine, and eye diseases (42 cases). The committee subscribe 50 guineas annually to the hospital, and receive 200 letters of recommendation for the use of school children.

In addition, a number of children are treated at the official school clinic, at which 4,567 attendances were made in 1927. Of the children 58 attended for detailed examination of their eyes, and at the end of the year all except six had obtained spectacles.

During the year 22 children found to be suffering from defects were treated privately by their own doctors. This statement suggests that the vast majority of the abnormal conditions found in school medical inspection would have gone untreated but for activity of the school medical and nursing staff.

The two whole-time school nurses, besides attending at the school clinic, "follow up" children found defective in medical inspections, and inquire into the illness of children reported to be absent on medical grounds; their afternoons are largely spent at the schools in inspecting for the detection of uncleanliness. In 1927 they made 1,530 home visits.

The school medical work includes also the allocation of delicate children to the open-air school, and collaboration with the tuberculosis officer as to children with tuberculosis, and as to the examination of children coming from families in which a case of tuberculosis has been notified.

On the work of voluntary agencies in promoting the health of the school child see page 278.

For the dental work of the Cambridge Education Committee see page 274. A whole-time dentist is employed for this work.

Since 1911 Dr. Mabel Gurney has been personally responsible for the school medical work done in the public health department of Cambridge, and this gives significance to the following striking summary of the improvement secured, which Dr. Laird gives in his last Annual Report:—

Compared with the period commencing in 1911 the improvement of the children is remarkable, and as regards cleanliness and general appearance is a complete revolution. At all ages examined the children are taller and heavier, of better physique, freer from defects, better clothed and infinitely cleaner than their predecessors of 20 years ago. A poorly-fed or poorly-clad or really dirty child is exceptional. Skin diseases, especially impetigo and ringworm, are greatly reduced, ringworm indeed being for quite long periods entirely absent. There were no cases of this troublesome disease in the schools at the end of the year under review. There is almost as complete a change in the attitude of parents to medical inspection. In the early years of the work objections to inspection arose in about 20 per cent. of the cases, now they are practically unknown. At first, few parents accepted the invitation to accompany their children, now over 70 per cent. of the children have their mothers with them. This is almost as large a number as can conveniently leave their homes for this purpose.

The County.—In the county outside Cambridge there are 132 schools, one-third of the scholars in each of which are medically examined each year. The county M.O.H. is the school medical officer, Jessie Gellatly, M.D., being his chief assistant. Dr. Philip, the tuberculosis officer, as already mentioned, acts also for the borough of Cambridge. There is a whole-time school dentist, a part-time bacteriologist, and a part-time ophthalmic surgeon. The superintendent of the County Nursing Association (voluntary) is paid to act as the inspector of midwives for the county. She also supervises the work of the part-time health visitors and school nurses, who are district nurses.

Here, as in the borough, the gratifying increase in attendance of mothers when children are examined medically was noted. Defects are notified to the parent. School nurses make monthly visits at home and in school to the children thus noted, to ensure that the necessary treatment has been obtained, and they report as to progress of treated cases. In 1927, 15,949 home visits were made by the nurses. Dr. Gellatly, furthermore, made during 1927 some 5,785 re-examinations of children noted for treatment or observation, to ensure remedial action whenever possible.

The forms of treatment given by the Education Committee comprise:—

1. Contribution to Addenbrooke's Hospital for treatment of diseases of the nose and throat, X-ray treatment of ringworm, and for other general medical and surgical work.
2. Clinics for defective vision; provision of spectacles.
3. Travelling dental clinic.
4. Assistance in travelling expenses for treatment.
5. Provision of malt and cod-liver oil in the schools for cases of malnutrition.

Travelling clinic arrangements have been made, the more remote schools being grouped as occasion arises and examinations made at a centrally situated school. For this purpose children are driven in the school medical officer's car when necessary.

DENTAL TREATMENT

Cambridge.—Mr. W. B. Grandison, the official school dentist, inspected and examined 5,582 school children during 1927, of whom 3,593 were found to require dental treatment and 2,876 were treated. The number re-treated during the year was 1,301. Thus nearly 80 per cent. of those needing treatment received it.

The Report for 1927 is the twentieth annual official report on officially organised dental treatment for school children in Cambridge. This town was an early pioneer in realising the need for remedial measures for the teeth of school children, and in acting on this knowledge.[1] No other town, I think, can show equally prolonged activity in dental hygiene and treatment on a large and now almost a complete scale. The procedure adopted at each school is as follows :—

Having obtained the whole-hearted co-operation of the teaching profession, the dental inspection of the elementary school children in Cambridge is carried out with the maximum of efficiency and the minimum of time. The procedure is as follows :

1. A date is arranged, convenient both to the head of the department and the dental officer.
2. The dental charts are distributed to the children by the teachers, either before or on arrival of the dental officer.
3. Children without charts (i.e. infants or children from other schools, either within or without the borough) receive same, with their names, ages, previous school (if any), etc., written in pencil.
4. An uninterrupted inspection of the teeth of the children is

[1] Dr. Laird, the M.O.H. of Cambridge, contributed a valuable account of "School Dentistry in England" to *Public Health*, September 1921. This gives useful comparative information as to other parts of the country.

then carried out, the teachers assisting by so regulating the children that the dental officer is constantly employed until the inspection of the department is complete.

The accompanying statement shows the quantitative proportion between treatment and need for treatment. Treatment failed to be given to 717 children, or 23·2 per cent. of the total number found requiring treatment. The only compulsory charge made for treatment is for orthodontic and crown work.

NUMBER AND PER CENT. OF CASES IN WHICH THE REQUIRED DENTAL TREATMENT WAS NOT GIVEN TO ELEMENTARY SCHOOL CHILDREN IN CAMBRIDGE, 1927

Reason for Non-treatment	Number	Per Cent.
Definite refusals in writing ..	502	16·4
Repeatedly absent when called for .	76	2·5
Parents preferred to enlist the services of private dentists ..	104	3·3
Postponed by request of parents, occasionally supported by medical certificate	17	0·5
Postponed by dentist on reasonable grounds	18	0·5
Total number untreated ..	717	23·2

In the following diagram are compared dental conditions of school children in 1909 and in 1927. The comparisons relate to children of fairly equal age distribution.

The diagram shows in three series of columns the dental condition of school children in 1909 and 1927. The corresponding condition in 1914 is shown in the intermediate column in each series. The proportion of unsavable teeth has greatly decreased, while the proportion of temporary and permanent teeth which are sound has correspondingly increased. These results have been achieved by protracted effort in which teachers and voluntary workers have co-operated with the education authority's official salaried whole-time dentists, and in which educational talks to parents and others have borne their share.

This work, like that in the county, is being carried out with the steady approval and financial support of the authority which represents the local taxpayer. There has been no objection or obstacle on the part of the local medical or dental profession. The latter, in fact, appears to have welcomed the enterprise of local authorities in carrying out this work, as dealing with classes of patients who in

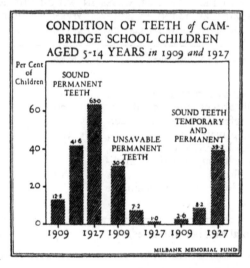

CONDITION OF TEETH *of* CAM-
BRIDGE SCHOOL CHILDREN
AGED 5-14 YEARS *in* 1909 *and* 1927

MILBANK MEMORIAL FUND

private practice cannot pay a dentist enough to make it "worth while". (As to payments for official work, see also p. 199.)

The County.—Much of what has been already written applies also to the county. Every school in the county is visited twice annually, first for routine dental inspection, and a few weeks later for treatment, the school nurses meanwhile interviewing reluctant parents. Every child from 5 upwards is examined. Usually the dental treatment is done on the school premises, the school dentist conveying his apparatus on his automobile. Local anæsthetics, but not general anæsthesia, are employed. This system has been in vogue since 1913, and is now complete. The great majority of the children are under dental supervision during the whole of their school life. It is noted in the school medical officer's Annual Report that from about the age of 7 years onwards there is a decline in the proportion of children in need of treatment. The policy of annual re-examination is adopted to ensure further treatment when required.

In 1927 there were 25 per cent. of refusals to accept dental treatment. Much time and effort are expended by the school nurses to prevent this percentage from being still higher. In 1927 the nurses paid 1,773 home visits to unwilling mothers to persuade them "to permit their children to receive what is practically a free gift of dental treatment, the maximum charge being 6d. (about 12 cents) regardless of the number of teeth requiring attention". (Extract from Annual Report.) Dr. Robinson is of opinion that the recent inclusion of dental treatment as an additional benefit given by many Approved Societies under the National Health Insurance Act has led parents to take a more enlightened attitude towards their children's teeth.

In the year 1927, 9,018 children were examined by the school dentist, 3,748 were found to need treatment, and 2,711 were treated.

Voluntary Agencies and Official Medical Work

Voluntary agencies play an important rôle in Cambridgeshire in preventive as well as in curative medicine; and in nearly every instance there is close co-operation between the officials and voluntary workers, the latter being helped materially from the resources of the communal purse.

Addenbrooke's Hospital in Cambridge, founded in 1719, is the great general (voluntary) hospital for the whole county and a wider area. It now has 190 beds and is an intrinsic part of the Medical School of Cambridge. In 1927 its total income was £30,343 derived from voluntary gifts, subscriptions, bequests, and official sources.

During 1927 the hospital received 3,102 in-patients, of

whom 612 were medical, 1,582 were surgical, 223 were gynæcological, 104 were ophthalmic, and 581 were ear, nose, and throat.

During the same year 10,979 out-patients attended this hospital, a number equivalent to 1 in 12 of the total population of Cambridgeshire.

Of its total income above £908, or 3 per cent., was paid by the County Council for the gratuitous treatment of venereal patients by the hospital on behalf of the Council.

A large proportion of the aural and throat work and some of the ophthalmic work of the hospitals are similarly done on behalf of the Borough and the County Council.

In 1918 the Borough Council arranged with the hospital to reserve 10 beds for difficult cases of parturition, and to admit children found in the course of their child welfare work to need hospital treatment. Such cases include marasmus, ophthalmia neonatorum, and epidemic diarrhœa, but not the common communicable children's diseases. For maternity cases the charge is 7s. per day, together with the surgeon's fee. Each child is charged 5s. a day. The hospital also undertakes the treatment of capital ringworm.

For the County Council similar arrangements have been made with the Addenbrooke's Hospital.

Apart from these official payments, patients are treated without payment in the hospital, a subscriber's letter as a rule being the passport for treatment.

Use of Voluntary Nursing Associations

In Cambridge there is a District Nursing Association and for the county there is a County Association (with affiliated district nursing associations) which leaves few villages without the help of a nurse-midwife. The Annual Report of the Borough and District Nursing Association for 1927 quotes the trite but very true statement that "the more efficiently a district is nursed, the healthier it becomes". The object of the association is to "provide efficient and gratuitous nursing for the poor in their own homes". The four nurses of the Nursing Association for the town attended 619 cases in the year, making 14,814 visits. By arrangement with the Borough Council they undertook the home nursing of cases of measles, whooping-cough, ophthalmia neonatorum, influenza, and pneumonia. The Town Council pays 8d. per visit, 11d. for two visits to the same case in one day, or, in the event of there being more than one case in a house, 4d. for each case after the first.

The Cambridgeshire County Nursing Association has 38 affiliated district associations, including a staff of 12 Queen's nurses, 7 other nurses, and 22 district village nurses. These nurses do a large amount of home visitation for the County Council, in addition to their work as nurses for the sick (p. 264). The County Superintendent of Nurses is substantially an official of the County Council.

Assessment of Charges for Medical Services

This is always a difficult problem. The principle almost universally governing action in England and Wales is that necessary treatment must be given, and must not be hampered by preliminary conditions as to payment, which may mean neglect of disease. This is a broad general statement, substantially true, but to which exceptions could be quoted.

In deciding whether medical aid given by them shall be paid for by the recipient, the Cambridge Town Council is much helped by a voluntary organisation, the Cambridge Central Aid Society.

This is a federation of local voluntary agencies, including the Cambridge and County Surgical Aid Association and the local branch of the Invalid Children's Aid Association. The objects of the society are set out in the following words of their Annual Report:—

The main objects of the society shall be the improvement of the condition of the people of the borough of Cambridge by such means as:—

(*a*) Encouraging in all the spirit of independence, and a sense of duty, alike as individuals and as members of a family, and of the community.

(*b*) Ascertaining the facts relevant to social improvement and the principles and methods of action most fitted to secure the same.

(c) Spreading this knowledge among all persons employed or interested in social work, whether official or voluntary, which affects the condition of the people, and endeavouring to influence public opinion thereon.

(d) Uniting in a common policy those who, by public service or private action, are minded to work for social betterment.

(e) Promoting such an organisation of charitable effort as will secure due investigation and fitting action for the benefit of all who need assistance, whether in the shape of sympathy, counsel, or practical help.

(f) Bringing into friendly co-operation, for the assistance of those in need of their aid, all suitable agencies and persons.

(g) Training suitable persons in the best principles and methods of social and charitable work, and providing centres of information, study, and experience.

(h) Undertaking or furthering enterprises likely to raise the standard of life and conduct in the community and among individuals, or helpful in the organisation of charitable effort.

The enunciation of principles of voluntary help for distress given above cannot be bettered; and it is advantageous to the public that voluntary workers imbued with these ideals are in touch with the work demanded from public official authorities for the treatment and prevention of disease. The work of the above-named society, of the voluntary child welfare centres, and of the superintendents and nurses of the Cambridge and County Nursing Associations are all forms of preventive social work. The question of a special profession of social workers in relation to public health work has scarcely arisen in England. The need is largely met by workers of societies such as those named above, except in the special instance of hospital almoners; and in general it has been found that health workers can also give a satisfactory report on the economic and social circumstances of the families visited by them.

In the county the M.O.H. determines the amount of payment to be made and advises the committee of his Council; but the above society negotiates with the patient and subsequently recovers any sums promised to be paid for midwifery.

As a rule the demands for payment for medical aid are limited and on a very small scale.

At child welfare centres early diagnosis without treatment is the rule; and through them private practitioners have many patients transferred to them who would otherwise be neglected. Nevertheless, there is manifest throughout England an attitude of watchfulness on the part of the general medical practitioners in respect of treatment at these centres at the public expense.

Midwifery work stands in a special position. The larger portion of this work has passed into the hands of midwives; and the supervision and control of these midwives by local authorities have been found to be necessary in the public interest. The arrangements for paying doctors called in by midwives at the public expense give a certain amount of remunerative work to them which in the absence of this provision would sometimes be done gratuitously by them.

The tuberculosis work again occupies a special position. There is an increasing willingness of private practitioners to use the official tuberculosis officer as a consultant in their cases. The fact that one-third of the population are medically insured, and private "panel" doctors are paid on a *per capita* basis whether their tuberculous patients are under their care or are attending an official dispensary, makes for smooth working of official and private arrangements.

The venereal disease clinics provide gratuitous treatment for all comers, and this arrangement is generally accepted.

CHAPTER XVI

GLOUCESTERSHIRE[1]

THE county of Gloucester is chiefly agricultural, with patches in which coal-mining and relatively small textile industries are pursued. A full account is given here of its medical administration, because—owing to the initiative of its county M.O.H., Dr. J. Middleton Martin—this county has evolved a partial system of co-ordinated public medical services, which furnishes valuable indications for other communities.

This co-ordinated service presents the following features:

1. It utilises existing agencies for co-ordinated and co-operative work, including voluntary[2] general hospitals, cottage hospitals (voluntary), and general practitioners engaged in private practice in the county;

2. It is based on the large voluntary hospitals in or near the county, these forming the centres for difficult cases and the source of consultant and expert advisers; and

3. It abolishes or reduces the number of *ad hoc* tuberculosis dispensaries, child welfare centres, and school clinics, replacing them by general local centres for these and other activities, including consultations by visiting consultants from populous centres.

Further reasons for describing the experience of this county in detail are that:—

4. Its scheme of co-ordination and co-operation has met with the entire approval of the private practitioners in the county, as represented by the local branch of the British Medical Association.

5. And perhaps this is most important of all, the scheme has been formulated and is carried on by the chief local public health authority in the county, and has become

---

[1] Date of investigation, January 1929.

[2] The word "voluntary" is used throughout to signify that the institution thus described is not maintained by any governmental body, but is supported by gifts and subscriptions of the charitable, and governed by a committee elected by subscribers.

an intrinsic part of the official public health machinery. Only by this means could it possess the elements of continuity of life, or have a prospect of success. This is a general proposition applicable to all organised communities. At the same time the scheme is an admirable illustration of voluntary work in an official setting.

The Private Practice Committee of the Council of the British Medical Association, in an Interim Report on the general problem of the sphere of private practice in the work of local authorities (Supplement to the *Brit. Med. Journal*, November 3, 1928) passed the following among some other provisional recommendations:—

That wherever possible all medical advice and treatment at local clinics should be given on a part-time basis by private practitioners, whether it is within the sphere of general practice or whether it is of a specialist character.

This is a good indication of the opinion of the general body of the medical profession in Great Britain; a subject which is more fully considered in Chapter II.

This resolution was considered at a meeting of the Gloucestershire Branch of the Association at which 53 members were present. The following summary of its proceedings is taken from the *British Medical Journal*:—

The meeting felt that the highly efficient and successful scheme of treatment inaugurated by Dr. Middleton Martin, the county medical officer of health, fulfilled the conditions which the association proposed should be established. In the opinion of the branch this scheme was an ideal method for a local authority to adopt in a county area to meet its obligations in respect of treatment. It was thought that the essential principles of the Gloucestershire scheme should be incorporated in all treatment schemes in the country. These principles, briefly summarised, were: (1) All ordinary work was done by general practitioners on a part-time basis. (2) All special work was done by the recognised consultants practising in the county on a part-time basis (with the single exception of the tuberculosis officer). (3) A strong medical advisory committee made itself responsible for all medical questions and was the negotiating body with the administrative committee, on which its chairman had a seat. The ophthalmic surgeon on the committee stated that it had been proved that the scheme, instead of lessening the opportunities of the consulting ophthalmic surgeon in the district, had definitely increased the amount of work available; while it was true that a certain number of private patients were absorbed by these public services, this loss was more than compensated for by the new work brought in. The throat, nose, and ear specialist, and the representatives of general practitioners, agreed that this applied to all the work done under the scheme.

A fuller note on the scheme is given at the end of this chapter. It has been written specially for me by Mr. Howell, the chairman of the County Medical Advisory Committee, and may be accepted as a judicial statement of the attitude of the local medical profession to the extended public medical service of the county of Gloucester.

Before describing this scheme in detail, we must place the county of Gloucester in its position as an element in the local government of England, and describe its ordinary public health activities. The geographical county of Gloucester comprises the administrative county and, in addition, two county boroughs: Bristol, with an estimated population in 1927 of 385,700,[1] and Gloucester,[1] with an estimated population in the same year of 53,560. The local, including the financial, administration of these two cities is entirely separate from that of the administrative county. In this respect county boroughs differ from New York City in its relation to the State of New York, or Chicago to the State of Illinois. This separation does not preclude voluntary joint committees for special purposes; thus the city of Gloucester has joint arrangements with the administrative county for police, and for schemes respecting tuberculosis and mental deficiency.

The city of Bristol has 13,100 persons per square mile, while in the administrative county the number per square mile is 268. Gloucestershire is sparsely populated. In 1921 it had 0·9 persons per acre, as compared with 8·4 in Middlesex and 2·0 in Surrey. These two counties are near London.

The entire population of Gloucestershire,[1] including Bristol and Gloucester, was 757,651 in 1921.

[1] The census (1931) population of the administrative county of Gloucestershire was 335,801, of Bristol 396,918, and of Gloucester 52,937.

Local Government in Gloucestershire

Within the administrative county there are 14 urban and 22 rural areas, each with its own local government, supervised in some respects by the County Council, and more generally by the Ministry of Health. Each of these 36 areas has its own M.O.H., though in some instances one M.O.H. acts for several districts. Thus for the 36 constituent sanitary areas of the administrative county there are 19 medical officers of health, of whom 5 devote their whole time to their public work; the remaining 14 are local medical practitioners in the district for which they are sanitary officers. As in the rest of Britain, the M.O.H. cannot be removed from office without the concurrence of the Ministry of Health.

Care of Mothers and Infants

Throughout England and Wales there has hitherto been some overlap between the duties of the local or district medical officers of health and of the county M.O.H. and his medical assistants. The control of the acute infectious diseases rests almost entirely with the local officers, and the hospital provision for acute infectious diseases is made by the district councils, or combinations of these. This is now being improved, and the County Council is required to arrange suitable combinations for hospital provision.

Births are notified within 36 hours by the midwife or doctor in attendance to the M.O.H. of the county, who apportions them for visits by the nurse attached to the district concerned.

In 1927 the number of births in the administrative county was 5,224. The work of visiting the homes concerned is organised, except for Cheltenham, by the County M.O.H., and in 1927, 78,928 such visits were made, or an average of 17 or 18 for each birth. Some of these visits were made to the homes of "toddlers", children between 1 and 5 years old.

The scale of this work is steadily increasing. If the number of visits in the year 1917 be stated as 100, the number in 1927 was 589. The births in the earlier year were 4,786, as compared with 5,001 in 1927.

Visiting on this liberal scale has been facilitated by the fact that district nurses in the greater part of the county are also health visitors (p. 298). In only three districts are there whole-time health visitors, who do not undertake district nursing.

Maternity and Child Welfare Centres.—There are 30 centres in the county. Most of them are conducted by voluntary local committees and workers, with a paid medical officer[1] and nurse. They are usually accommodated in a village hall, with a separate room for the doctor, and in the larger centres another room where the toddlers can be kept amused while the mothers hear a health talk, etc. At these centres no medical treatment is supposed to be given; if this is needed, the children are referred to the usual doctor of the family or they can be recommended to an out-station for treatment; or, if in-patient care is needed, the child can be sent to a hospital.

Hospital Treatment for Infants.—Under the orthopædic scheme (p. 309) children come under observation much earlier than in the past, sometimes shortly after birth. These cases are reported by midwives and health visitors. At present hospital treatment is limited to orthopædic cases and to the groups mentioned below. It is being increasingly utilised. In 1926, between the ages of 3 months and 5 years, 140 children were referred to the orthopædic surgeon at the Cheltenham General Hospital, of whom 8 became in-patients; in 1927 the numbers were 176 and 19 respectively.

In-patient treatment has also been arranged in a few instances for severe cases of marasmus and rickets. At a number of homes, hospitals, etc., arrangements have been

[1] He is a local medical practitioner.

made for the hospital treatment of infants with ophthalmia neonatorum.

Provision of Milk.—The early history of infant consultations and child welfare centres is largely concerned with the supply of appropriate milk (*gouttes de lait*). As time went on, it was realised that, in the absence of meticulous precautions, this supply was apt to favour the adoption of artificial feeding. There remained, however, instances in which artificial feeding of the infant was unavoidable, and other instances of pregnant and nursing mothers who suffered from deficient nutrition. For these, allowances of milk have been included in the items for which 50–50 grants from the Ministry of Health have been available.[1] The giving of milk is now—except in distressed areas or in local instances of exceptional poverty—largely abandoned.

There can be no doubt that adequate nourishment must be ensured. The only doubt is as to the general advisability of supplying the milk from child welfare centres, in which hygienic advice is the predominant feature. In Gloucestershire all applications for milk must be made through the health visitors, and grants are made for a month after being endorsed by the Chairman of the Maternity and Child Welfare Committee of the County Council. In 1927 the number of applications for milk (including extensions) was 1,818, as compared with 2,500 in 1926. This provision is hedged in by special inquiry in each case. About £800 was spent in 1927 in supplying milk gratuitously in suitable cases.

There is a considerable coal-mining centre in the county (Forest of Dean), as well as textile industries in the Stroud valley, both of which are in a depressed condition. It is especially in the coal-mining centre that milk is provided. It is made a usual condition of receiving milk that the child for whom it is supplied shall be brought regularly to a child welfare centre for observation.

Closely related to child welfare work is that of—

[1] As to the block grants superseding special grants from 1930 onward see page 33.

SUPERVISION OF MIDWIVES

This is undertaken by the Superintendent of the County Nursing (Voluntary) Association and the eight county health superintendents (official), whose relation to each other is indicated on page 299.

In January 1929 the County Council appointed a whole-time doctor (female) to be responsible for supervising midwives and to act as chief administrative officer of the child welfare centres.

The midwives, who number altogether about 250, are generally provided by local nursing associations, and they function as district nurses for ordinary cases of illness as well as for confinements. In 326 of the 354 parishes in the county the midwives are in the service of district nursing associations (population aggregate 294,648); in 15 parishes (population 27,805) independent midwives practise; and in 13 parishes (population 6,893) there are no resident midwives. The nursing associations have done valuable work in "planting" a nurse-midwife in areas in which, without their help, she could not earn a livelihood. The fees received by the midwife range from 15s. (for subscribers) to 35s. to 40s. (for non-subscribers).

The supply of midwives is helped by obtaining money for training young women (by bazaars, etc.), and by a small subsidy from the County Council.

In 1927 midwives attended 65·1 per cent. of all the births in the county. These midwives are all visited by a health superintendent during the year. On an average each midwife is visited at least four times annually. If morbid conditions or complaints respecting her practice draw attention to a midwife, she is visited more frequently. The visits thus made are not merely of an "inspectorial nature". Advice and help are looked for by the midwives and readily given by the superintendents. In particular, the latter have helped in developing antenatal work by the certified midwives. Occasionally, but rarely, disciplinary action is needed.

For consultations required by doctors, the medical fee

is three guineas (about $15) within five miles of the consultant's house, 3s. 6d. (84 cents) being allowed in addition for each mile or part of a mile over five miles. To promote antenatal work the Maternity and Child Welfare Committee of the County Council has helped by obtaining calipers and selling them to midwives at wholesale prices; and midwives have been instructed in their use by the health superintendents. Some hospital provision has been made for difficult confinement cases.

OFFICIAL TUBERCULOSIS ARRANGEMENTS

The organisation of tuberculosis public work presents difficulties of overlap between the County Council and local sanitary authorities. These have been overcome in Gloucestershire and commonly elsewhere by the willingness of the part-time medical officers of health of districts in the county to hand over most of the work to the county administration.

Notifications of cases of tuberculosis are received from private practitioners by each local M.O.H. Copies are transmitted to the county M.O.H. The fact that some of these local medical officers are also engaged in private practice would make official investigation in cases occurring in the practice of other doctors a task requiring tact and discretion.

The copies of notifications are distributed by the county M.O.H. to the health visitor nurse of the appropriate district, who obtains information as set out on a detailed schedule. After this has been reviewed by the county's tuberculosis officer, a copy is sent to the local M.O.H. of the district from which information of the case was received, marked as to any matter requiring consideration. Disinfection is left in the hands of the district officials.

Home visits are made by the nurse with varying frequency according to circumstances. As a rule they are only made by the tuberculosis officer when a consultation is requested.

There are two tuberculosis officers for the county, both resident at the Tuberculosis Sanatorium, Standish House:

Dr. W. Arnott Dickson, as its Superintendent, with an inclusive salary of £1,000, with house and other expenses; and Dr. E. D. D. Davies, with a salary of £450 and board and lodging. There is a third resident medical officer at the Sanatorium at a salary of £250.

The tuberculosis officers attend weekly at six dispensaries and periodically visit six out-stations (p. 302). They also see patients in their homes who are unable to attend at one of these places, and they hold frequent consultations with the usual medical attendants. Thus in 1927, in addition to the work set out below, the tuberculosis officers had 298 consultations, saw 412 patients at out-stations, etc., and paid 191 home visits in the county. The new cases reported, the new cases coming within the purview of the official dispensaries, and the number of attendances made at these dispensaries are shown in the diagram (page 291) in which the number for the initial year 1917 is given in each case as 100. These relative figures can be changed into actual numbers by reference to the following table:—

	1915	1927
No. of new cases of tuberculosis reported to the M.O.H. ..	679	411
No. of new cases attending at dispensaries	921	677
Total attendance at dispensaries.	4,741	5,579

The diagram indicates that the total of discovered cases of tuberculosis follows roughly the same lines as the number of dispensary cases. More cases attend the dispensary than are notified, giving evidence of its utilisation for diagnosis of suspected cases. The fact that attendances increase and their increase is great while fewer new cases occur is further evidence of the public appreciation of the facilities offered.

At the tuberculosis dispensaries persons are seen on the recommendation of their medical attendants.

Contacts with notified cases of tuberculosis are usually examined at schools by the school medical inspector.

If patients attend the tuberculosis dispensary without the known concurrence of their private practitioner, they are examined, and a special letter is then sent to the latter with a report on the case.

The tuberculosis officers in their periodic visits to the

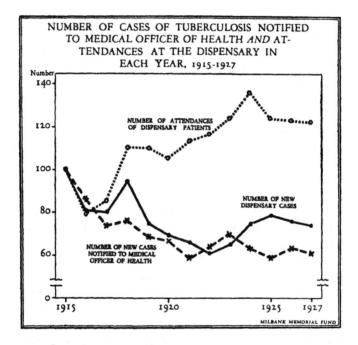

NUMBER OF CASES OF TUBERCULOSIS NOTIFIED TO MEDICAL OFFICER OF HEALTH *AND* ATTENDANCES AT THE DISPENSARY IN EACH YEAR, 1915-1927

MILBANK MEMORIAL FUND

out-stations (see p. 302) consult with the medical officers of these stations in regard to children.

Besides the sanatorium treatment in the county sanatorium, 37 beds are provided for advanced pulmonary cases in the Gloucester and Stroud isolation hospitals. From time to time these cases are reviewed by the tuberculosis officer. The work of home-visiting of tuberculous patients is undertaken as part of the duties of the 8 county superintendents and 127 district nurses of the county (see p. 298). In

1917 the number of these visits was 4,578; in 1927 it had increased to 9,636.

Patients living at home who have open tuberculosis are sometimes supplied with a shelter, which is placed in the garden or any available open space.

In 1927 the number of shelters in use was 114.

THE CONTROL OF VENEREAL DISEASES

The circumstances in which the gratuitous confidential treatment of venereal diseases is given to all desirous of accepting treatment at the public expense are described on page 233. So far as Gloucestershire is concerned, the diagram on p. 293 shows the remarkable success of the treatment centres. These are stationed at general hospitals (see map on p. 302). While the number of new cases is not increasing, the average number of attendances per patient shows striking improvement, and there has been a great increase in the number of specimens submitted for gratuitous examination (Wassermann tests, and search for spirochætes and gonococci).

Private practitioners are nearly all willing that patients, without class distinction, should receive gratuitous treatment at these centres. The modern treatment of venereal diseases has become in large measure an expert concern; but private practitioners in Gloucestershire as elsewhere who are competent for this work are supplied gratuitously at the expense of the County Council with arseno-benzol preparations to be used in their private practice. This is in addition to the free use of the pathological facilities in diagnosis already indicated.

MEDICAL WORK IN SCHOOLS

· In describing this work in Gloucestershire the following historic note is pertinent.

The Inter-Departmental Committee on Medical Inspection and Feeding of Children attending Public Elementary Schools, 1905 (Cd. 2779, Para. 51, p. 12), drew attention to the system of medical inspection which was carried on by

Dr. Martin in the Stroud District of Gloucestershire between the summer of 1904 and the spring of 1905, as being the only experiment of the kind which had been attempted.

The official school service of the county is administered

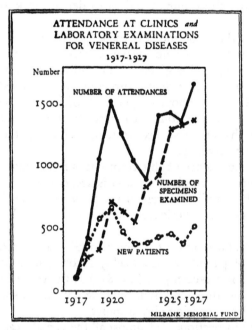

ATTENDANCE AT CLINICS *and* LABORATORY EXAMINATIONS FOR VENEREAL DISEASES 1917-1927

In this diagram, the first number under each heading is stated as 100, and the numbers for each of the years 1917-27 in proportion to this. To convert these relative into absolute numbers, 71 new cases attending the clinics in 1917 = 100, 258 total attendances = 100, and 75 specimens examined = 100.

by the County Council, except in the municipal borough of Cheltenham.

The county M.O.H. is the administrative school medical officer for the county's educational area, and has associated with him one male and one female doctor, devoting their whole time to the work, and three additional doctors who are also medical officers of health of sanitary districts in the county. These school medical inspectors examine the school children who are contacts of tuberculous patients notified in the county.

There are also three whole-time dental surgeons who make independent inspections of school children. Further facts as to school nurses and as to dental work are given later.

The methods of medical inspection and treatment are similar to those in Cambridgeshire, except that much of the treatment required is given in out-stations (p. 302).

Three whole-time dental surgeons are employed by the County Council. About 60 per cent. of the children examined by them are found to need treatment, and about seven-tenths of these are treated, either by the school dentists or privately.

In the experience of this county it is found that if dental treatment is to be given on a satisfactory scale to children, it must be supplied largely at the public expense. This has been the general experience of school authorities throughout England.

Free dental treatment is given in Gloucestershire to the children of parents whose weekly income, after deducting rent, does not exceed 50s. (say $12) in the case of a father, mother, and three children. Suitable adjustments are made for families in varying circumstances.

All the inspections and almost all the dental treatment are undertaken in the schools attended by the children. In the early days of these activities an interval of 10–14 days was allowed between inspection and treatment, to encourage parents to take advantage of the treatment given in certain cases in special centres. This interval has now been abolished, while the proportion of children to whose treatment parents consent has improved. The accommodation for treatment at schools is far from ideal; the dentists carry a very compact equipment from school to school in motor-cars, and the standard of work done is good. The nominal fee of 6d. (12 cents) per treatment is remitted in the great majority of the cases. Wherever the head teacher from his knowledge considers that something should be paid, the fee is taken.

OTHER ARRANGEMENTS

The special arrangements for orthopædics are indicated on page 309.

It is not proposed to describe arrangements made for the care of blind, deaf, mentally defective, insane, and epileptics, as for these conditions problems of the relation between private and public assistance, and between private and public medical attendance offer few difficulties. Nor will space permit me to give details of the work of medical inspection in secondary schools, i.e., in schools other than elementary, which has recently been inaugurated and which follows on lines parallel to those for children in elementary schools.

The existence of the Sickness Insurance Act for one-third of the population over 16 years of age undoubtedly favours the willingness of private practitioners to accept the official medical services at these ages, while relative poverty in many children reduces risk of friction when these are treated by official agencies.

MEDICAL SERVICES FOR THE DESTITUTE

In the public administrative machinery of Gloucestershire for education and the prevention and treatment of disease, only the work of the 36 local sanitary authorities and of the County Council has been described. But until April 1930 there were also the poor law authorities with fundamentally important duties of alleviation and treatment of destitution and of the disease commonly associated with it.

These duties now devolve on the County Council, which thus becomes more nearly the complete parliament for all county public affairs. At present there are 14 workhouses in the county, with some 700 infirmary beds for the sick. These in the main are residential homes for aged persons and other destitute and disabled persons. They always give also some provision for the sick, especially for patients suffering from advanced and incurable diseases, for whom provision is not made at general (voluntary) hospitals.

Nearly all the insane are treated in asylums at the public expense, and of the official sick and infirm over one-fourth are treated in the poor-law workhouses and their infirmaries. The total beds in these institutions in January 1926 were 2,145, of which 715 were described as infirmary beds. The quality of this provision for the sick is below that of voluntary hospitals; and one of the earliest reforms now needed is their overhauling and the provision of nursing and other medical needs up to modern standards. Their geographical distribution helps to make many of these infirmaries medical centres and hospitals for the surrounding population; and, by simple adjustment between these and existent voluntary cottage hospitals, it will not be difficult to expand the present scheme for co-operative medical services (p. 299), making also increased use of the larger hospitals in Bristol and Gloucester for consultative purposes and for cases of special difficulty.

Besides the institutional treatment under the poor-law, each parish or union of parishes has a district medical officer, whose duty it is to attend any sick person living at home, concerning whom the doctor has received the authorisation of the official relieving officer. In emergencies this is not required. In the administrative county there are 252 medical practitioners (including a large number in the city of Gloucester, many of whom practise also in the county area). Of this number 212 engage in medical practice. Of the 212 the number engaged in attending patients under the National Insurance Act is 174, while 75 are poor-law or district medical officers. Thus 82 per cent. of the doctors in practice attend insurance patients, and 35 per cent. attend poor-law patients. Inasmuch as both of these are forms of officially organised practice, they are paid for partially (insurance) or wholly (poor-law) at the expense of national or local official funds. Dr. Martin[1] has suggested that special

[1] "Poor Law Reform and Public Health," by J. Middleton Martin, M.D. Cantab., *British Medical Journal*, August 28, 1926.

appointments in every area of a district medical officer for the poor should be abandoned:—

He says:—

It would not entail very great changes if some arrangement were made whereby domiciliary medical attendance on poor-law persons were distributed among all doctors willing to accept them as they do insured persons. Indeed, it would appear that the time has arrived when the anticipation of the Royal Commissioners of 1905 (made three years before the National Insurance Act) may well be realised—namely, "we hope that, ultimately, it may be possible to dispense altogether with the service of the district medical officer and that his duties will be shared among medical men practising in the district".

This course would have great advantages over the present arrangement and would put the 8,500 so-called poor-law persons on the same footing as the 140,000 insured persons, and would remove once for all the distinction or stigma of "poor law" so far as medical assistance is concerned.

In putting such a proposal into operation there are two practical difficulties. The first is the varying periods for which persons on the border-line of necessitous would require medical care, and the second is the distribution of the funds available for such care. Both these difficulties are, however, of a diminishing quantity, as the probability is that, with the full development of health insurance, the number requiring what is at present called poor-law medical assistance will decrease; as an example it may be mentioned that an insured person is entitled to medical benefit on the insurance basis when he ceases to be an insured person and becomes an old-age pensioner, in future at 65 instead of 70 years of age, and the remuneration for such medical attendance is provided from insurance funds, presumably including the share of the State contributions.

If this were to be brought about, the differences between poor-law and insurance domiciliary medical practice would disappear. On this point see also page 94.

PATHOLOGICAL FACILITIES

Certain gratuitous pathological facilities are provided at the public expense without any limiting conditions to all medical practitioners, private and public, in the county. Specimens are examined on behalf of the County Council in the laboratories of the Bristol University and the Gloucestershire Royal Infirmary. The number thus examined is shown below for a few years :—

Yearly Average	Diphtheria	Enteric Fever	Tuberculosis	Cerebro-spinal Fever	Others	Total
1905–14 ..	1,553	49	207	—	—	1,809
1915 ..	1,713	31	369	6	—	2,119
1919 ..	506	20	569	2	8	1,105
1927 ..	2,649	50	2,445	5	6	5,155

COUNTY PROVISION FOR NURSES

In Gloucestershire, as in most counties, a County Nursing Association organises home nursing for the poorer inhabitants. It is controlled by a voluntary committee, usually of ladies; and in each local area there is a branch or district nursing association for local needs. Private practitioners find the services of these nurses invaluable. Nearly all the county association's nurses act also as midwives. For their nursing work—usually a daily or twice-a-day visit, not continuous attendance—the nurses have a scale of charges which is commonly remitted for poorer people. The nurses are supported largely by the voluntary subscriptions of the well-to-do, and cases introduced by these subscribers are attended free. For subscribers' cases midwifery fees are reduced.

In Gloucestershire there are 120 associations affiliated with the Gloucester County Nursing Association; there are five associations affiliated with other county associations; and there are five associations not affiliated.

The nurses of these 130 associations serve 326 out of 354 parishes in the county, covering an area of over 700,000 acres out of a total area of 785,000 acres, and a population of 295,000 out of 329,000. There is at least one nurse for each local association.

As already stated, the County Council—following its general policy of utilising existing agencies—has appointed the district nurses as part-time health visitors, and pays their associations for the health work done by them. The Council itself employs eight whole-time superintendent nurses to supervise the health visiting of the district nurses; and, so that there may be complete co-operation between the voluntary and official workers, the County Nursing Association has appointed these eight official superintendents as assistants to their Superintendent of Nurses. The advantage of this arrangement is that the superintendents when visiting midwives (see p. 288), or when visiting local nurses in their capacity as health visitors, can function in a double capacity. The gift of their work constitutes a substantial subsidy to the funds of the County Nursing Association. The County Council also gives an annual grant of £400 for the training of district nurse-midwives. Legally they are only entitled to do this in aid of midwifery work.

The borough of Cheltenham in these and in most other respects has its independent public health organisation.

The visits made by these nurses (see p. 285) have a real hygienic value; the mother is nearly always ready and even anxious to discuss her child's case with the visitor, and to accept her advice as to further visits to the centre, or as to consulting a private practitioner. The visits establish a personal relationship between mothers and nurses which is of great value. They assist in promoting resort to antenatal consultations, and in helping to secure early medical assistance in any illness.

For visits to cases of measles and some other illnesses the Nursing Association charges the modest fee of 1s. 3d. (about 30 cents) per case (not per visit), which is paid by the County Council. In 1925, 1,196 visits were paid to the homes of 232 cases of measles; and in 1927, when measles prevailed less, 393 such visits were made to 93 children.

THE COUNTY SCHEME FOR THE EXTENSION OF MEDICAL SERVICES

As set out on the opening page of this chapter, Dr. Martin, the County M.O.H., has obtained successful co-operation from voluntary hospitals and from the private medical practitioners of the county for various branches of medical work, carried out wholly or in part at the public expense, and has thus reduced the scope of narrowly specialised *ad hoc* clinics. The success attained in ensuring the co-operation of the general medical profession is especially noteworthy. The scheme in its present stage of development only comprises a part of the county within its activities, and in this part does not—nor does any known scheme—meet the complete medical needs of the population.

The general problem, towards the solution of which this county scheme represents a definite advance, was made the subject of an inquiry and report by a Consultative Council of the Ministry of Health, with Lord Dawson of Penn as its chairman. (Cmd. 693, May 1920.) In this report it is stated that a plan of services had been agreed on in 1918 in Gloucestershire under the guidance of Dr. J. Middleton Martin which had met with the approval of all the doctors in the county, and which "was not dissimilar in its aims" to the one set forth in the Consultative Council's report. It differs in maintaining intact the control of the representative local authority. The Gloucestershire scheme has been organised by the chief statutory health authority in the county, and although voluntary helpers are invoked in each department, its finances and general control are in the hands of the permanent health authority. The Gloucestershire County Council, while securing the expert assistance of advisory medical committees, retain their own administrative and executive control.

The diagram on page 301 shows the relationship between the different elements of the Gloucestershire scheme.

In April 1920 the scheme was approved by the Ministry of Health, having been adopted by the County Council in the preceding July. It speaks much for the skill and assiduity of Dr. Martin, the executive medical officer of the scheme, and of Dr. W. Arnott Dickson, its clinical medical officer, that a scheme involving the active co-operation of so many organisations and persons is now successfully at work.

Hospitals.—The scheme is based on three large general hospitals, each related to a geographical division of the county, and on certain special institutions for tuberculosis, etc. In deciding on these divisions, regard necessarily was had to the geographical position of existing hospitals and

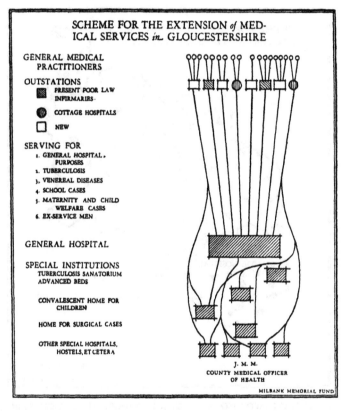

SCHEME FOR THE EXTENSION *of* MEDICAL SERVICES *in* GLOUCESTERSHIRE

GENERAL MEDICAL PRACTITIONERS

OUTSTATIONS

PRESENT POOR LAW INFIRMARIES.

COTTAGE HOSPITALS

NEW

SERVING FOR
1. GENERAL HOSPITAL, PURPOSES
2. TUBERCULOSIS
3. VENEREAL DISEASES
4. SCHOOL CASES
5. MATERNITY AND CHILD WELFARE CASES
6. EX-SERVICE MEN

GENERAL HOSPITAL

SPECIAL INSTITUTIONS
TUBERCULOSIS SANATORIUM ADVANCED BEDS

CONVALESCENT HOME FOR CHILDREN

HOME FOR SURGICAL CASES

OTHER SPECIAL HOSPITALS, HOSTELS, ET CETERA

J. M. M.
COUNTY MEDICAL OFFICER OF HEALTH

MILBANK MEMORIAL FUND

to readiness of means of communication. Local hospitals have a treble relation to the work. From them consultants and experts are available for special services; at them pathological specimens are examined for the medical practitioners in the county (see p. 297); and, in addition, patients requiring hospital treatment are sent to these hospitals.

Out-Stations.—The hospitals are related to institutions called out-stations, which are centres for consultation and treatment for patients living at home. Eight of these out-stations are conveniently situate at cottage hospitals, and these serve also for the indoor treatment of certain classes

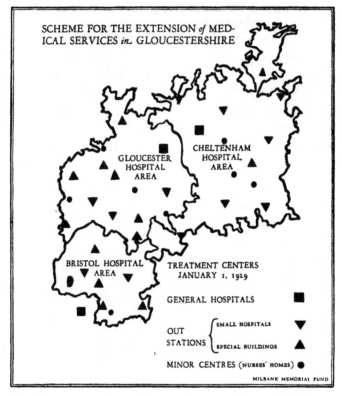

of patients; two also serve as tuberculosis dispensaries, and two are in buildings erected for this special purpose.

In one instance, at Thornbury, a poor-law institution is already used for treatment purposes under the scheme, throat operations being performed in it. This is a beginning of utilisation of poor-law arrangements, which will figure largely in future medical public administration.

The medical work at the out-stations is carried on by a

rota of general practitioners, assisted by consultations with
the tuberculosis officers of the county and by specialist
consultants from general or special hospitals. No change
occurs in the rota in a less period than six months.
The structural arrangements of out-stations are simple.
The same consulting-rooms are used for medical and dental
purposes.

Scope of the Scheme.—The out-stations form a partially
successful attempt to break down the conception that for a
special disease a separate institution is needed. This means
saving in capital and current expenditure.

Geographically the out-stations already organised serve
more than half of the entire county, and further additions
are being made. The County Council (January 1928) have
decided on further extensions, and within three years the
whole county will be served by out-stations. There are wide
areas of sparsely populated country in the county, in which
it would be uneconomical to provide out-stations; some
provision is proposed for these districts by arranging for
the treatment of minor ailments at a room in the district
nurse's home. The same rooms will be utilised for medical
consultations.

County councils and other local authorities can only
raise capital and incur current expenditure for medical
expenses for which there is exact statutory sanction, or
which is authorised by regulations issued by a Central
Government Department, either the Ministry of Health or
the Board of Education. Thus the County Council, the
authority organising the scheme, can only authorise payment for patients who can legally be treated at the public
expense.

The statement which follows in close type is taken chiefly
from Dr. Martin's Report.

1. *School Children*
The Board of Education have limited the conditions eligible
for treatment at the public expense to the following groups:
    (*a*) Minor ailments. Blepharitis, conjunctivitis, and other
        external eye disease; ringworm, scabies, and other skin

conditions; septic wounds and burns; uncleanliness
associated with pediculosis; otorrhœa, abscesses, etc.

(*b*) Defective eyesight.

(*c*) Defective hearing.

(*d*) Various conditions of the mouth, nose, and throat, including adenoids and enlarged tonsils.

The memorandum of the Board abstracted above adds that
it is impossible entirely to exclude conditions of a more
general nature, but there are affections and ailments which
the Board would not deem suitable for treatment unless it
were shown that adequate treatment at a reasonable cost
could not be otherwise obtained. In actual fact, if public
opinion and the Board of Education reflecting it desired to
extend the schedule of conditions for which treatment may
be supplied at school clinics to conditions other than those
enumerated above there would be no legal difficulty. But
until private practitioners can be more fully utilised there is
much to be said for giving special attention to the treatment
of conditions which are likely to be neglected if school aid
is not forthcoming. This applies especially to minor skin
ailments, to defects of vision requiring spectacles, to
adenoids, and to dental caries.

2. *Maternity and Child Welfare Cases*

The conditions eligible for treatment under this heading will
be chiefly those from which children are found to suffer on
entering the elementary schools, by which time often permanent
defects have developed. Amongst them may be mentioned
defects of the eye, nose, and throat, skin diseases, malnutrition.
By this means defects are discovered and treated, which might
otherwise escape detection until the child is medically inspected
at school.

3. *Tuberculosis*

This group embraces, more particularly, patients of any age
referred by the tuberculosis officer for intermediate treatment
and observation, and includes pre-tubercular cases (especially
contacts with tubercular cases) amongst school children.

4. *Orthopædic Cases*

For those cases, whether amongst children at, or below,
school age, special arrangements will be made, and it is desired

that full particulars of any patient shall be sent to the county medical officer of health promptly, so that all defects may be brought under treatment at as early a stage as possible.

All these groups represent abnormal conditions for which the County Council is entitled to expend its funds. It has been necessary to make a regulation that the medical practitioner in charge of an out-station, who is responsible for treatment, shall take precautions that no infants and school children be treated at the expense of the Council, who are outside the scope of the scheme.

Children are reported to the out-stations:—

(1) By the county tuberculosis officer for continued observation. It is the duty of the medical officer of the station at intervals to collect and group cases (contacts and others) for examination by the tuberculosis officer on his visit to the station.

(2) The school medical officer and school nurses refer children to the out-station for treatment for minor complaints and visit the station to confer with its medical officer. Head teachers of schools furthermore refer suitable cases to the school medical officer to obtain a voucher authorising treatment at an out-station.

(3) The district nurses of the county, who in their limited area act in the triple capacity of health visitors, school nurses, and tuberculosis nurses, are asked to ensure that each sick person receives treatment, and to refer cases eligible for treatment at the public expense to an out-station in the portions of the county possessing one.

The out-stations are also utilised for the following purposes:—

(a) For the use of consultation services of physicians for infants and children with possible rheumatic hearts;

(b) For the examination by ophthalmic surgeons of children referred by the County Association for the Blind;

(c) For the examination of insured persons by ophthalmic surgeons.

All the costs of use of the out-stations are paid by the County Council excepting (c); for these cases the out-station is lent free of charge, but the physicians collect their fees for insured persons from the Approved Societies to which the insured belong. The County Association for the Blind refunds to the County Council the fees for their cases at the rate of 7s. 6d. per examination.

The following statement of *Cost per Attendance* at each station incidentally shows the reduction per attendance with increase in number of patients :—

	1922		1923		1924		1925		1926		1927	
	s.	d.	s.	d.	s.	d.	s.	d.	s.	d.	s.	d.
Total cost—per attendance ..	15	6	10	5	7	11½	8	0	6	1	7	10¾
Medical officers —per attendance at out-stations ..	4	3½	2	10½	2	1¾	2	0¼	1	6	1	7¾
Specialist services cost per examination .	12	0	11	1¼	9	6	8	8½	8	5	7	4¾

The following statement shows the scale of fees payable by the County Council for the various grades of help given in the different branches of the scheme :—

Medical Officer of Out-Station
> £1 1s. for the first hour or part of an hour and 10s. 6d. for each subsequent half-hour. This averages about £80 per annum per Medical Officer.

Hospital Staff (Ear and Throat Surgeon and Ophthalmic Surgeon)

	£	s.	d.
Examination at ordinary			
Out-patient department, per case	0	7	6
Visiting fee for out-stations, including 4 cases	2	2	0
Each case above 4	0	5	0
Mileage allowance, per mile, one way	0	3	6
Operations (including anæsthetic) per case ..	1	2	6

Physician (Rheumatic Heart Survey)

For two sessions on one day	5	5	0
For one session on one day	3	3	0
Mileage allowance, per mile, one way, after first five miles	0	3	6

Consultant for Obstetric Difficulty and Puerperal Pyrexia.

Orthopædic Surgeon	£	s.	d.
Consultation fee, per case	3	3	0
Mileage allowance, per mile, one way, after first five miles	0	3	6
Inclusive fee for quarterly visits seven out-stations	160	0	0

Fees Paid by Patients.—For ordinary treatment, the assistance is given free to children of families comprising father, mother, and three children, and with an income under 50s.

Travelling Expenses.—In needy cases these are also paid by the County Council.

Appropriation.—About November in each year a detailed estimate is prepared of the probable cost of the services for the next financial year, April 1st to March 31st. So long as this is not exceeded, the Medical Services Committee are authorised by the County Council to carry out all the work covered by the estimate.

WORK OF GENERAL PRACTITIONERS IN THE SCHEME

The work at each out-station is carried on by medical men practising in its vicinity. All doctors are eligible for the work, but the Medical Services Committee (see p. 308) have decided to appoint only those recommended by the Medical Advisory Committee. When there is more than one doctor eligible for the work, each of these undertakes it for six months at a time. By this means it has been possible to avoid professional friction and to secure the active co-operation of practitioners.

Although county councils are under an obligation to provide for the treatment of venereal disease in any person applying for treatment, it has only recently been found practicable to have the routine treatment of venereal diseases at the out-stations. Sentimental considerations, as well as unnecessary fear of infection, had rendered this inexpedient.

The doctors employed at each out-station have the right to exclude any patient applying for treatment who is above a certain financial status. Usually before treatment is begun at the out-station, cases are referred to the family medical attendant, if there is one. This is not done consistently in cases obviously suitable for immediate treatment (as visual defects, skin affections) or where distances to be travelled are great. The income limit usually adopted is that the person applying is below the standard of a family of man and wife with three children earning 50s. a week or more, or an equivalent amount in other cases.

MANAGEMENT OF THE SCHEME

The general conduct of the scheme is controlled by the County Council through its Medical Services Committee, of which the chairman of the County Council is also chairman. It includes representatives of the Maternity and Child Welfare Committee, Education Committee, Public Health Committee—all official committees of the County Council; and further representatives from the Joint Committee for Tuberculosis, in the formation of which the County Council and the Council of the city of Gloucester combine for joint tuberculosis provision. The chairman of the Medical Advisory Committee has been co-opted on this committee without a vote.

On medical points this committee is advised by a Medical Advisory Committee of 22 members, formed of members of the consultant staff and medical officers in charge of the out-stations. Their duties comprise: (1) ensuring that treatment given at the out-stations is effective, and (2) advising the Medical Services Committee on difficulties arising in medical matters.

This committee is elected by a postal vote of the medical officers of the out-stations. The county medical officer of health and the tuberculosis officer, who is the clinical officer for the scheme, are members of this committee, which meets as required. It considers matters referred to it by the Medical Services Committee, and can initiate recommendations to the latter committee.

The Hospitals in the Scheme

The situation of the larger institutions, of the cottage hospitals, and of poor-law infirmaries is shown in the outline map on page 302.

It will be noted that the workhouses and the voluntary cottage hospitals are much more convenient of access than the three voluntary general hospitals, on the co-operation of which the scheme is based.

The general hospitals which are co-operating are Bristol Royal Infirmary and General Hospital, the Gloucester Royal Infirmary, and the Cheltenham General Hospital, which altogether have over 300 beds. In addition, certain cases needing specialist treatment are sent to the Cheltenham Eye, Ear, and Throat Hospital, the Gloucester Children's Hospital, the Bath Ear, Nose, and Throat Hospital, and the Stratford-on-Avon Hospital (ear, throat, nose and vision cases only).

Some 18 hospital physicians and surgeons and about 60 general practitioners are interested in, and take part in, the working of the scheme. In addition, services are rendered by members of the staff of Radcliffe Infirmary, Oxford, for eastern parishes in Gloucestershire, the lines of communication in this direction making this arrangement desirable.

It may be added that the members of the hospital staffs concerned are satisfied with the existing official arrangements for sending patients to them and would like to see them extended. It is hoped to arrange shortly for period-ical visits of special physicians and surgeons at each of the out-stations for consultative purposes.

Orthopædic Defects

The working of the orthopædic portion of the scheme for extended medical services is described in the Annual Report of the County M.O.H. for 1927. In that year 316 patients were treated. Every effort is made to get cases at an early stage. Cases of congenital club-foot have been received within a few days of birth. Of the total cases 109 were received in the first two years of life. For such cases a large percentage of manipulative cures can be obtained. Fifty-eight cases of flat-foot and 46 cases of infantile paralysis were treated during the year, and the proportion of cases in which deformity is prevented increases as the work extends.

RELATIONS WITH GENERAL PRACTITIONER

The views of the general practitioner are stated on page 283. These are supplemented by the letter of the chairman of the Medical Advisory Committee, which is appended to this chapter.

CONCLUDING REMARKS

The description of a largely successful effort to secure the co-operation of the medical profession as a whole in the medical branches of public health work is, I think, of general interest. Besides describing this scheme I have given in rather full detail particulars of the general public health administration of the county, which is fairly typical for a somewhat sparsely populated area with a few large towns in or near it. Quite apart from its special scheme of extended medical services, Gloucestershire shows active public health and medical work by public authorities, and this work may be regarded as fairly exemplifying provincial and chiefly rural administration in England. Some counties have more advanced administration in certain particulars; while similarly they may not have equally satisfactory arrangements in other particulars. Local initiative and variation of local needs and standards imply such variations.

A NOTE ON THE

GLOUCESTERSHIRE SCHEME FOR THE EXTENSION OF MEDICAL SERVICES

THE Cheltenham General Hospital Staff were wholeheartedly in favour of the scheme from the outset with one exception, and he remains an uncompromising opponent to this day. The Gloucester Infirmary Staff, after a short period of criticism and consideration, supported it, as also did the Staff of the Stroud Hospital, with one exception. He consistently opposed it for some time, and at every meeting of the Medical Advisory Committee that he attended seized any opportunity to animadvert on the scheme, basing his censure on infinitesimal benefits to be derived from it.

At first it must be admitted that the cost of the scheme, for various reasons, but chiefly that it was new and out of the experience of its pioneers, was high and the attendance small. In process of time the cost was very much reduced absolutely, and owing to the large increase in attendances the relative cost per case decreased in a very striking way.

The uncompromising attitude of the member of the Cheltenham Staff threatened to wreck the scheme at its very outset, for he was an essential part of the machine: this was the most dangerous crisis which the scheme encountered. However, it was happily surmounted by the appointment of another consultant who was in favour of the scheme, who threw himself with such enthusiasm into the work that his example had great influence in bringing about the smooth working of this special department in other parts of the county: in fact, it saved the scheme.

With regard to the attitude of the general practitioners, it may be said that, at the General Meeting called to consider the scheme, for the most part they candidly expressed themselves as suspicious; it was another encroachment on private practice; where was it all going to end? the expense would be enormous and the results to be obtained ridiculously small; Dr. A's patients would be treated by Dr. B during his tenure of office at the out-station, an intolerable intrusion, etc., etc. These arguments were obvious and foreseen, and the replies were ready. The appointment at this meeting of a Medical Advisory Committee to the Medical Extension Services Committee of the County Council, consisting of equal numbers from amongst themselves and the staffs of the General Hospitals, and the confidence this gave them that their interests would be looked after, not only as between one practitioner and another, but as between the practitioners and their employers—the County Council—soon broke down what was never a serious opposition, but merely a hesitation to take the leap into the dark.

This Medical Advisory Committee was the fruit of experience with a similar Advisory Committee to the Executive Officer of the Cheltenham War Hospital. This hospital had 1,200 beds, a consultant staff of six, and about 20 "medical officers", and the committee was elected at a General Meeting, a small one of three or four consultants and an equal number of medical officers. This committee pooled all monies received and distributed them equally, portioned out the work, drew up standing orders for the medical working of the hospital, arranged holidays and so on, and worked admirably. Hence the suggestion of such a committee to the General Meeting, so many of whom had already had experience of the excellent working of the above.

At first the Medical Committee met fairly frequently, and a fresh election took place annually, resulting almost invariably in the re-election of the old committee, except where changes were inevitable through death, removal and so on. For the last few years, so smoothly and satisfactorily has the scheme worked, that in the absence of any serious question to discuss, it has rarely been necessary to call a meeting. The committee gives advice to the County Council on all matters of medical organisation; the qualification of practitioners for appointment to out-stations; deals with complaints as to late attendance (one only), incapacity of out-station officers (one); fees for work, suggested clinical inquiries; and their recommendations have been accepted without exception by the Medical Services Committee of the County Council. The chairman of the Medical Advisory Committee was invited to a seat (without a vote) on the Medical Services Committee.

To sum up: a short period of hesitation and suspicion was soon followed by a recognition of the advantages of a scheme, which was peculiar to this county, for carrying out statutory medical treatment. Now it may be confidently stated that the scheme has the warm support of all the doctors in the county, with individual exceptions—some four in number out of over 200.

JNO. HOWELL, C.B.E., F.R.C.S., M.B.
Chairman, Medical Advisory Committee

March 6, 1930

CHAPTER XVII

COUNTY OF DURHAM[1]

THE administrative county of Durham illustrates some special methods of medical attendance for its industrial population, and shows the great extent to which public health administration, in the hands of the County Council and their M.O.H. (Dr., now Sir Eustace Hill),[2] has been able successfully to supplement the deficiencies of private medical care, and of the widely prevalent contract practice for miners and their families.

The geographical county of Durham contains, in addition to the county administrative area, five county boroughs—Darlington, Sunderland, Gateshead, South Shields, and West Hartlepool. These centres of large industrial activities, including shipping, are not included within this report.

The administrative county has an area of 632,280 acres, with a population close on a million. In 1921 it was 955,344.[3]

Physically, the county consists of undulating beautiful country, traversed by several rivers, with coal-mines somewhat widely distributed, thus diminishing their devastating effect on scenery. In some parts of the county an elevation of over 2,000 feet is reached. The parts of the county where mines exist are densely populated. Other parts are agricultural and moorland, and are sparsely peopled.

The administrative county consists of four non-county boroughs, having populations in 1925 varying from 68,000 to 17,000; of 27 urban districts, with populations varying in the same year from 1,884 to 35,370; and of 14 rural districts, with populations of from 3,937 to 62,450. Each of these boroughs and districts has separate government for elementary sanitary work and for the control of infectious

---

[1] Date of investigation, September 1929.
[2] Dr. Hill retired in April 1930.
[3] The census (1931) population of the administrative county of Durham was 924,050, of the county boroughs in Durham 561,928.

diseases; but the greater medical services, except the school medical service in the boroughs of Durham city, Hartlepool, Jarrow, and Stockton, and the urban districts of Felling and Hebburn, are in the hands of the County Council. As it is in these special services that the problems of interrelation between doctors and public authorities arise, we can now confine our attention chiefly to the work of the County Council and allied voluntary agencies.

The medical position in Durham county is profoundly modified by the mining industry. At the census of 1921, 140,960 males, or nearly 15 per cent. of its total population of men, women, and children, were engaged in coal- and shale-mines. There is little industrial non-domestic employment of women in the county.

The present statistical position of the county can be seen from the following data supplied by Dr. Hill.

The county birth-rate in 1924–28 was 22·7, as compared with 36·1 per 1,000 of population in 1892–96. After the same interval of 32 years the death-rate had become 12·2, a decline of 34 per cent.; the death-rate under one year of age per 1,000 births had declined from 163 to 92 (i.e. 43·5 per cent.), the death-rate from infantile diarrhœa had declined 54 per cent., from enteric fever 97 per cent. (to one per 100,000 population in 1924–28), and from pulmonary tuberculosis 37 per cent. (to 84 per 100,000 in 1924–28).

The later figures given above imply vast improvement in sanitary and social conditions. In securing this improvement public health and education authorities and many voluntary social workers can all claim a share. The County Council have been fortunate in having Dr. Hill as their chief adviser during 37 years, and there has been, therefore, consistent and wise medical counsel for a council which has shown its appreciation of the importance of sanitary-medical reforms.

The personnel of the county health department given below indicates the extent of its medical activities:—

PERSONNEL OF THE COUNTY HEALTH DEPARTMENT
(*Not including Clerical Staff*)

The County Medical Officer.
The Deputy and Assistant County Medical Officer.
1 Central Tuberculosis Medical Officer.
5 District Tuberculosis Medical Officers.
1 Whole-time and 3 part-time Clinical Venereal Diseases Medical Officers.
1 Senior Welfare Medical Officer.
9 Whole-time and 4 part-time Assistant Welfare Medical Officers.
1 County Health Inspector.
1 Superintendent Health Visitor.
2 Assistant Superintendent Health Visitors.
84 Permanent and 2 temporary Health Visitors.
1 Midwives Inspector and 1 Assistant Inspector.
3 Medical Superintendents of County Sanatoriums.
1 Assistant Medical Officer of County Sanatoriums.
3 Matrons of County Sanatorium.
Nursing and Domestic Staffs at three above-mentioned Institutions, which vary from time to time.
1 Medical Officer, Richard Murray Hospital.
1 Matron, County Maternity Hospital.
1 Matron, E. F. Peile County Convalescent Home.
Nursing and Domestic Staffs at County Maternity Home and County Convalescent Home, which vary from time to time.

NURSING IN THE COUNTY

It will facilitate understanding of Durham's public medical machinery if I first describe the work of Durham County Nursing Association. Its objects are to promote the provision, development and increased efficiency of district nursing and midwifery throughout the county, while not interfering with the liberty of action and finances of the district nursing associations within the county. It arranges for the training of "village nurse-midwives" (definition given below), and their supply to the district nursing associations which cannot afford to employ more highly-trained nurses.

There are 80 affiliated districts in the county, employing 127 nurses; and during the year 1928–29 these made 395,220 visits to 18,351 cases, of which 14,929 were general, 702 were attended for maternity nursing, and 2,720 confinements were attended by midwives.

Of the total 127 nurses, 78 are fully-qualified nurses, who are also qualified midwives; 34 are qualified midwives with a shorter period of training as nurses ("village nurse-midwives"). Nine-tenths of the entire county is covered by the work of these nurses. A few collieries still employ nurses not yet affiliated to the county association.

These nurses visit and nurse tuberculosis patients needing actual bed-side nursing and assist in persuading tuberculosis patients to attend the 11 tuberculosis centres in the county. The hygienic visiting of tuberculosis cases is undertaken by the County Council health visitors. In a few sparsely populated areas this work is combined with bed-side nursing.

The County Nursing Association acts as the agent through which the County Council gives grants to the various district nursing associations for their local midwifery work, for the work of maternity nursing, and for the nursing of cases of infectious disease which are treated at home.

The County Council encourages district nursing associations to appoint qualified midwives for their area, making a grant of £30 per annum for each district nurse acting as midwife and maternity nurse. The council also undertakes to make up the deficit in the salary of whole-time approved midwives appointed by district nursing associations. Returns of number of cases and receipts are required.

In addition, a grant of £10 is given by the County Council to each district nursing association for nursing infectious cases. The rest of the expense of district nursing is defrayed from local subscriptions and from payments made by patients. The total grants given by the County Council in the year 1928–29 amounted to £2,937, of which one-half is derived from national and one-half from county public funds. The system is thus an admirable combination of personal contributions by beneficiaries, supplemented by voluntary gifts of the well-to-do, and by county and national money. The county owes much to Miss Simpson, the superintendent of the County Nursing Association, who secures admirable co-operation between the voluntary and official agencies.

MIDWIFERY IN THE COUNTY

The voluntary County Nursing Association takes an active part in the midwifery service of the county, which may now be described.

The births in the county in 1928 numbered 20,040, of which about 49 per cent. were attended by midwives. Of this number, as already stated, 2,720 were attended by midwives of the district nursing associations, of whom there are 112 in the county. Over 200 additional midwives in the county are engaged in private practice.

Every midwife is entitled to send for any local medical practitioner chosen by the patient, whose standardised fee for this service must be paid by the County Council. The latter may recover it, or part of it, from the patient. The midwife is required to notify to the county M.O.H. each call for medical aid, and in 1928 medical help was sent for in 3,502 cases, of which 242 were still-births; 27 were deaths of mothers; 204 were deaths of infants; 65 were cases of artificial feeding; in 57 cases the midwife had assisted in laying out the dead; and in 103 cases there was risk of infection.

The fees obtained by midwives for their services, which include attendance for ten days after parturition, are 21s. for each case attended by a midwife of a nursing association. "Bad debts" for this work are rare.

Each patient when booking for attendance with a district nurse-midwife has her urine examined, and this examination is usually repeated several times. The association cases (2,720 in 1928) received 11,360 antenatal visits.

Between 1921 and 1925 the percentage of births notified by midwives, and therefore presumably attended independently by them, increased from 29·0 to 42·5 per cent. of the total births. In the same period the fees paid to medical practitioners called in to help midwives on an uniform

official scale increased from £1,694 in 1921 to £3,502 in
1925, i.e. more than doubled. Evidently midwives are now
calling in the aid of doctors more frequently than in earlier
years. Dr. Hill states that the proportion of medical calls
varies in different districts from 6 per cent. to 50 per cent. of
the total cases attended by midwives. It is probable that in
some districts "the patient has not an absolutely free choice of
doctor, but is unduly influenced by the midwife". It is also
likely that in some districts medical aid is unnecessarily
requisitioned.

These facts bear on the *relation between midwives and doctors*.
The salaried nurse-midwife of the district associations
receives from £170–180 per annum, if she is a fully-qualified
nurse; otherwise from £130–150. She is not allowed to book
an excessive number of cases. She is competent to diagnose
presentations by abdominal palpation. Breech presentations
thus diagnosed during pregnancy, as well as cases of
albuminuria, are sent to a private doctor or to an antenatal
centre. In several districts the formation of a district nursing
association has been opposed by the local doctor, in fear
that his midwifery practice would suffer; in other instances
the association has been welcomed by the local doctor,
whose ordinary medical work is immensely helped by having
in the midwife a nurse available in any of the many surgical
and medical cases where the doctor needs one.

It should be added that a large proportion of the fees
lost by doctors in attending confinements through the
increasing resort to midwives has been recovered in fees for
attendance when called in by midwives. I heard of instances
in which the doctor's income from midwifery cases is
stated to have been actually increased since midwives took
over his cases. In most instances this would scarcely hold
good.

The county nursing superintendent's salary is partly paid
by the County Council, as she acts as county supervisor of
the midwives in the county, who work under the nursing
associations.

In the districts in which there is no nursing association,

the County Council provides whole-time midwives to the number of 21. They are paid a salary of £120–150, with additional fees for antenatal visits. These midwives and the midwives in independent private practice are supervised by the county midwives' inspector.

The puerperal mortality in Durham is somewhat above the average for England, and it has shown no marked decrease. It is possible that the stationary position is partially explicable by more accurate certification in recent years. There is a marked difference between the mortality in cases attended by midwives and those attended by doctors in favour of the former, although complicated cases subsequently receiving medical care at home or in hospital are reckoned as midwives' cases. The explanations of this may more appropriately be discussed under a general heading. One very competent practitioner in the county of Durham informed me that he had given up midwifery, and considered that official supervision of unfavourable cases and the largely advertised Governmental inquiries had "frightened the lives out of doctors". He also voiced the point, which must occur to all, that if the younger doctors obtain no experience in normal midwifery, how can they become competent to assist midwives in complicated cases?

At five institutions in the county—three maternity homes, and two hospitals—women are admitted for their confinement. In 1925 the number confined in these institutions was 691, or about 3 per cent. of the total births in the county.

The payment required for each patient confined in one of these institutions is shown below. It is based on the weekly total family earnings. A large proportion of the total cost of these patients falls on the County Council, in part because a large proportion of families are partially exempt from payment owing to low wages, and in part because of the difficulty in collecting charges not paid beforehand. In 1928–29 hospital provision for parturition cost the County Council £7,250.

Revised Scale of Fees for Patients Admitted to County Maternity Homes

To arrive at the net weekly income, the earnings for four weeks immediately preceding the date of application are to be averaged, and 5s. per week is to be deducted for rent and 5s. per week for each child under 14 years of age and for each other member of the household who is not a wage-earner.

In the case of a person unemployed at the date of application, if appreciably before the expected date of confinement, the fee to be paid shall be reviewed at the date of admission.

Net weekly income—			Fee payable—		
Not exceeding £2	0	0	Maternity benefit (£2) or free.		
„ 2	2	6	„	„	*plus* 2/6 per week
„ 2	5	0	„	„	5/0 „
„ 2	7	6	„	„	7/6 „
„ 2	10	0	„	„	10/0 „
„ 2	12	6	„	„	12/6 „
„ 2	15	0	„	„	15/0 „
„ 2	17	6	„	„	17/6 „
„ 3	0	0	„	„	20/0 „
„ 3	2	6	„	„	25/0 „
„ 3	5	0	„	„	27/6 „
„ 3	7	6	„	„	30/0 „
„ 3	10	0	„	„	32/6 „
Over 3	10	0	Three guineas weekly		

The County Council provides a trained emergency nurse to attend in their homes patients suffering from puerperal pyrexia, etc. It has also made provision for the service of obstetric consultants for such cases and for difficult midwifery cases.

Maternity and Child Welfare Work

Midwifery work, as seen in the preceding section, is carried out in Durham by a combination of official and voluntary agencies, supplementing the ordinary work of the doctors and midwives who engage in private midwifery practice; and this supplementation is needed in the economic and social circumstances of Durham, and to some extent throughout Great Britain. What is usually known as Child Welfare Work—with some additional antenatal care of expectant mothers—is organised almost entirely on official lines, and occupies a large staff of doctors and health visitors (public health nurses). There is a senior welfare medical officer, Dr. Mary Howie, with nine whole-time assistant welfare medical officers, doing very valuable work under their skilled chief; and associated with these is a superintendent health visitor, Miss Hodgson, who has two assistants and a staff of 84 whole-time health visitors, whose work is also admirably organised.

In a few districts part-time health visitors are employed.

Of the 16,874 births registered in the County Council's administrative area for child welfare work during 1928, about 50 per cent. were notified by midwives and presumably attended by them. Nearly all these homes were visited by the health visitors. In addition to these first visits, 27,942 revisits were made during the first year, and 84,204 revisits to children aged 1–5 years. In addition, health visitors paid 2,244 first visits and 19,611 revisits to cases of tuberculosis; they also paid 17,536 home visits to school children. These numbers are in addition to the large number of attendances at various clinics and schools.

The welfare doctors are occupied chiefly in giving medical hygienic advice at 60 centres scattered throughout the county. A few centres have been staffed by private practitioners, but difficulty has arisen in these instances, owing to the unwillingness of other practitioners to allow the children of their private patients to attend the centre and because of the urgent medical calls in private practice, which occasionally interfere with attendance at the centres. For antenatal work there is, furthermore, much natural unwillingness of rival medical practitioners to accept consultations at the centre.

At the end of 1928, 3,600 expectant mothers were on the registers of antenatal centres. This work, which is in its early stages, is additional to the antenatal work done for mothers booking for admission to maternity homes.

At the infant consultation centres a doctor attends at each session, and infants are seen by her at least monthly, the nurse seeing and weighing the infants at intermediate visits, and referring them to the doctor if unfavourable conditions develop. At many of the centres children aged 1–5 equal the number of infants in attendance.

As the procedure at the child welfare centres in Durham is similar to that elsewhere, I do not describe it in detail.

No systematic medical treatment is given. When this is needed mothers are referred to a private doctor or to a hospital. Much cod-liver oil is distributed, for which some payment is exacted; and occasionally grey powder (hydrarg. cum creta) is given when it is known that the mother in the circumstances would not consult a doctor. I was informed that—contrary to specific instructions—doctors sending patients to a centre in a few instances received no letter from the welfare doctor in return. On the other hand, there was ample evidence that private doctors often neglected to acknowledge letters sent to them respecting patients. It was also clear that from both antenatal and child welfare centres doctors receive patients who but for the centres would have failed to secure medical care. Gradually co-operation between private doctors and the official doctors of the centres is improving, and illness is being treated and prevented to a steadily increasing extent.

In Durham an exceptionally large amount of cod-liver oil and dried milk is given at the centres. A private doctor, with whom I conversed, was strongly of opinion that an average pitman earning 35s. a week, even when living in a low-rented house belonging to the colliery employing him, could not be expected to buy this oil. That there has been great decline in severe rickets in recent years is universally agreed.

A large part of the miners of Durham have been out of work in recent years, and one means of relieving distress has been the giving of dried milk to mothers and their infants. Large sums have been expended on this supply. During the four quarters July 1928–June 1929, the cost of dried milk given at centres on behalf of the County Council was £29,389. In addition, some assistance in this direction has been given from a National Coal Relief Fund. There is no evidence that the distribution of dried milk for infants and young children has led to diminution of breast-feeding of infants. It appears probable that the substitution of dried milk for condensed milk in the feeding of children has had a large share in producing the more favourable diarrhœal experience in recent years.

It will be noted that as a rule none of the county health visitors undertake also the nursing of the sick. Dr. Hill strongly opposes the view that this combination is good. The health visitor has sometimes to report sanitary defects, which the district nurse as a friend of the family might not do. Thus in 1927 health visitors reported to district medical officers of health 1,718 cases of overcrowding and 1,059 instances of sanitary defects. The health visitors visit mothers and infants, pre-school children, and tuberculosis patients, and attend the various child welfare centres, where they have considerable duties in regulating the giving of supplies of dried milk. There are separate school nurses, who attend the school clinics, but home visiting in respect of ailing children is undertaken by the health visitors, the Education Committee paying an annual sum (£2,600) to the Health Committee for these services.

Supplying dried milk undoubtedly gives health visitors and welfare doctors, in the circumstances of Durham, a very advantageous means of frequent supervision of children. No milk is given unless the welfare doctor signs the application form.

The appended rules displayed at each centre show the general conditions of this distribution; and rigid inquiry as to family earnings and income is made in each application, so that abuse by those able to pay is unlikely. Renewals of supply give further checks on the supply.

Rules for the Supply of Dried Milk at Centres

1. No dried milk to be supplied unless ordered by the doctor at the centre.
2. No child to be allowed dried milk unless the centre is attended at least once a month.
3. No baby under 3 months old will be allowed more than 2 lbs. dried milk fortnightly, unless ordered by the doctor.
4. No child to be supplied with more than 3 lbs. dried milk fortnightly, unless ordered by the doctor.
5. Children over 12 months old to be supplied with not more than 2 lbs. fortnightly.
6. The identity paper must be produced and the amount of dried milk should be noted on the paper each time.
7. No mother to be supplied with dried milk for another mother unless the pink paper is produced.
8. Nothing in the way of cod-liver oil or drugs, etc., to be supplied unless ordered by the doctor.

A shrewd practitioner interviewed by me was certain that the supply of "cheap milk" was largely responsible for attendance at the centres. He agreed that half the children attending were entitled to this supply, in view of the state of family finances.

Summing up the child welfare work, I appreciated the force of the conclusion reached by Dr. Mary Howie, the chief welfare doctor, that in the circumstances of Durham "you will never get the medical practitioner to do this preventive work". They would be unwilling to keep records, unable to attend the centres regularly, and unwilling to spend their time in treating the minor ailments, in the hygienic treatment of which welfare doctors and health visitors are daily engaged.

School Medical Work

The school medical work in Durham need not be described in detail, but a few illustrative items may be given. Owing to prolonged industrial depression, the further development of the school medical services has been delayed.

The extent of the medical work may be inferred from the following statement of staff and expenditure:—

SCHOOL MEDICAL INSPECTION SERVICE
Year ending March 31, 1930

	£
School Medical Officer (Dr. Hill)	100
i.e. in addition to Dr. Hill's salary as County M.O.H.	
Deputy School Medical Officer	800
11 Assistant School Medical Officers	7,100
2 School Oculists	1,300
1 Part-time School Oculist	150
3 Dental Officers	1,750
1 Part-time Dental Officer	210
8 School Nurses	1,530
Health Visitors (Contribution)	2,600

Estimated total cost of the medical service for the above year, including the above items of expenditure:—

	£
Elementary Education	28,198
Higher Education	3,074
	31,272
Less Receipts	300
	£30,972

In 1928, 43,652 school children were medically inspected at routine examinations of the three groups of entrants, intermediates, and leavers, and, in addition, 18,522 medical reinspections and special inspections were made. Of the first group 21·7 per cent., of the second group 26·7 per cent., and of the third group 25·0 per cent. were found to require medical treatment.

The only conditions which are treated by the County Council's doctors themselves (except dental) are minor ailments, including uncleanliness.

In this group 7,121 children were treated, chiefly by the official staff. This group included ringworm, impetigo, other skin diseases, external eye diseases, and many others.

In a few centres there are minor treatment clinics for such cases, at which school doctors and school nurses attend at fixed times. One of these seen by me at Bishop Auckland was evidently doing admirable work for ailments which would otherwise have been neglected, and for which medical aid apart from this clinic would not have been obtained.

This clinic was held in premises which also served as a

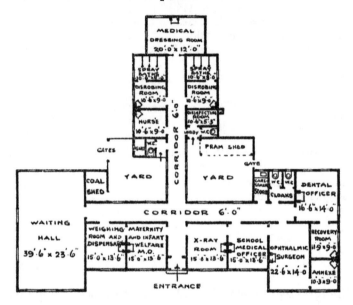

GROUND FLOOR PLAN.

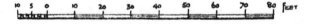

centre for ophthalmic and like work; while in separate sections of the same building were rooms reserved for the welfare doctors' clinics, and for the tuberculosis dispensary.

The diagram above shows one of the Durham school

clinics, which, it will be seen, has separate rooms for maternity and child welfare consultations, but not in this instance also for tuberculosis.

Dental clinics form a partial exception to the statement that no major treatment is directly undertaken by the County Council. In 1928 the number of children dentally inspected was 22,170, of whom 15,673 required treatment, and 9,614 were treated. In addition, 3,099 were re-treated as the result of periodical inspection.

In addition, 6,761 cases of defective vision, including errors of refraction and squint, were treated by the county oculists. This is in addition to treatment carried out for minor external eye conditions.

Diseases of the throat and nose received operative treatment under the County Council's scheme in clinics or in hospitals in 754 instances. I was informed by a private practitioner that the school medical service had been a great boon, in that he could now secure the treatment of his tonsils and adenoid cases, for which previously the parents would not secure expert help. The usual plan adopted is to send these children to certain specified voluntary hospitals, the County Council paying the fee in accordance with the scale arranged by the British Medical Association. In another part of the county there was some evidence of feeling on the part of doctors, that they were thus occasionally deprived of patients.

Tuberculosis Work

The arrangements for control of tuberculosis do not require full description. The following particulars will suffice. Free facilities for examination of sputum are made, the County Council contracting with the Bacteriological Department of the College of Medicine, Newcastle-on-Tyne, for this purpose; and similar arrangements are made for other diseases. The details are summarised below. All these specimens are examined gratuitously for medical practitioners at the expense of the County Council, i.e. of the general public.

BACTERIOLOGICAL WORK IN 1928

No. of specimens examined for—

Tubercle bacilli	2,857
Enteric fever	26
Diphtheria	1,199
Spirochætes	37
V.D. Wassermann	2,383
Gonococci	1,347
Others (Comp. Fixation test, C. Sp. Fluid, etc.) ..	45

In 1928 there were available 493 institutional beds for tuberculous patients, and 251 cases were the subject of radiographic examinations. In the year 1,202 pulmonary and 992 cases of non-pulmonary tuberculosis were notified to the M.O.H. by doctors.

Some further details must be given of dispensary arrangements.

During the year 2,750 new patients were received, of whom 1,346 proved to be non-tuberculous. In addition, 906 contacts were examined. At the beginning of the year there were 6,039 persons on the dispensary registers.

District nurses made 2,276 visits to consumptive patients in the year for sick nursing. These visits are additional to those made by health visitors.

The work of the tuberculosis officers in dispensaries is chiefly consultative. As a rule patients are only received when sent by private practitioners or school doctors. For these special reports are sent to the consulting doctor, if necessary with the result of a radiographical examination; and arrangements are made for institutional treatment as needed. A leading private practitioner told me he regarded the dispensary for his district as a "perfect godsend". He was always certain of a prompt answer to a letter asking for a consultative opinion on any of his patients.

I was unable to ascertain to what extent the domiciliary treatment of tuberculosis, under the chiefly contract conditions of medical treatment in the county, presents unsatisfactory features.

VENEREAL DISEASE WORK

This also is similar to that in other areas in England. Gratuitous treatment for all applicants without distinction is given at four centres situate in general voluntary hospitals in Newcastle, Sunderland, Durham, and Stockton. At these hospitals 1,479 new cases were treated in 1928, of which 336 were syphilis, 653 gonorrhœa, 7 soft chancre, and 483 were found to be non-venereal. The average number of attendances at the clinic per new case was 27·5.

As in tuberculosis there is no evidence of friction with private practitioners. One of the best-known general practitioners in the county interviewed by me was very emphatic on this. In his opinion doctors in private practice did not want this work; and even if they did want it, they were not, as a rule, in his view competent to give treatment of the special character and the protracted duration which was provided at the V.D. clinics. It should be added that the whole-time venereal disease surgeon of the County Council sends particulars to private practitioners concerning each case referred to a V.D. clinic.

Private practitioners, as elsewhere, are entitled to receive free supplies of arseno-benzol preparations for the treatment of their private patients if they desire this and can show that they are competent to give intravenous injections. This privilege is rarely used. In 1929, up to the end of August, no applications for this purpose had been made.

There is said to be relatively little venereal disease in Durham.

The readiness of doctors to send patients to the V.D. clinics and of patients to go to them independently, is in part ascribable to the conditions of privacy in which treatment is carried out, and to the quality of the medical care at the clinics. The fact that the majority of sick persons in the county are treated under a system of contract between doctors and insurance authorities or between doctors and employers of labour in mines is also an important factor in this direction.

The last-named consideration applies also very largely to the official medical provisions in tuberculosis dispensaries and child welfare centres. It is, therefore, necessary, in order to have a complete survey of medical arrangements in Durham, to state in conclusion the main features governing domiciliary medical attendance in the county.

DOMICILIARY MEDICAL ATTENDANCE

The extremely important aid given to such attendance by the district nurses with which nearly every area is provided by voluntary associations has already been stated.

So also for midwifery work, the division of this between doctors and midwives has been indicated; and it is to be noted that not only does the County Council make substantial contribution towards the provision of midwives, but also towards securing maternity nurses for patients medically attended.

The hygienic work of the small army of health visitors employed by the County Council is an important contribution to preventive medicine and to a hygienic home life. The school nurses of the County Council secure by their missionary work among parents a large amount of medical treatment by private doctors or at hospitals, which otherwise would be neglected.

Durham is mainly an industrial county, and at least one-third of its total population aged 16 years and upwards is insured for domiciliary medical attendance under the National Insurance Acts. The conditions of this service, as in the rest of Great Britain, are on the basis of a *per capita* payment for each insured person who enrols his or her name with the doctor chosen by the insured person; and the treatment given is that within the competence of an average general practitioner.

There is much further contract medical work in Durham. Long before the national system of sickness insurance began, the miners of Durham were insured *inter alia* for medical attendance on themselves and their families, usually on a *per capita* basis, a fortnightly deduction being made from each miner's wages for this purpose. The rate of payment to doctors varied in different mines and groups of mines. At intervals there were struggles by doctors to obtain less unsatisfactory terms of payment with varying results; but the system as a whole was in evil odour. The introduction of the National Insurance Act greatly improved the conditions of work of doctors in mining areas. They have more recently been further improved; and it is certain that in many parts of Durham doctors could not earn a livelihood in present conditions unless their patients were beneficiaries under the National Insurance Act.

Even when miners are out of work and the usual deduction from their weekly wages for insurance cannot be made, the *per capita* payment of the doctor is uninterrupted, and the treatment of his insured patients continues. While it is true that doctors in pre-insurance days commonly gave medical treatment gratuitously for their mining patients when they were out of work and were paying no weekly contributions, the present position is greatly improved, both in monetary conditions of medical treatment and in security against its cessation.

The contract medical work for colliers in the past included medical care for the collier's wife and family; and payments for wife and family are still made by miners outside the conditions of the National Insurance Act, the amounts being deducted fortnightly from wages. At present a flat rate of 1s. fortnightly is required from each miner, irrespective of size of family. It was formerly much less than this, and reference to the columns of the *British Medical Journal* of former years will show the activity of the British Medical Association in securing the present more favourable tariff.

In one particular instance, the Horden Colliery, some 15,000 miners and their families are concerned in the medical arrangements made. My information concerning this mine was obtained from Alderman Hedley Mason, J.P., who is also the chairman of the Public Health Committee of the County Council. Some further particulars are here given as to this colliery.

The Horden Colliery

The medical arrangements of this colliery are made by the Horden Colliery Lodge of the Durham Miners' Association, of which Mr. Mason is the secretary. The appended detailed sheets show the weekly deductions made from each miner's wages for various purposes:—

Horden Colliery
Name: Married Man (Hewer)

Offtakes—	"A" Week Amount		"B" Week Amount	
	s.	d.	s.	d.
Fire coal	0	6	—	
Water..	0	8	—	
Explosives	0	9	—	
Electric light..	1	9	—	
Unemployment Insurance	0	7	0	7
Health Insurance	0	9	0	9
Picksharper	—		0	3
Doctor Martin	—		1	0
P.R. Fund	—		1	6
Sick Fund	—		0	2
Band..	—		0	1
Weigh Fund..	1	0	—	
Reading-room	—		0	2
Building Fund	—		0	6
Hospital	—		0	4
D.M.A. Super.	0	2	0	2
Welfare Levy..	0	1	0	1
Total	**6**	**3**	**5**	**7**

A and B are given, as some of the deductions are made fortnightly. An amount of 9d. is deducted each fortnight from a coal hewer's wages for explosives, and of 1s. 9d. for domiciliary supply of electricity. The first-named charge is in connection with piece-rate working. A workman is fined 6d. for every safety-lamp glass broken by him, 2d. if there is more than 22 lbs. of dirt in any tub of coal. Workmen, if Roman Catholics, are allowed to pay 1s. a week out of wages to the R.C. priest.

Two shillings a week is deducted weekly from the earnings of each workman who received poor-law relief during the national coal crisis of 1926 (E.U. Relief).

D.M.A. relief was arranged by this Lodge for young and unmarried workmen who were not eligible for poor-law relief at the same period. Two shillings weekly is deducted under this heading.

D.M.A. super is a deduction of 2d. weekly made to ensure a pension of 4s. a week for miners ceasing work at the age of 60. This is a voluntary local fund, supplementary to national old-age pensions.

There is an additional voluntary contribution of 1d. weekly for local welfare work.

It will be noted that the statutory deductions from wages weekly are 7d. for insurance against unemployment, and 9d. for insurance against sickness.

In connection with this colliery five doctors are employed for the miners and their families. They are paid on the usual basis of 1s. a fortnight for each family. This is additional to the *per capita* payment to doctors under the National Insurance Act. The above amount does not include vaccination, which is done gratuitously by the public vaccinators. For midwifery a charge of 21s. to 30s. a case is made. The colliery has a small hospital of its own, but the colliery doctors send most of their more serious hospital cases to the General Hospital in Sunderland.

Besides the deductions already made, every miner voluntarily pays 4d. fortnightly as a contribution to voluntary hospitals, and is thus, in a sense, entitled to treatment in them.

Contract medical service in Durham, as elsewhere, comes under two chief headings :—

1. The National Insurance Act, under which one-third of the total population insures *inter alia* the ordinary services of a private practitioner.

2. Poor-law medical attendance carried out by salaried

district doctors, who also engage in private general medical practice. This is supplemented by infirmary treatment when required. Persons unable to secure medical treatment otherwise are entitled to parochial help.

In Durham County there is also:—

3. The universal system of contract attendances on the wives and children of miners, already illustrated.

Here and there in the county:—

4. Arrangements like those for colliers' families have been made by means of medical clubs, organised by doctors in association. The rules of the Jarrow and Hebburn "public medical service" may be taken in illustration. Its work is limited to those families whose head is insured under the National Insurance Act.

Subscribers can choose their own doctor, and change their doctor at any time. The conditions of subscription are as follows:—

Per week.

For Subscribers 16 years of age and over (Adults)	
entered alone on card	6d.
One Adult and One Child	7d.
One Adult and Two Children	8d.
One Adult and Three or more Children	9d.
Additional Adults (each)	4d.
On Cards where no Adult is entered:—	
One Child	4d.
Two Children	5d.
Three or more Children	6d.

These terms are identical with those for similar clubs in Newcastle, Gateshead, and elsewhere.

If a person becomes a subscriber while actually ill, he is required to pay a special entrance fee of 10s. Apart from this there is no special condition of admission to the club for dependents of insured persons. The subscription includes the cost of drugs; the limitations of treatment are similar to those under the National Insurance Act.

The existence of these clubs, and the rapid spread of periodical payments to associations which thus partially ensure treatment in voluntary hospitals are significant indications of the trend of events for medical attendance on the mass of the people.

A further point of interest arises. What has been the influence on out-patient treatment at general (voluntary) hospitals of the contract systems of domiciliary medical attendance in the county? We have seen that so far as concerns the special departments of medical service for which the County Council are responsible (especially child welfare tuberculosis and venereal disease), but little difficulty has arisen. There has been but little friction and a vast amount of co-operation, this co-operation doubtless having been aided by the fact that the contract doctor suffers no financial loss when his patient consults a medical officer of the special county official services.

Although I have no exact figures, it would appear that the same holds good for the large hospitals under voluntary management. Their out-patient departments are even more congested than in the past; in part because private practitioners wish to obtain the advantage of consultations with a specialist, and in part because patients themselves may desire advice independently of their private doctors. There is evidence that contract medical practitioners are relieved of part of their contract work not only by attendance of patients in the out-patient departments, but also as a result of in-patient treatment in voluntary general and special hospitals. This relief must in many instances be welcome to the practitioners concerned.

CHAPTER XVIII

THE BOROUGH OF SWINDON[1]

SWINDON is a town with 65,000 inhabitants,[2] situated in the county of Wiltshire, a county chiefly agricultural in character. In this county the population averages 0·3 person per acre, and of its population aged 12 and over, 224 per 1,000 are agricultural workers. The urban population of the county (133,224) is comprised in eight municipal boroughs and five other urban districts. The rural part is divided into 18 rural districts. Each of the above 31 districts has separate government, so far as elementary sanitation is concerned. For poor-law administration there were formerly 17 unions, which did not as a rule coincide with the sanitary areas, but from 1930 onwards the care of the poor has been taken over by the County Council of Wiltshire.

The borough of Swindon has several independent factories and other industries; but in the main its prosperity depends on the local engineering construction works of the Great Western Railway, in which a majority of Swindon's adult male population is employed. From this relation to the Great Western Railway has arisen a very interesting medical scheme of treatment, in which at least two-thirds of the total population of the town are actively interested: and it is this scheme which gives special interest to the medical experience of Swindon. On the side of official public health administration, several interesting developments also deserve mention; and the interrelation between these and the Great Western Railway Medical Fund Society presents features having suggestive bearings on general medical policy.

The population of Swindon lives in small two-storied houses not closely congested in area, and most of them in fairly good repair. Housing conditions may therefore be

[1] Date of investigation, February 1929.
[2] The census (1931) population of Swindon was 62,407, that of the administrative county of Wiltshire (including Swindon) 303,258.

said to be exceptionally satisfactory. Half the population of Swindon own the houses in which they live. The wages earned at the railway works vary from £2 12s. 6d. to £8 10s. a week, the majority of family incomes being nearer the lower limit. There are few families in Swindon in which less than £3 a week is earned; and, speaking generally, there is very little poverty, and unemployment is exceptional. The Great Western works supply steady work year by year for the majority of the population.

The Great Western Railway Medical Fund Society was established in 1847, and has had a continuously prosperous career. Membership of the society is not compulsory on workers at the G.W.R. works, but it is almost universal, both for single men and for married men and their families. The society gives medical attendance to its members and their families, but not any financial sickness benefit. Money benefits since 1912 are supplied by the National Insurance Act, and for medical insurance work the medical staff of the G.W.R. Fund act like "panel" doctors engaged in private medical practice, undertaking medical care of each member, sick or well, at an annual charge of 9s. (a little over $2).

The G.W.R. Fund Society's scheme gives much wider medical benefits than those under the Insurance Act. The latter gives only such medical attendance as is within the competence of the average medical practitioner, to which some societies have added partial dental treatment, convalescent homes, contributions for a few hospital beds, and spectacles.

The contributions payable by each member are deducted by the G.W.R. Company's staff from the weekly wage; and the G.W. Railway helps the society in various other ways—as by taking a part (unfortunately too small) in the management of the society, by helping in capital expenditure, by giving a free supply of fuel, gas, and electric light for the premises of the society, and by undertaking repairs of their premises.

The contributions directly payable to the society are shown in the accompanying table:—

WEEKLY FEES FOR MEMBERSHIP IN THE GREAT WESTERN
RAILWAY MEDICAL FUND SOCIETY

Type of Patient	Single Men Over 16	Married Men
Panel (insurance) patients[1]	3 pence	6½ pence
Non-panel patients	5 pence	8½ pence

It will be noted that the above contributions do not cover the entire cost of insurance under the National Insurance Act. Further weekly sums are paid by insured men by stamps affixed to their insurance books, to enable them to receive the monetary benefits under that Act in case of sickness.

The medical benefits insured by the society are shared by the entire family of the insured, including all children living at home, up to the age of 16. Retired workers and their widows can continue membership on reduced terms.

Members requiring medical help are expected to attend the dispensary of the society if well enough to do so. They must live within four miles of the offices of the society if they require home attendance in sickness. The number of contributing members is about 17,000, and these and their families, making a total of about 45,000 beneficiaries, are attended by the doctors of the society. Less than 1 per cent. of the G.W.R. workers contract out of the medical benefits given by the society.

There is a flat rate of contribution for all members. A few higher officials of the Railway Company utilise the medical service of the staff; but as a rule the members of the society are those who come within the scope of the National Insurance Act.

The medical staff consists of practitioners who devote

[1] For these the society receives an additional payment of 2d. a week from the local insurance committee, in consideration of its undertaking their medical care as insured persons.

their whole time to the work of the society; and their testimony is that arrangements from a medical standpoint are mutually satisfactory for themselves and for their patients. The fact that eleven doctors and a chief dentist with qualified dental assistants are employed gives opportunities for intercommunication and consultation in difficult cases; and for emergency and night-work it is found practicable to have a rota, which greatly relieves the rest of the staff. The rules of the society give one doctor to 1,500 paying members; but in view of the large amount of dispensary work, and the need in modern medicine for more protracted examination and for consultations, this rule may need revision.

The medical staff consists of a medical superintendent and consultant, Dr. Percival Berry, who receives an annual salary of £1,400; a consulting surgeon and assistant superintendent who receives the same salary, and nine assistant medical officers who receive salaries varying from £700–£900. All the staff are expected to devote their whole time to their official work, the only exception being that of the consulting surgeon, who is allowed outside consultative and operative work. It is doubtful if this exception is in the interest of the society. There is also a consulting radiologist, who is paid per case, and a consulting pathologist, who does a vast amount of work for the inclusive annual sum of £400. There are four whole-time dental surgeons receiving salaries of from £450 to £800. The hospital attached to the dispensary has a matron and nurses.

Dispensary attendances are made by the medical staff from 9.30 a.m. to 7.30 p.m. in definite order, which ensures regular attendance of a physician and a surgeon at the same hour. Home visits must be arranged for before 10.30 a.m. except in emergencies.

The time-table is so arranged that any member can consult any of the medical staff at the dispensary except the consulting surgeon without leaving his work, and therefore without losing pay. New ophthalmic clinics provide similar evening facilities. The work of the nine assistant medical officers consists partly in treating patients at home and

partly in consultations at the dispensary. The proportion
between these two may be gathered from the two accompanying tables. The increase in special calls is deprecated,
implying some non-adherence to rules for requesting a visit.
The number of attendances at the dispensary in 1928 was
100,828, as compared with 93,614 in the previous year. The
magnitude of the dispensary work is shown in the second
part of the table below. This means that an average of
323 patients are seen at the dispensary each week-day.

VISITS MADE BY THE NINE ASSISTANT MEDICAL OFFICERS OF
THE GREAT WESTERN RAILWAY MEDICAL FUND SOCIETY
AT SWINDON TO THE HOMES OF PATIENTS, 1927–29.

Type of Visit	1927	1929
First calls at patient's home	16,949	15,881
Special calls at patient's home.. ..	2,701	3,088

VOLUME OF WORK AT THE DISPENSARY OF THE GREAT WESTERN
RAILWAY MEDICAL FUND SOCIETY AT SWINDON, 1928

Sessions	Attendances by Doctors	Patients Seen
Morning consultations	2,252	48,829
Evening consultations	1,124	44,350
Midday consultations	307	6,431
Sunday consultations	106	1,168
TOTAL	3,789	100,778

For home-visiting work within four miles of the dispensary
the sphere of activity is divided into nine areas, each having
its own medical officer. For home treatment, members and
their families living in a given area can only be visited by
the medical officer allotted to this area, who normally lives
in it. This cuts across the free choice of doctor given in
"panel" practice under the National Sickness Insurance Act.

In Swindon the absence of this free choice leads to remarkably little trouble. There is little or no evidence of dissatisfaction. It does not involve complete allocation to a single doctor, for—

1. When a "special call" has to be made, it is sometimes arranged for another doctor to visit, if any dissatisfaction has been expressed.
2. Whenever a patient desires to see another doctor, the Chief Medical Officer offers to see the patient with the doctor in attendance. If this does not satisfy the patient, the Chief Medical Officer interviews both the doctor in attendance and the doctor whose attendance is desired (both are on the staff of the society), and with the approval of these two arranges for the desired change.
3. The patient, whenever able to attend the dispensary, can be treated by any one of the nine doctors in attendance. I understand that this opportunity to change doctors is seldom utilised.

Except when the rare adjustment mentioned above is made, the districting system is rigidly enforced. If a patient moves from district A to district B, he automatically changes his medical attendant. A doctor is always on duty at the dispensary for special calls.

Evening and Sunday work are also undertaken at the dispensary. The dispensing is carried out by a staff of eight dispensers. No restrictions on drugs are made. The drug bill appears to be excessive. In 1928 it was £4,874. Of cod-liver oil and malt, 79¼ cwt. were consumed, and of liquid paraffin, 562 gallons.

MIDWIFERY

During 1928 the medical staff attended 103 confinements at the members' houses, and 40 at the Maternity Home. It is a rule that the medical staff shall not book a confinement unless a duly-qualified midwife has been engaged; and a charge of 10s. is made for each case, which goes into the funds of the G.W.R. Fund Society. It will be seen (p. 346) that very material help is given by the municipality to the wives of members of the G.W.R. Fund Society as to others, in the care of pregnancy and parturition. The same may be said in regard to the treatment of children of members of the society.

THE DENTAL DEPARTMENT OF THE DISPENSARY

The four dentists on the staff are kept busy daily from 9 a.m. to 7.30 p.m., Saturdays 9 a.m. to 12.30 p.m. Appointments can be made to avoid waiting. During 1928 there was an increase of over 10 per cent. in conservative work—fillings, scaling, etc. The local public health and education authorities of the Borough and the County Council (for within and without the borough) also provide much dental treatment for school and younger children and for mothers; and some insurance societies under the National Act give dental benefits. Notwithstanding these auxiliary agencies, the figures below show that, apart from the society, much-needed treatment would fail to be secured. Dentures are provided at a low charge, and there is a small charge for teeth extractions. There is active co-operation between the dental and medical services of the society. In 1928, patients made 19,430 dental visits to the dispensary; 1,530 dentures were provided, and 2,405 permanent fillings were made.

SPECIAL PATHOLOGICAL WORK

The pathologist, Dr. Knyvett Gordon, whose laboratory is in London (93 miles distant), reports that—

During the year 1928, 803 specimens from members of the Medical Fund were examined:—

Surgical	103
Blood films	142
Vaccines	125
Miscellaneous	433
Total	803

Grand total since August 1922 .. 4,523

The increase under the heading "Miscellaneous" is accounted for chiefly by chemical examinations of the blood in cases of diabetes under treatment in the clinic and hospital of the society.

There is no limit to the pathological aid available, and, where necessary, Dr. Gordon visits Swindon to consult on cases. In other instances patients are sent up to his laboratory, the G.W.R. giving free passes for the journey. The Railway gives the same facilities when expert services or further treatment are required at certain hospitals in London and elsewhere, to which the society subscribes.

During 1928, 1,984 free railway passes were issued to members on a medical certificate that the journey was required for consultation or for treatment. The availability of consultant facilities, and especially of unlimited pathological help, contrasts very favourably with the usual lack of such assistance in the medical work of the National Insurance Act.

HOSPITAL TREATMENT

The Medical Fund Society has its own hospital with 36 beds. The maintenance of this hospital costs the society about £14,000 a year, exclusive of the contribution made by the G.W.R. Company in the form of cleaning, lighting, heating, and repairs. The hospital is a temporary building, and very shortly the question will have to be faced of rebuilding or, as an alternative, of amalgamation with and extension of the Victoria Hospital, a separate institution in Swindon, which is supported by voluntary contributors. Only surgical cases are treated in the society's hospital. No medical beds are available except at the Victoria Hospital, over admission to which the medical staff of the society have no lien. This is a defect in the provision made by the Fund.

During the year 570 patients were admitted to the G.W.R. Fund Hospital: 1,794 X-ray examinations were made. Both the out-patient department and the wards are crowded. There is a long list of waiting patients, and the possibilities of special consultation with medical and other colleagues which exist in a satisfactorily organised general hospital are incomplete. If this hospital were to be scrapped, and its annual cost of some £14,000 devoted to securing adequate indoor medical and surgical treatment for the members of the society and their families in the Victoria Hospital, with its greater possibilities of satisfactory team work, the society would have made a long stride towards securing ideal medical conditions for its members.

The preceding statement does not exhaust the benefits secured under the society's organisation. It is responsible for large washing baths and a laundry, for swimming baths and Turkish baths, to which members and their families are admitted on reduced terms. The public have access to these. They form part of this history of the society; but it would be well if these non-medical activities were shed, and they were handed over to the Swindon Corporation or to some trading body.

The benefits include also the use of invalid chairs, the provision of spectacles, surgical appliances, trusses, etc., and hearses for funerals. Usually the first appliance of each description is supplied free. The only charge for use of a hearse is for horse hire.

Patients are sent to convalescent homes, only half the cost of maintenance being charged. The same applies to tuberculosis sanatoria.

For the treatment of children of members attending the elementary schools who are suffering from, and need operations for, enlarged tonsils and adenoids, an arrangement has been made with the County and Borough Education Authorities. The full amount payable for each child, according to the regulations of the Board of Education, is paid to the society, less 25 per cent. of the amount which is expected from the parents.

GENERAL OBSERVATIONS

The scheme outlined above is one of great interest in medical practice. It has continued for many years, and it shows that, under a system of voluntary insurance, it is possible to secure satisfactory and fairly complete medical treatment under a single organisation for a large population. Swindon obviously is exceptionally favourably placed for this purpose, as a great railway company is the chief employer of the community, and this company lends its prestige and gives much help to the organisation.

Perhaps the chief interest of the scheme, in addition to its embracing nearly all branches of medicine and supplying consultative services, is the fact that without unlimited family choice of doctor the people are satisfied. There is no evidence of failure in the personal relations between doctor and patient. The scheme is also satisfactory to the large medical staff concerned, and, so far as I could ascertain, the relationship of this staff to outside medical practitioners is not unsatisfactory.

The deficiencies of indoor hospital treatment already mentioned can be met in the manner already indicated, economically and with increased efficiency. A further criticism must be made. The control of the society rests with a committee elected by the members. The G.W. Railway is represented by vice-presidents of good standing, and a chief official of the company is president; but the management of the society is left entirely in the hands of a committee of members of the society, which does not include the chief medical officer of the Fund.

Given the above reforms, the society, in my judgment, has before it a future career of enhanced importance and usefulness, and one of great value as showing how, under a voluntary insurance organisation, it is practicable to ensure adequate medical treatment for every member of a working man's family.

THE OFFICIAL MEDICAL SERVICES OF SWINDON AND THE COUNTY

Swindon is a municipal borough, having a mayor and corporation elected by the direct vote of the ratepayers. It is not a county borough, and therefore has not completely separate public health administration in regard to the diagnosis and treatment of tuberculosis, and the diagnosis and treatment of venereal diseases. These are organized by the Wiltshire County Council for the whole of the administrative county, including the borough of Swindon. Swindon has a separate education authority, which is solely responsible for the medical care of its school children. It is also responsible for maternity and child welfare work, excepting the supervision of midwives. It will be convenient to describe this local work somewhat fully. The relationship of the borough M.O.H. (Dr. Dunstan Brewer) with the county M.O.H. (Dr. Tangye) is like that of the corresponding officers in Cambridgeshire. Medical aid is sought by midwives in about 26 per cent. of the total confinements attended by them. Of the doctors' fees (£669) for which the County Council was responsible in 1927 about 34 per cent. was recovered from the patients. In two sanitary areas in the county the County Council gives subsidies to supplement the earnings of two local midwives to ensure their continuance in practice.

MATERNITY AND CHILD WELFARE WORK

The Town Council accords to all children under school age the same medical services as are given to school children. This has enabled the public medical services for all children to be unified under the control of the M.O.H., who is also chief school M.O. He has working with him on the medical side two whole-time assistant medical officers, and, in addition, two whole-time dental surgeons, a part-time ophthalmic surgeon and a part-time aural surgeon. There are three health visitors and four school nurses, all of them fully-qualified nurses, who also hold the certificate of the Central Midwives Board.

The maternal side of the work is rapidly developing. Antenatal clinics are held, which Dr. Brewer prefers to name "women's consultation centres" to avoid the suggestion that they are primarily concerned with morbid conditions.

The *Maternity Hospital*, which is a municipal undertaking, during 1927 received 233 patients, for 52 of whom the County Council was responsible: 62 per cent. were attended by midwives. In 29 no delivery took place. In 59 cases medical aid was asked for by the midwives. Only one case of puerperal fever occurred, and six cases of puerperal pyrexia (i.e. a rise of temperature to 100·4° F. or its recurrence). No maternal deaths occurred. Patients choose their own midwifery attendant.

A new maternity hospital is being erected by the Borough Council, which will have 25 beds for mothers and 6 beds for infants suffering from diseases of infancy. The patients admitted to the Maternity Hospital pay in accordance with the scale set out below:—

SWINDON MATERNITY HOSPITAL

SCALE OF FEES

1. *Where the Maternity Benefit is Payable under the National Insurance Act.*[1]

(*a*) Where the income is less than 12s. 6d. per head per week. — The full maternity benefit up to a maximum of £2.

(*b*) Where the income exceeds 12s. 6d. per head per week, but is less than 15s. per head. — The full maternity benefit up to a maximum of £2 plus 5s. per week.

(*c*) Where the income exceeds 15s. per head per week, but is less than 17s. 6d. per head per week. — The full maternity benefit up to a maximum of £2 plus 10s. per week.

(*d*) Where the income exceeds 17s. 6d. per head per week. — The full maternity benefit up to a maximum of £2 plus £1 per week.

2. *Where the Maternity Benefit is not Payable.*

A minimum fee of £1 per week, or part of a week, in all cases.

The above fee may, however, in exceptional cases, be remitted or reduced at the discretion of the chairman and vice-chairman of the Health Committee, the chairman of the Maternity Sub-Committee, and the medical superintendent.

An antenatal clinic is conducted by the assistant M.O.H. (Dr. Violet King).

---

[1] This benefit is 40s. for the wife of an insured man, or double this amount when the wife is also an insured person under the Act. The second possible benefit is not considered in the charges of the Maternity Hospital, as shown above.

CHILD WELFARE WORK

There are three centres in the borough at one of which any treatment which is needed is undertaken. Two of the centres are "run" by health visitors, the treatment centre by the M.O.H., or the lady assistant M.O.H. It is estimated that more than 90 per cent. of the young children in the borough attend these centres; 8,335 home visits were made during 1927, including 815 first visits and 3,674 revisits to mothers and children, 168 visits to expectant mothers, and 3,421 visits to children aged 1–5 years.

During the year milk was distributed to children at a total cost to the Borough Council of £140.

Special importance attaches to the chief child clinic, which is kept open all day, a doctor being always in attendance. The mothers in the borough have acquired the habit of bringing their children here at all hours of the day for counsel as to whether medical advice or more than immediate medical advice is indicated. No responsibility is taken for any case for which domiciliary or hospital treatment is indicated. For these the centre acts as a prompt clearing-house, ensuring immediate medical first-aid and guidance for further action. The treatment centre is also a school clinic, and it is understood that any child up to 16 years old may be brought to it and receive attention. This work goes on without friction with medical practitioners in the borough. They gain by the prompt reference to them of patients needing daily attention. In practice the cases chiefly treated at the centre are those which otherwise would remain untreated. It must be remembered that for three-fourths of the population of Swindon, there are no family doctors, the doctors of the G.W.R. Fund Society providing all the domiciliary treatment that is given.

The infant mortality rate in Swindon is very low. In 1928 it was only 38, and in 1927 was 47 per 1,000 births. For the county as a whole it was 50 and 51 in 1926 and 1927 respectively.

Dr. Brewer rightly attaches importance to the all-day

clinic in securing this low death-rate. The fact that there is almost no serious poverty in Swindon must also be borne in mind.

The arrangements for the treatment of venereal diseases do not call for comment; nor those for tuberculosis, except the comment that closer co-operation is desirable between borough and county medical staffs, and an extension of hospital provision for bed-ridden cases of consumption.

THE HOSPITAL TREATMENT OF PNEUMONIA

Primary pneumonia and influenzal pneumonia are compulsorily notifiable in England; and Dr. Brewer holds that "the notification of pneumonia is the first essential of temperate epidemiology". He adds:—

The law only requires influenzal and primary pneumonia to be notified, but fortunately it is not possible to decide without somewhat elaborate tests whether pneumonia is primary or secondary (if, indeed, either term means anything); so that the pneumonia complications or forerunners of epidemic diseases are in fact notified.

The local isolation hospital has admitted cases of pneumonia for several years. During 1927, 202 cases of pneumonia were notified. Of these, 63 were removed to the hospital, and 14 died, while 139 were treated at home, and 44 died. Taking the total cases for seven years, hospital-treated cases had a case mortality of 18·0 per cent., and home-treated cases of 34·7 per cent. Even if we allow the possibility of selection of cases (some severe cases being thought too ill to be moved), and of unequal age distribution of cases, it appears probable that hospital treatment, in well-spaced wards with ample ventilation, greatly favours recovery.

THE MEDICAL CARE OF SCHOOL CHILDREN

As child welfare increases in efficiency, its influence on school hygiene becomes more evident; and as public medical organisation advances, the unwisdom of separating the school child from the rest of the population becomes

more evident. Dr. Brewer states this point in his Annual
Report:—

The "entrant" to a school can now be expected to be free from
any condition which is either preventable or curable. . . . The
work of the School Medical Officer is not to start, but to
continue.

Evidence of this auspicious trend is beginning to appear in
the medical examination of school children; and especially it
is becoming more common for diseased tonsils and adenoids
to have been treated before school-life begins. Early treatment of dental disease is still only realised for a minority of
toddlers.

The chief conditions treated at school clinics were contagious and non-contagious skin diseases, ear, throat, and
nose diseases, wounds and injuries, external eye diseases,
infectious diseases, and some others; 520 errors of refraction
were dealt with. Treatment of chronic ear discharges by
ionisation was largely practised. The two dentists of the
education authority inspected 5,815 children, of whom 4,125
were found to require treatment, and 3,624 were treated,
1,388 further children being re-treated as the result of
periodical examination.

Payment is supposed to be required for medical and dental
treatment, but not in such a way as to inhibit or restrict
treatment; and in fact it is found that collection of the
nominal fees charged costs more than the money value.
For the treatment of orthopædic patients, costing some 50s.,
parents are asked to give from 1s. to 3s. a week.

OBSERVATIONS

From the above sketch it will be seen that the municipal
and county official arrangements for treatment supplement
the work which is done by the G.W.R. Medical Fund for its
members and their wives and children. There is a considerable range of treatment in which there is theoretical need of
both medical and financial adjustments between official and
non-official agencies. This applies to the treatment of tuber-

culosis and venereal disease, to maternity cases, to antenatal and postnatal care, and to the care of all children.

Advantage would accrue from periodical discussions between the medical heads of each of these spheres of medical activity, to ensure that the relative departments are being worked with the maximum efficiency in relation to each other.

The municipal work in the hospital treatment of pneumonia compensates largely for the great deficiency of voluntary hospital beds for serious medical patients in Swindon.

The municipal all-day treatment and consultation centre for children of all ages is an excellent institution; and it is satisfactory to find that it can be carried on with little or no opposition on the part of private medical practitioners. It will have increased value when it has become possible to secure as general a system of medical and dental inspection for toddlers as is now in practice for children of school age.

For my comments on the work of the G.W.R. Fund Society, see page 344.

CHAPTER XIX

COUNTY BOROUGH OF BRIGHTON[1]

BRIGHTON is a good illustration of a county borough in which the governing body (town or county borough council) has always taken an enlightened view of its responsibilities, and has promoted reform and permitted its chief health officer to experiment repeatedly in the direction of improved and extended medical control of disease. In 1908, at the end of my 19 years' experience as its M.O.H., much progress had already been made; and under the guidance of its skilful and far-sighted M.O.H., Dr. Duncan Forbes, Brighton has taken a leading share in the national extension and elaboration of medical provision for the needs of the public.

In 1908 Brighton's population was 129,065; now it is close on 150,000.[2]

Brighton, throughout its history, has been autonomous in most respects; and in its official, general and medical arrangements as a county borough it is completely independent of the administrative counties of West and East Sussex, which are contiguous with it. This, until April 1928, was only partially true as regards poor-law medical administration; for a considerable part of the borough was within the poor-law Union of East Steyning, which comprises also the abutting borough of Hove and some rural districts. Now the poor-law administration of the county borough of Brighton has become coterminous with its area for public health administration.

Brighton's sea-side position enables one to see why the voluntary medical charities of Brighton serve for a wide area of Sussex, and not merely for the two boroughs of Brighton and Hove.

The provision for the sick poor for Brighton in its poor-

[1] Date of inquiry, May 1929.
[2] The census (1931) population was 147,427.

law infirmary, and by home treatment, does not differ markedly from that in other parts of England, though the institutional treatment of the destitute in the infirmary now ranks high in efficiency.

The voluntary hospitals of Brighton serve also the surrounding districts, for which Brighton is the natural focus.

The following table shows the institutions in which 753 or 39 per cent. of all deaths occurred in 1928. Official institutions are printed in italics.

INSTITUTIONAL DEATHS, BRIGHTON, 1928

	Residents	Non-residents
A. *Deaths in Brighton Hospitals :*		
Royal Sussex County Hospital ..	140	116
Royal Alexandra Hospital	37	42
Throat and Ear Hospital	1	1
Sussex Maternity & Women's Hospital	10	10
New Sussex Hospital for Women ..	7	9
Sanatorium ⎰ Pulmonary Tubercle ..	12	—
Other tubercle	1	1
Other diseases	13	4
Brighton Poor Law Institution	426	17
French Convalescent Home	—	2
Red Cross Hospital	2	6
B. *Deaths of residents in outside Institutions:*		
Brighton County Borough Mental Hospital .	52	—
Other Mental Hospitals	5	—
Shoreham Poor Law Infirmary[1]	22	—
Other Hospitals and Homes	25	—

The deaths in the various hospitals enumerated above are only those of inhabitants or of visitors to Brighton (i.e. temporary residents who have a definite home elsewhere).

A further indication of the hospital provisions for

[1] Serving part of Brighton officially prior to April 1928.

Brighton and for patients beyond it (omitting beds for mental patients) is given in the following table :—

	Number of Beds	Number of In-patients in 1928	Number of Out-patients in 1928
Voluntary:			
Royal Sussex County Hospital	225	3,070	16,582
Royal Alexandra Children's Hospital	98	1,430	1,504
New Sussex Hospital for Women	50	604	2,062
Sussex Eye Hospital	30	356	4,988
Throat and Ear Hospital ..	22	1,354	1,599
Sussex Maternity Hospital[1] ..	35	465	994
Official:			
Brighton Fever Hospital and Tuberculosis Sanatorium	{ 100 73 }	804[2]	—
Brighton Smallpox Hospital ..	14	12	—

The second table does not show the number of beds in the Brighton Poor-law Infirmary. These now total 625.

There is, in addition, in Hove a valuable hospital (Lady Chichester Hospital for Women and Children) at which cases of early nervous breakdown are treated.

A large proportion of the sick poor who are not in receipt of poor-law relief are treated at the Brighton Dispensary, a voluntary institution, at which patients are received on the recommendation of subscribers, a fee of 1s. being required on registration.

Patients are seen at the dispensary or at home according to need by the medical officers of the dispensary.

PROVIDENT HOSPITAL TREATMENT

In recent years, on the initiative of the late Dr. Gordon Dill, a successful provident scheme for Sussex has been

---

[1] Including 18 Maternity beds reserved for Brighton midwifery patients.
[2] Not including patients from school clinics admitted temporarily and kept in for a day or more after operation for tonsils and adenoids.

organised for ensuring to subscribers hospital and specialist help. This is an—

association of subscribers who, by means of fixed annual payments, endeavour collectively to meet the cost of such hospital services as those of them, who are sick, may require during the year. After making the necessary reservations for administration expenses, the scheme distributes yearly the whole of the amount collected by way of subscriptions among the hospitals, proportionately to the actual work done by each.

In the words of the report on the scheme:—

The key-note of the scheme is co-operation: hospitals co-operate by agreeing to accept, in place of payment by patients, their share in the distribution of the funds which the scheme finds itself able to make to them: the contributors co-operate to help the hospitals within the limit of their means, and to lighten the burden of those among their number who need hospital treatment.

Thirteen hospitals co-operate in this scheme, of which nine are situate in Brighton and Hove. All persons—

who are residents of Sussex are eligible for membership, provided:—

1. That their incomes are within the following limits:—

£250 per annum in case of single persons.
£300 per annum in case of married persons without children under 16.
£350 per annum in case of married persons with children under 16.

2. That they, or their dependents, are not attending hospital, or to the best of their knowledge and belief are not in need of any of the hospital services specified at the time of making their applications.

The subscriptions payable to ensure the benefits are:—

12s. per annum if paid in one sum in advance.
13s. per annum if paid by weekly instalments of 3d., or by monthly instalments of 1s. 1d.

Those who elect to pay by instalments are required to complete their full subscription before being eligible for benefit during the first year of membership only. After that period they will always be eligible for benefit as long as their instalments are paid up to date.

The subscriber ensures the benefits to:—

The subscriber himself, his wife and children, under the age of 16, living with him and supported by him; and, in the case of an unmarried subscriber, the brothers and sisters under the age of 16, as well as the parents with whom he or she lives, if they are solely and entirely supported by the subscriber.

The subscription exempts the contributor and his family:—

(a) from the necessity of producing a hospital letter from a subscriber;

(b) from any inquiry as to means;

(c) and from payment for hospital treatment, as set out below:—

Urgent cases receive immediate treatment. Admission to hospital of other patients is subject to the usual hospital regulations.

Necessary dental treatment is given, but not dentures.

Eye treatment, including refraction work, is undertaken; and patients obtain 15 per cent. reduction of prices of lenses from recognised opticians.

When recommended by the consultant doctor, electrical treatment, X-ray examinations, and massage are provided. Pathological facilities are also free.

Each patient is required to bring a letter of recommendation from his own doctor when he pays his first visit to the hospital, except in cases of accident or emergency.

The treatment of children suffering from the following diseases who attend elementary schools is not included in the benefit, as the education authorities in each district undertake this.

1. Diseases of the nose, throat, and ear (including the removal of enlarged tonsils and adenoids).
2. Defective eyesight.
3. Teeth (conservative treatment of).
4. Certain skin diseases.

If any charge is made by education authorities for treatment of these conditions, this is remitted for children whose parents contribute under this scheme.

The above outlined statement gives the general gist of the

Sussex Provident Scheme. It already has 47,454 beneficiaries, of whom 27,840 are dependents of subscribers; and in 1928 it contributed the sum of £38,500 to the co-operating hospitals, of which £19,090 went to the Royal Sussex County Hospital, £4,603 to the Children's Hospital, and smaller sums to various special and local hospitals. A sum of £375 was given to the Board of Guardians for treatment of subscribing members in the Brighton Infirmary, and of £107 to Educational Authorities in remission of charges for treatment of school children. In addition, £1,322 was refunded to subscribers who were charged for treatment in non-co-operating hospitals.

The amounts paid to voluntary hospitals represent only a portion of the total cost of treatment in these hospitals of subscribing members of the scheme: but they form a welcome aid to the hospital funds, which otherwise would bear a large proportion of the burden of treatment of these subscribers without any charge or with a small charge difficult to collect.

Sickness Insurance arrangements resemble those elsewhere.

OFFICIAL TREATMENT OF DISEASE

Particulars are given on page 374 of the official arrangements for treatment of school children in Brighton. Other official medical arrangements for medical diagnosis and treatment may now be briefly summarised.

1. As in nearly every part of England, diphtheria antitoxin is supplied gratuitously to any private medical practitioner asking for it. In addition, children are immunised against diphtheria free of charge at the infant welfare centres and in residential institutions. At the Guardians' residential school 150 out of the 228 children have been thus protected, and all the children in two other residential institutions.

2. Similarly gratuitous examinations of pathological products from cases of infectious or suspected infectious disease are made, and the number thus examined in 1928 is shown below:—

	Throat Swab, K.L.B	Sputum	Blood (Widal)	Tinea
For private practitioners ..	1,272	476	4	—
In work of M.O.H.	1,928	—	—	—
In work of School M.O.H. ...	71	—	—	24
In work of Tuberculosis Officer	—	195	—	—
In work of Fever Hospital and Sanatorium	3,772	311	16	—
In work of Voluntary Hospital	466	—	—	—

In addition, the following specimens were examined at the expense of the Local Authority, aided by the Central Government's Grant for venereal diseases :—

(a) At the Treatment Centre for V.D.: 36 specimens for spirochætes; and

(b) Sent to the special Laboratory at the County Hospital: 1,905 specimens for gonococci, 12 for spirochætes, and 1,735 Wassermann reactions.

It is not altogether satisfactory to find that during the year only 78 V.D. specimens (coming from only 13 private practitioners) were sent for examination, the rest being from hospitals, including the special V.D. Centre. It must be remembered, however, that the institution of V.D. clinics has meant that the treatment of active cases of V.D. is now probably undertaken at these clinics to a preponderant extent. But there remain many cases of doubtful disease (miscarriages, still-births, etc.), in which the laboratory would give valuable aid in scientific treatment.

3. The services of the M.O.H. are placed at the disposal of every medical practitioner to assist in the diagnosis of suspected infectious disease or in the investigation of suspected food poisoning. His services are also available for special tests, and for the taking of specimens of blood and cerebro-spinal fluid in the homes of the patient.

4. A large proportion of the total infectious diseases occurring in the borough are treated in the Borough Fever

Hospital. The proportion thus treated in 1928 can be seen from the following statement:—

Number of Cases	Notified to M.O.H.	Treated in the Fever Hospital
Smallpox	2	2
Diphtheria	265	243
Scarlet fever	188	132
Enteric fever	13	11
Puerperal fever and puerperal pyrexia	72	11
Ophthalmia neonatorum	22	2
Pneumonia	86	—
All other notifiable diseases, excepting Tuberculosis	13	3

No charge is made for any infectious case treated in the municipal hospital.

5. Although tuberculosis is considered separately in later paragraphs, it is convenient to give here the number of tuberculous patients treated institutionally at the public expense during 1928. These patients for the last 30 years have been treated successfully and without cross-infection in detached wards of the Borough Fever or Isolation Hospital. The number of cases of pulmonary tuberculosis admitted to this sanatorium in 1928 was 84, of other forms of tuberculosis 17; the average stay in weeks of the former being 17·7, of the latter 25·0 weeks. These numbers should be compared with the following numbers: In the town 226 cases of pulmonary and 57 cases of non-pulmonary tuberculosis were notified during the year; and the number of deaths under these two headings were 112 and 24 respectively.

This treatment of cases of pulmonary tuberculosis in the Isolation Hospital of the Public Health Authority is in addition to the extensive treatment and care of destitute and advanced cases of tuberculosis in Brighton's Poor-law (now Municipal) Infirmary. The proportion of total consumptives thus segregated in its infirmary amounted to

20 per cent. as early as 1904, as measured by the proportion of deaths of consumptives occurring in this institution. This represents much more than 20 per cent. of the total infection from such patients, as during the later stages of the disease patients remaining in the domestic circle not only discharge more massive doses of infective material, but are also less competent to dispose of it without serious risk to relatives and nurses. I may add that in 1904 the average stay in the infirmary of each consumptive patient was 221 days, a very large proportion of his total infectious life.

6. We may now briefly outline the extent and character of the three special medical services which hitherto—in addition to the treatment and prevention of acute infectious diseases and the treatment of lunatics—have formed the chief medical activities of public health authorities in Brighton and elsewhere. Shortly, in addition, the duty of medical treatment of all the destitute will be transferred to them from the abolished Boards of Guardians.

These services are—

Maternity and Child Welfare Work,
Tuberculosis Work, and
Venereal Disease Work.

PUERPERAL MORTALITY

The experience of Brighton in recent years is seen below, as compared with that of the county as a whole:—

PUERPERAL MORTALITY PER 1,000 BIRTHS

	Sepsis		Other Causes		Total	
	England and Wales	Brighton	England and Wales	Brighton	England and Wales	Brighton
1911–15 ..	1·42	0·76	2·61	1·32	4·03	2·08
1916–20 ..	1·49	0·94	2·61	1·84	4·10	2·78
1921–25 ..	1·40	1·09	2·50	1·57	3·90	2·66
1926 ..	1·60	2·55	2·52	3·06	4·12	5·61
1927 ..	1·57	1·06	2·54	2·66	4·11	3·72
1928 ..	1·79	0·99	2·63	1·48	4·42	2·47

The comparison here made is with the average experience of the entire country, which expresses the smoothed-out experience of many areas of divergent experience; while in that of Brighton is represented the experience of a limited child-bearing population, in which a few deaths gravely alter the puerperal death-rate. Approximately the national mortality from supposedly non-septic complications of child-bearing is almost stationary; and it is the same for sepsis, except in the three last years recorded in the table. In Brighton, on the other hand, sepsis and other causes of puerperal mortality were more prevalent for several years; this has been followed by recent improvement.

As a large part of the midwifery work in Brighton is done in, or from, a charitable institution, the Sussex Maternity Hospital and its Wellington Road Branch, one naturally first examines the records of that institution. It was during the war that the first rise in the figures occurred, at a time when the doctors were overworked and more work and responsibility were left to the midwife staff at the hospital than in ordinary circumstances. Unfortunately, after the war, on the midwifery side, the medical staff did not resume a sufficient control of the work, and the mortality figures increased until a climax was reached in the late spring and early summer of 1926, when nine hospital patients died from puerperal sepsis. This led to an inquiry into the working of the hospital by the medical officer of health. On his recommendation administrative changes were made which have led to a decided improvement.

The lying-in hospital has 24 maternity beds, to which complicated cases and women badly housed are admitted from Brighton and mid-Sussex. Sixty-nine were admitted at the expense of the Town Council during 1928. These were kept in the hospital on an average for 16 days. The Council pays 7s. 6d. a day for each of these patients, nearly half of this being refunded by the patients, either directly or indirectly under the Sussex Provident Scheme (p. 354). The total net cost to the Town Council last year was £211.

Twelve midwives are on the staff of the Maternity

Hospital, and during 1928, 31 pupils were trained for the certificate of the Central Midwives Board.

In 1928 the births in Brighton numbered 2,023, of which 144 were illegitimate. These represent a birth-rate of 13·6 per 1,000 of population. In accordance with annual legal requirements, 56 midwives notified their intention to practise in the town. Of this number only 22 were nominally in private practice, and 12 either did not practise or only for a short time. With two exceptions all the midwives are "qualified" after examination by the Central Midwives Board.

In 1928, of the total 2,161 births in the borough, 866 were attended either as hospital or home patients by midwives of the Sussex Maternity Hospital, which is a training centre for midwives administered by a voluntary charity. A charge of 15s. or 21s. is made for each case attended at home. In these cases medical aid was called for in 265 cases (30 per cent. of the total cases).

Midwives in private practice are entitled to call in a doctor to assist them in emergencies, and the local authority is required to pay the doctor's fee, in accordance with an authorised scale. The doctor is chosen nominally by the patient. In 1928 the Town Council paid £164 for these services rendered by doctors on 111 occasions, of which some £91 was recovered from patients.

TWO ANTENATAL CENTRES

(1) The Municipal Antenatal Centre was established for the convenience of the private midwife. Naturally some of these are unwilling to send their patients for antenatal examination to the Sussex Maternity Hospital, from which, at low fees, many women are attended in confinement in their own homes. At the municipal centre 196 patients sent by private midwives were seen by the whole-time municipal woman doctor, their attendances numbering 543.

(2) The larger antenatal centre is that held at the Sussex Maternity Hospital, at which all patients booking for

attendance from the hospital must attend. At this clinic 1,972 examinations were made in connection with 1,011 confinements.

CARE OF INFANTS AND TODDLERS

The infant mortality in 1928 was only 51 per 1,000 births, that for England being 65.

Of the 2,023 infants born in 1928, 1,474 were visited by the health visitors, an average of five visits being made to each infant. In addition 5,796 children aged 1–5 were visited during the year.

Five health visitors are employed by the Council, one of these giving part-time to tuberculosis work. These made 17,855 visits to infants and mothers during 1928, including 379 to expectant mothers.

There are five infant welfare centres at various points in the town, each open on one day weekly. At these the average attendance per session in 1928 was 57 for mothers and 67 for children under 5. The number of mothers who attended during the year was 1,997, of infants (0–12 months) 1,410, and of children (1–5 years) 1,136. It will be noted that the number of infants who thus received medical counsel was equal to 70 per cent. of the total infants born in the year. Most of the infants and toddlers attending these centres are seen first by the health visitor (a certified nurse), who keeps the lady doctor fully occupied during a long afternoon in examining and advising concerning children who are indisposed or who are not gaining weight normally. A certain amount of treatment is done for minor ailments, for which a private doctor would otherwise not be consulted. As seen by me, great care was taken in detecting cases which called for domiciliary medical attendance, as, for instance, a case of bronchial catarrh—verified after careful auscultation of chest and back. The mother of this patient was advised as to her responsibility for obtaining a doctor.

In the work of the child welfare centres there appears to be no friction with medical practitioners; though as seen in our general English review, the relative position of the centres and of practitioners is one of watchfulness rather than of complete sympathy.

From these centres both mothers and children with dental disease are referred to the official dental clinic; and during 1928, 710 attendances at this clinic were made by 116 mothers and 50 children under 5 years of age.

The infant welfare medical officer gives an annual lecture to the students training at the Municipal College for elementary teachers; and during the year each of the senior students at this college attended a welfare centre twice, to familiarise herself with the actual work done. There are two voluntary crèches in the town partially subsidised by the Council.

Other activities include the provision of milk for expectant and nursing mothers and delicate children (cost £122 in the year), dried milk (£11), dentures (over £6), confinement fees (£5), and home-helps (£59). In addition, malt and cod-liver oil were given costing £115. The various forms of help enumerated above include also help given at school clinics and to tuberculous patients. Half of the cost of the milk and oil was paid by parents.

"Home-helps" are working women chosen by the mothers to help them in domestic work during the lying-in period. This form of help has proved of great value for mothers who cannot command domestic aid.

TUBERCULOSIS WORK

The death-rate from tuberculosis in Brighton in 1928 was 0·81 per 1,000, of which 0·75 was pulmonary. The new cases notified during the year were—pulmonary 1·67, non-pulmonary 0·54 per 1,000 of population.

As bearing on the general problem of institutional treatment (p. 222), it should be noted that in 1928, 70 of the total 112 deaths from pulmonary tuberculosis occurred in public institutions, over 62 per cent. of the total. Of these, 34 occurred in the Poor-law Infirmary. As Dr. Forbes remarks in his Annual Report:—

By segregation of the advanced cases, which are the most highly infective, much is done to prevent the spread of the disease.

At the official tuberculosis dispensary during 1928—

> 429 new cases were examined,
> 925 old cases were re-examined,
> 123 X-ray examinations were made, and
> 79 laryngeal examinations.

In addition, 368 patients were examined by the tuberculosis officer at the sanatorium, their homes, or elsewhere.

Of the new cases during the year, 283 were sent by private doctors,

> 17 were seen in consultation with doctors,
> 20 examined at the request of the patient or relatives,
> 87 were contacts or others,

examined by arrangement of the inspector (for males) or the health visitor (for female patients), as the result of their visits to the homes of notified cases. The degree of co-operation of private doctors shown by these figures is exceptionally good.

Brighton possesses valuable arrangements for home visiting and for monetary or other assistance for consumptives.

The Queen's Nurses (a voluntary organisation) are utilised for giving home nursing to the poorer consumptives. During the year 79 patients were thus attended, 6,659 visits being made to these, or an average of about two visits weekly to these patients.

The tuberculosis officer gives personal tuition to these nurses on their work, to secure the value of their hygienic teaching. Reports are received as to the needs of patients. Bedsteads are lent, when necessary, to enable the patient to sleep in a separate bed.

By aid of a charitable bequest, known as the Hedgcock Bequest, many forms of auxiliary help can be given. The total expenditure under this fund in 1928 was £689, the largest items of help being under the headings of milk, aid towards the cost of living, and aid while the head of the family was in the sanatorium; but in other cases assistance was given for rent, boarding out of the baby, training in commercial work, boots and clothing, etc.

No payment is exacted from any patients, of whatever social position, who accept treatment in the Borough Sanatorium; and consultations at the Tuberculosis Dispensary, whether patients are sent by a private doctor or apply for diagnosis independently, are similarly gratuitous.

VENEREAL DISEASE WORK

The treatment of venereal diseases at the public expense is arranged at the Sussex County (Voluntary) Hospital, this centre being utilised for patients from the rest of Sussex as well as for Brighton patients. Three-fourths of the expenditure on this treatment is paid from the National Exchequer, the remaining fourth being paid by various public health authorities according to the use made of the V.D. clinic by patients coming from their respective areas. The treatment is arranged so that the home address and name of each patient are known only to the medical officer of the V.D. clinic. He is an expert in these diseases, who is also engaged in private practice.

During 1928, 370 Brighton new patients applied for treatment at this clinic, of whom 168 were found to be suffering from non-venereal complaints. Female patients form only one-third of the total patients. For syphilis the number of the two sexes is equal; for gonorrhœa male are seven times as numerous as female patients. During the year 211 patients were treated at this centre for the first time who came from outside Brighton. The total 581 new patients and patients who were continuing attendance from a previous year made 19,803 attendances at the clinic. For these patients 2,689 doses of arseno-benzol preparations were given, and the patients received in the aggregate 402 days of in-patient treatment during the year. The number of pathological specimens examined is stated on page 358. Sections of liver are examined for spirochætes from still-born infants on the doctor's request. Up to the end of 1928 this had been done in 173 cases. Of these 6·9 per cent. showed spirochætes. The midwife is paid 4s. for each still-born infant brought by her to the Public Health Office.

THE HISTORY OF MEDICAL INSPECTION AND TREATMENT OF SCHOOL CHILDREN IN BRIGHTON

The stages by which the medical treatment of school children in Brighton needing to be treated has been developed have a more than local interest. They illustrate in an accentuated form the course of events in some other parts of England; and the only conclusion possible from a consideration of the following outlined history is that, given perseverance and tact, it is possible to establish, without continued opposition of the general medical profession, a partial system of public treatment of defects in school children which, apart from such provision, would be neglected. Medical practitioners gain in their private practice by the official measures taken to detect disease in children attending school.

The attempt to treat some of the more obvious cutaneous contagious diseases in school children began about 1906, when a school clinic was held weekly by the then M.O.H., with the help of the single school nurse then provided! To this clinic severe cases of pediculosis of the head, especially cases complicated by eczema and enlarged cervical glands, also cases of impetigo, of ringworm, of blepharitis, etc., were sent by school teachers, and these were treated. Usually parents paid a small sum for ointments supplied. The work developed, but it did not become systematised until after the general enforcement of medical inspection of schools from 1908 onwards.

The subsequent stages in the evolution of a satisfactory scheme can be summarised from the annual reports of Dr. Forbes, who became M.O.H. in 1908, and under whom the work of school hygiene has developed to its present highly organised and successful position.

When, in 1908–9, the first group of children were examined under the new system, the parents of those requiring medical attention were advised to consult their private medical attendants. But difficulties arose:—

1. Many families had no regular medical attendant.

2. In many other families, although a doctor was occasionally employed, monetary circumstances rendered parents very unwilling, or even unable, to seek his advice, except for urgent need.

3. A high proportion of the defects found in school children were of a character not usually treated by general practitioners.

The first two groups do not need special observation, except to say that as a rule some form of assistance, as by hospital treatment or otherwise, was needed.

The last group included in particular:—

(a) Children suffering from ringworm of the scalp. Ringworm was sometimes treated by practitioners, but with relatively small success.

(b) Mouth-breathers, requiring removal of tonsils or adenoids, or both.

(c) Children requiring spectacles.

For the first class [(a) above] parents were commonly unwilling to continue private treatment for a prolonged period, and not infrequently this treatment failed to be satisfactory. The unwillingness of parents to incur expense was increased by the fact that the condition did not affect the child's health unfavourably.

So far as the second and third classes were concerned, Dr. Forbes points out that most of the affected children were patients of doctors having large practices among the poor; that they would require specialised treatment, of a character nearly always unfamiliar to the doctors in such practice; and that their parents could not pay adequately for these services.

What, then, was to be done?

A meeting of the medical men of Brighton and the district was called in November 1910, on behalf of the local branch of the British Medical Association. Between 60 and 70 attended this meeting, but apart from doctors in dispensary and hospital practice, few of those having the largest practices among the poor were present.

The scheme adopted for recommendation to the Brighton Education Authority was one prepared by the parent British Medical Association, based on their policy at that time for the whole country, which was embodied in their resolution (Minute 97) as follows:—

The duties of the school medical officers and their assistants should be confined to necessary inspection and report; and that the treatment of those children found defective should not be undertaken by them.[1]

It proposed a special centre for treatment of children found to have defects.

This centre, as proposed, would be managed by a committee of medical men elected by the general body of Brighton practitioners and responsible to the Brighton Division of the British Medical Association. No provision was made for representation of the Brighton Education Authority or its medical officer on the Committee of Management. The intention was that the authority would "control" the clinic exactly as it would "control" a whole-time officer, the substitution of a committee for one or more officers in their view constituting no difference. The staff of the school clinic would be settled by the Committee of Management, in accordance with principles approved by the Division of the B.M.A. and the Education Authority. A rota of practitioners was proposed. It was arranged that the consent of the patient's own medical man should be obtained, or that it should be definitely ascertained that the parents were unable to pay for treatment before treatment at the clinic was begun.

[1] A chief argument in arriving at the conclusion embodied in the above resolution was that treatment should be done by those whose life-work it is, and who could transmit to the school children the experience gained in their general work, and conversely their clinical experience in school work to the general public. Their view undoubtedly was that, although there are all grades of efficiency and of inefficiency in both general practice and among school doctors, the best general practitioner is more efficient than the best school doctor.

These were the proposals of the organised medical profession, as represented by its association. Evidently, however, others were concerned before a practical plan could be followed. If the patient's parents were willing to undertake treatment privately, the problem became one merely of discovery of defects in the course of medical inspection at the school; and nowhere did there emerge organised opposition to such medical inspection, undertaken on behalf of the Education Authority. But when parents were unwilling or unable to undertake the needed treatment, alternative measures were not a question affecting merely the medical profession. The views of the Board of Education, the national controlling authority on educational matters, had to be regarded, as well as those of the local education authority, representing directly the views of the Brighton ratepayers— whose children needed treatment.

The local authority could only act with the approval of the Board of Education, which defrayed one-half of approved local expenditure on medical inspection and treatment: and this Central Board had issued instructions that the local authority must in the first place take advantage "of the benefits of whatever existing institutions, such as hospitals, infirmaries, and dispensaries, are reasonably available in each district".

The hospitals thus available in Brighton for the treatment of enlarged tonsils and adenoids, or for the prescribing of spectacles, were:—

> The Sussex County Hospital,
> The Throat and Ear Hospital,
> The Eye Hospital,
> The Children's Hospital,

all supported out of voluntary charitable funds; but in each instance the committees of these hospitals stated that they could not enter into any special arrangement with the Brighton Education Committee for the treatment of school children. This being so, the Education Committee during

1911 became ordinary subscribers to the hospitals, and thus obtained letters of recommendation.[1] During that year they subscribed £89 5s., and obtained, as an equivalent in out-patients, 550 letters of recommendation for the above hospitals and for the Dental Hospital and the Brighton Dispensary. The hospitals, with one exception, were willing to treat school children up to the end of 1911, but stated that "after that date they would, except in special cases, decline to treat school children attending the primary schools of the Brighton and Hove Education Authorities and found on medical inspection by the medical officers of the said authorities to be suffering from otorrhœa, enlarged tonsils, adenoids, errors of refraction, skin diseases, or defective teeth".

The possibility of general use of voluntary hospitals and dispensaries having been thus excluded, the Brighton Education Committee had the choice of the scheme proposed by the organised local practitioners, or an alternative scheme proposed by their chief school medical officer, who was also M.O.H. (Dr. Forbes).

The 1910 scheme of the practitioners meanwhile was modified, and in 1911 it was as follows:—

	Number of Cases	Doctor	Salary per Annum
			£
Skin and scalp cases ..	150 per week	1	50
Ringworm, X-ray treat-			
ment of	200 per annum	1	50
Defective vision	350 per annum	1	50
Tonsils and adenoids ..	300 per annum	1	50
Anæsthetists	—	1	50
			£250

[1] Voluntary hospitals at that time generally gave to their subscribers letters of recommendation which admitted for treatment—in-patient or out-patient —the persons recommended by the subscriber, the number of letters being proportional to the amount of the subscription. This practice happily is falling into desuetude.

An increase in these figures beyond 15 per cent. was to be paid for in proportion. The organised doctors undertook to obtain applications for these posts from doctors of standing and experience, from whom the authority could appoint those whom they thought most suitable, each appointment being made for a year, renewable or not as the authority might determine. The hours of work were not to exceed on an average two hours per week for each post.

The above scheme provided only for treatment of those children already found, apart from this scheme, to need treatment. The alternative scheme of the M.O.H. provided for medical inspectors to discover defects by inspection and treat those specified in the above table at a total cost of £650; and early in 1912 the Brighton Education Committee, after full consideration, decided in favour of the second scheme, which provided for inspection and treatment by two whole-time official doctors, with the assistance of a part-time surgeon for removal of tonsils and adenoids.

It does not appear that the possibility of medical inspection by private practitioners was entertained. Without discussing this point here, it may be stated summarily that medical inspection by doctors engaged also in private practice has proved a failure in England, and has been very largely abandoned.

The next stage was unfortunate. The scheme proposed by the local branch of the British Medical Association was endorsed by the association itself, and an advertisement for two whole-time appointments of school medical officers proposed by the Brighton Education Authority was sent to the *British Medical Journal*, which refused to insert it. The position thus created was commented on by the late Dr. R. J. Ryle, then one of the most distinguished medical practitioners in Brighton, from whose letter to the *British Medical Journal*, June 22, 1912, I quote the following paragraphs :—

We are to know nothing but Minute 97, and are to care not at all whether or not the interests of the community are best served by this or some other scheme. The resolution (of the local branch of the B.M.A.) which condemned the appointment did so simply and solely *"because the terms of the appointment are contrary to the principles of the British Medical Association as laid down in Minute 97, etc."*

.   .   .   .   .

The Brighton Education Committee has, of course, a perfect right to select from among various possibilities whichever scheme it believes to be the best suited to its wants.

.   .   .   .   .

On the other hand, the association may fairly use its influence to secure that, whatever scheme is adopted, the doctor or doctors employed shall be properly paid. This done, any further action on their part surely becomes a merely impertinent interference with what is not the business of the association, but is purely the business of the education authority.

The senior school medical officer referred to above was appointed under the education authority's scheme. He was then expelled from the British Medical Association: and there is little doubt that the M.O.H. himself would have been similarly expelled and ostracised but for determined action taken by the Society of Medical Officers of Health. These events are recalled because they throw light on difficulties which may arise in countries which have not yet developed services of medical inspection and treatment of school children. In Brighton, as in the rest of Britain, there is now but little objection on the part of private medical practitioners to school medical work. Children are referred by the school doctor to their family doctor when this is practicable; and the morbid conditions chiefly treated at school clinics are those which, if not treated there, would in the vast majority of cases be neglected. It does not follow, of course, that this will always be so. The ideal of family medical practice is the best. It may become realisable even for the poor—who have not had it hitherto except very partially—if ever family medical attendance becomes organised on a provident or insurance basis, the family doctor then supervising satisfactorily the hygiene as well as the medical treatment of the families in his charge. Even then it would still be necessary—again possibly in the future on a provident basis—to have consultants for conditions in which specialised skill is required.

THE PRESENT POSITION OF SCHOOL MEDICINE IN BRIGHTON may now be outlined. It works with success and without friction.

Brighton has a population of 149,300, and an average attendance of 14,582 children at its elementary schools.

Dr. Forbes, the M.O.H., is the School Medical Officer; he has three full-time medical officers and two full-time dentists on his staff. There is also a part-time orthopædic nurse.

Routine medical inspections are made as in other areas. Of the 5,020 children thus inspected in 1927, 35·7 per cent. were found to be defective. Parents were present at the inspection in half the total cases. Children found defective are further examined and treated at a special school clinic, special days or hours being allotted for different conditions.

At this clinic is determined the fitness for return of children who have been absent from school. Many such cases are thus sent by teachers and attendance officers; not infrequently private doctors send cases, and parents often bring their children for advice independently.

The table opposite summarises the work done in a year at the clinic.

The "following up" of cases with a view to securing treatment and after-care is done by school nurses who visit children at home. These school nurses do important work in the detection of verminous conditions, ringworm, impetigo, scabies, and like conditions, and in securing their attendance at the Minor Ailments Clinic. In 1927 they made 61,058 examinations of such children; 5,643 children were discovered by them to be suffering from some one or other minor cutaneous condition.

At the school clinic treatment is provided for the following conditions: minor ear diseases, including zinc ionisation treatment for chronic otorrhœa; minor eye diseases, also testing of vision, retinoscopy, and prescribing of spectacles; skin diseases, including X-ray treatment for ringworm, orthopædic treatment, including massage, remedial exercises and electric treatment; dental treatment, and examination by the medical staff of all children who are to have teeth extracted under nitrous oxide anæsthesia. In addition, children applying for employment certificates are medically examined, as are also children applying for licences for employment in entertainments.

It is unnecessary to follow in detail the treatment given; but it will be noted that actual curative treatment of all the above conditions is carried through at the clinic.

	Number of Children	Number of Attendances
Skin Clinic	2,310	8,865
Eye Clinic (External Diseases)	304	1,020
Ear Clinic	565	8,423
Ionisation Clinic	29	255
Verminous Clinic	945	2,392
Inspection Clinic	2,233	3,222
Tonsils and Adenoids (Pre- and Post-Operative) and X-rays (Post-treatment)	679	745
Ringworm of the Scalp by X-rays ..	9	9
Refraction Clinic	299	584
Employment Cases and Theatre Licences.	209	209
Dental Clinic	3,516	6,008
Orthopædic Clinic	62	1,863
	11,160	33,595

The newly developed orthopædic work requires a separate note. The medical work of the Borough Council being under the chief administrative medical officer, the M.O.H., it has been practicable to unify work in tuberculosis, in dentistry, and now for crippled children of all ages. Congenital club-foot, cases of infantile paralysis, of flat-foot, rickets, birth palsy, and many other conditions are now seen by a specialist surgeon, hospital treatment provided when necessary, and curative exercises undertaken by the orthopædic nurse.

The dental work also calls for special remark. The aim of

the dental service is to secure an annual dental inspection of all children at school, and this is almost attained. The inspection is not a complete dental survey; but merely adequate to decide whether reference to the dental clinic is indicated. In 1927, 9,523 children were inspected and 46 per cent. referred for treatment. Of the 4,380 thus referred, 83 per cent. were actually treated. The number of fillings were 3,552, of extractions 4,774, of administrations of nitrous oxide 531, and of other operations 1,554. A very satisfactory position is being attained; the number of children leaving school in a perfectly healthy dental condition is steadily increasing. Of the final age group examined in 1927—

543 children had perfectly healthy mouths, as compared with 373 in 1926, and 245 in 1925.

These numbers must be related to the number similarly examined seven years earlier on entering school.

It should be added that an increasing amount of dental treatment is being done for children under school age and for expectant and nursing mothers.

The arrangements for treatment of school children in Brighton now receive much support from private practitioners, tonsil and adenoid cases often being sent for treatment. One practitioner sends as many as a hundred cases for treatment in the year. For an operation on tonsils and adenoids parents are expected to pay 6s. 6d.; this includes the administration of calcium lactate for three days before the operation.

THE BOROUGH OF HOVE

Mention has already been made of the contiguous borough of Hove, which is governed separately from Brighton. Hove has a population of 48,000, with a smaller proportion of poor than in Brighton. It has a whole-time M.O.H., Dr. A. Griffith, and a part-time school medical officer, Dr. L. A. Parry.

The experience of Hove is interesting in relation to medical inspection and treatment of school children. Those children requiring treatment for tonsils and adenoids are dealt with at local hospitals, the local authority paying for their treatment. Arrangements are also made for the treatment of dental and other defects.

Dr. Parry has been school M.O. for Hove for 21 years, and his experience is valuable as illustrating the possibilities of good work by a school doctor who is also engaged in private medical practice. He assured me, however, that the present excellent relationship between him and private practitioners in Hove had only been possible because his private practice was entirely among patients who were remote from the class whose children attended elementary day schools. Had this not been so, he affirmed his private medical practice would have been incompatible with satisfactory and adequate school medical work without friction.

Public Health Staff

The work of the Public Health Department of Brighton (population approaching 150,000) is under the general executive control of Dr. Duncan Forbes, the M.O.H. As elsewhere in England, his work forms a special division of the administrative work of the Town Council. The Town Council has a mayor or chairman, elected annually by the members of the Council. The Council itself consists of 76 members, of whom 57 are councillors elected by the rate-payers to represent the 19 wards into which the borough is divided; and 19 aldermen, elected by the councillors for a period of six years, and commonly re-elected during life. They are usually elected from the councillors, but may be chosen from without.

The detailed oversight of the work of the Council is entrusted to various committees, the *Health Committee* being responsible for all public health work except school medical work. Dr. Forbes is its executive officer. This committee has 15 members, elected from the 76 councillors and aldermen.

The Health Committee delegates the supervisory work for the blind to a sub-committee of 11, of whom 4 are co-opted. There is, in addition, the *Children's Care Sub-Committee*, which consists of 9 members of the Education Committee, and 5 further members who are not members of the Town Council, but are co-opted on the Education Committee because of their special interest in its work.

On the public health staff, in addition to Dr. Forbes, are three medical men and one medical woman. One of these is deputy M.O.H., one is resident medical officer of the sanatorium, one is tuberculosis officer, and one is medical officer for maternity and child welfare work.

The staff includes also six sanitary inspectors, one disinfector, two inspectors under the Factory and Workshops and Shops Acts, one food inspector, five health visitors, and one hospital matron, the nurses, etc., on the hospital staff.

All the above are whole-time officers. To these must be added the staff for school medical work, headed by Dr. Forbes and his deputy. This staff comprises two additional medical officers, two dentists, and five school nurses, all whole-time officers.

The staff of the Public Health and School Divisions of work comprise also ten clerks.

LONDON

TABLE OF CONTENTS

CHAPTER XX

LONDON

THE preceding local sections have been concerned with medico-hygienic public work in smaller towns and in rural counties. In order to obtain a bird's-eye view of these activities in the entire country, a somewhat full description of certain aspects of metropolitan administration must be added. This is necessary, furthermore, in view of the magnitude and complexity of public medical provisions in London, both by voluntary hospitals and allied organisations, and by authorities elected by the rate-payers of the metropolis. The story is somewhat difficult to follow because of the numerous authorities concerned, and because of the recent changes introduced by the Local Government Act, 1929. These changes are not yet fully operative; and in describing actual work one is compelled to describe work by authorities, whose functions are changing, or by an authority in the case of the Poor Law, whose functions have now been merged into the work of the London County Council. The relation of the work of the authorities concerned to that of the private medical practitioner will appear as we proceed.

THE GOVERNMENT OF LONDON

LONDON AND GREATER LONDON

At the census of 1931, the administrative county of London (London proper) had an enumerated population of 4,396,821, and an area of 117 square miles. There are several Londons, the one with which we are concerned from the public health point of view being the County of London, which forms one unit (divided into many subsidiary units) for purposes of general administration, including poor law, public health, and education. Among the other Londons are the main drainage area of London, containing 180 square miles, and the water area for control of public water supplies, containing 574 square miles. There are also metropolitan telephone, electricity supply, and traffic areas, which cover still wider areas. The police administration of London, which is not controlled by popularly elected representatives, but by the Home Office of the Government, includes in its scope the "Outer Ring", comprising with London proper a population in 1921 of 7,480,201 (Greater London). This outer population and large numbers coming from more remote communities benefit by the voluntary hospital provision of the metropolis.

The distribution of the population in the Outer Ring is further shown in the following table (census year 1921):—

Essex: East Ham County Borough	143,246
West Ham County Borough	300,860
Aggregate of other districts	454,232
Hertfordshire	59,155
Kent	198,291
Middlesex	1,253,002
Surrey: Croydon County Borough	191,375
Other Districts	395,517
TOTAL Outer Ring	2,995,678

In 1931 (census) the Outer Ring had 3,805,997 population.

London grows only in this Outer Ring. Between 1911 and 1921 the population of London proper declined 0·9 per cent., while that of the Outer Ring increased 9·6 per cent. This "swarming" of London outside its technical borders has created many administrative problems, and notwithstanding the large use of metropolitan voluntary hospitals by persons outside the metropolis—it has meant a considerable lack of hospital accommodation for the dwellers in London's "outside dormitories". The efforts to provide new voluntary hospitals, including cottage hospitals, have failed to meet the need adequately: and this explains in part the rapidly increasing use of poor-law infirmaries as general hospitals for persons who are not technically destitute (p. 60).

I do not attempt to outline the vital statistics of London, as these are readily accessible. Its population is recruited from every part of Great Britain and from other countries, and its vital statistics represent a composite result of both urban and rural life.

ADMINISTRATIVE DIVISIONS

London, for public health and general local administration, is divided into 27 boroughs and two cities which, in most respects, have separate administration, and in which the local taxation varies within wide limits. The two cities are Westminster and the City of London, which in most respects have the same relationship to the central governing body (the County Council) as the 27 boroughs; but the City of London, for historical and other reasons, has official privileges, with which we need not be concerned. Its population now is chiefly non-resident.

Prior to 1930 there were 25 poor-law administrative areas in London, the boundaries of these not exactly corresponding with those of metropolitan boroughs. Until April 1930 poor-law and general local administration have been under separately elected local bodies, but since the passing of the Local Government Act, the conditions set out on page 383 hold good.

LOCAL TAXATION (RATING)

Local taxation in each borough (called rates) is based on the assessable or rateable value of business premises and dwellings; and it follows that, as a rule, the boroughs which have the meanest houses have the poorest basis for taxation (rating) and the highest rates in proportion to their financial competence. For instance, in 1927 Bermondsey's rateable value was equivalent to £8 8s., while that of the City of Westminster was £64 4s. per person living in the respective areas. Other instances of differences in rateable values in pounds sterling per head of population in 1927 are as follows :—

Battersea	..	.. 6·6	Finsbury	.. .. 16·2
Bermondsey	..	.. 8·9	Holborn	.. .. 38·4
Bethnal Green	..	.. 5·1	St. Marylebone	.. 26·3
Stepney ..	..	.. 6·9	Westminster ..	.. 65·2
Chelsea ..	..	.. 16·5		

This unequal distribution of financial ability to pay the necessary costs of local government has been partially rectified by the metropolitan common poor funds, by which the poorer areas benefit at the expense of the richer. Furthermore, certain great expenses, as, for instance, those for elementary education and main sewerage, are more equally distributed throughout London. The cost of elementary education to ratepayers still presses very heavily in poorer boroughs.

Under the new conditions initiated in 1930, there will be further equalisation of the costs of public assistance. Its control comes under the London County Council, which will have the power to require the payment of an equal rate throughout London, while insisting on uniform principles of administration of relief in accordance with uniform regulations.

For governmental purposes bearing on medical problems, London had prior to April 1930 the following authorities :—

1. The County Council.
2. Borough Councils.
3. Metropolitan Asylums Board and Boards of Guardians.
4. London Education Committee of the County Council.
5. London Insurance Committee.

The third group of bodies has now disappeared. The London County Council's powers and duties have been increased and extended, modifications have occurred in the relationship of the borough councils to the L.C.C.,[1] while the functions of the Education and Insurance Committees remain substantially as before.

The above enumeration of metropolitan governing bodies is not complete. Among others the most important are the Metropolitan Water Board controlling the water supply of most of Greater London, and the Metropolitan Police, already mentioned. These need not be further mentioned, as they have little bearing on current medical problems.

[1] In this chapter L.C.C. is London County Council, M A.B. is Metropolitan Asylums Board.

LONDON COUNTY COUNCIL

The London County Council consists of 124 representative councillors, men and women, directly elected by the rate-payers of the metropolis every third year, and of 20 aldermen elected by these councillors from within the council or from outside. The County Council, among its other duties, is responsible for education and its medical work throughout London, for the treatment in hospitals of diseases treated at the public expense, for the organisation of schemes for the control of venereal disease, and for the control of midwives practising in London.

BOROUGH COUNCILS

Each of the 27 Borough Councils and the City of Westminster has 30 to 60 councillors (according to its population) elected by the borough rate-payers triennially: and in addition about one-sixth of this number of aldermen, elected for six years from within or without the council. The mayor of the borough is elected by the councillors and aldermen, and may be re-elected at the end of his year of office. He has no special powers, but acts as chairman of the council.

The City of London Corporation consists of 206 common councillors elected annually, and 26 aldermen, also directly elected by the citizens, but for life. Its head is the Lord Mayor. The head of the County Council, with its more extensive and far-reaching functions, is called its Chairman.

The Borough Councils and the two Cities carry on the ordinary scavenging, sanitary, and other work of a local authority, including child welfare centres and health visitors, tuberculosis dispensaries, and the investigation and control of acute infectious diseases, except their institutional treatment. The institutional treatment of tuberculosis and venereal diseases and of lunatics and feeble-minded, wholly or in part, is centrally organised for the whole of London. Some feeble-minded and harmless insane have been also treated in poor-law infirmaries by the Poor-law Guardians (now superseded by the Public Assistance Committee of the L.C.C.).

POOR-LAW GUARDIANS

A further note is needed of the extensive services of public assistance which are now taken over by the L.C.C. Prior to 1930 there were separate Boards of Guardians for the 25 metropolitan poor-law areas in London, each directly elected by the rate-payers. Each had its separate administration of relief, institutional (in part) and domiciliary (completely); and the variable standards of domiciliary relief in different unions and the differences in tests of eligibility to relief have caused much confusion and led to serious abuses.

Many of the poor-law hospitals had, as already seen (p. 97), evolved into first-class hospitals for the sick poor of London. In addition, there was the *Metropolitan Asylums Board*, which was established pursuant to the Metropolitan Poor Act, 1867. This Board consisted of 73 members, 55 elected by the Metropolitan Boards of Guardians for the 25 parishes and unions in London (population 4,541,000 in 1927), and 18 nominated by the Ministry of Health.

The M.A.B. possesses special interest from the standpoint of British democratic institutions for two reasons:—

1. It is an exceptional instance of indirect election (by Boards of Guardians who were elected by the rate-payers), the members of the M.A.B. thus elected being "diluted" by a large number of persons nominated by the Ministry of Health.

This exception has disappeared with the passing of the Local Government Act; and the duties of the M.A.B. are added to the already multifarious work of the County Council. The London County Council becomes an almost complete parliament for metropolitan government; water control and police being the two chief administrative departments still partially or entirely under separate control.

2. The history of the M.A.B. embodies the more liberal and humane policy in treatment of the sick which has gradually displaced the deterrence of older poor-law con-

ditions. This change is particularly shown in the provision
of hospital accommodation for fevers, diphtheria, and smallpox, which has been an important part of the work of the
Asylums Board. At first infectious patients sent to these
hospitals technically became paupers, but in 1883 all poor-
law restrictions and resultant civil disabilities were removed,
and gratuitous treatment of these cases became substantially
the right of every Londoner and his children. The same is
true, as we have seen (p. 212) throughout Great Britain,
treatment in an isolation hospital nearly everywhere being
free from individual or familial charges. Of course, there
remains the charge levied as a quasi-insurance policy in the
form of local rates. Poorer persons are not exempt from
payment for this insurance; for their weekly rental paid
to a landlord is placed at a figure which enables the latter
to pay the communal rate.

LOCAL EDUCATION AUTHORITY

The Education Committee of the County Council, which
is the Local Education Authority for London, is an instance
of unification of local governmental functions for the whole
of London similar to that effected in 1930 for the work
of the Boards of Guardians and the M.A.B. The first
School Board for London was elected in 1871, after the
passing of the first Elementary Education Act in 1870. In
1902 *ad hoc* school boards directly elected by the rate-payers
were abolished, and in London the powers and duties of
the School Board were transferred to the County Council.
Every elementary school has its committee of managers; but
the control of essential educational matters lies with the
Council's Education Committee.

A similarity may be traced between the history of payment
of fees by parents for their children's schooling, and payment for maintenance of these children in a fever hospital.
The small weekly fees charged for school attendance were
difficult to collect, and they were gradually discontinued:
and the Elementary Education Act, 1891, substituted a payment from the National Exchequer in lieu of the fees payable

by or for the children. The cost of elementary education and of maintenance in an isolation hospital is now partly a national and partly a municipal charge: in both alike communal safety and efficiency are regarded as justifying and in fact requiring this.

LONDON INSURANCE COMMITTEE

The London Insurance Committee is concerned with an important branch of medical administration, that of the relation between the insured and "panel" or insurance doctors who treat sick persons insured under the National Insurance Acts. This committee is not in the democratic sense a representative body, elected by rate-payers generally. It could scarcely be so, as the insured constitute only one-third of the total population. Nor are the members of the committee all elected by direct vote of the insured persons. The London committee consists of 80 members, of whom 48 are representatives of insured persons belonging to "approved societies" or who are "deposit contributors", 16, including at least 2 women, are appointed by the London County Council, 2 are elected by metropolitan medical practitioners, 3 are medical practitioners appointed by the County Council, and 11, including at least 1 medical practitioner and 2 women, are appointed by the Ministry of Health.

Owing to the extreme centralisation of sickness insurance administration in the insurance division of the Ministry of Health, the duties of this committee are limited, and its abolition has been recommended by a recent Royal Commission.

The above is a sketch necessarily in incomplete outline of the main machinery concerned in the government of London, so far as medical and public health matters are concerned. The relation of the different parts may perhaps be further elucidated by reference to the following diagrammatic scheme, which shows the position before the passing of the Local Government Act, 1930.

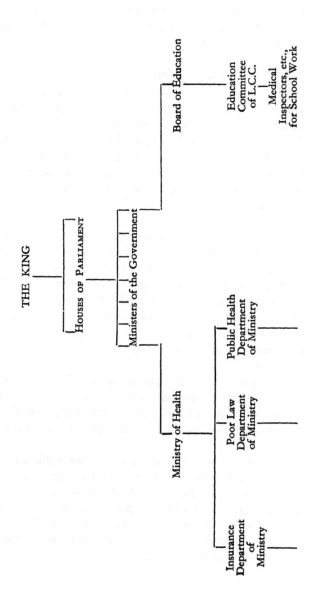

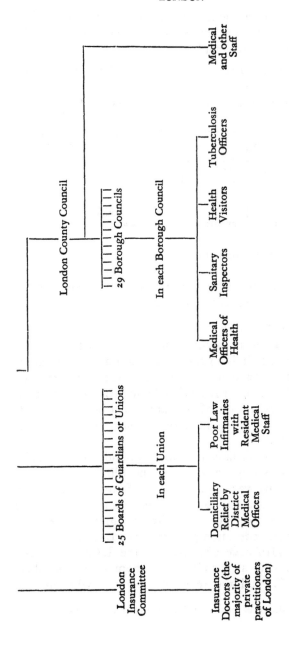

London County Council

29 Borough Councils

In each Borough Council

Medical Officers of Health — Sanitary Inspectors — Health Visitors — Tuberculosis Officers

Medical and other Staff

25 Boards of Guardians or Unions

In each Union

Domiciliary Relief by District Medical Officers — Poor Law Infirmaries with Resident Medical Staff

London Insurance Committee

Insurance Doctors (the majority of private practitioners of London)

In the next scheme the new arrangements are outlined, so far as the governing agencies are concerned. More detail is given in the next paragraph.

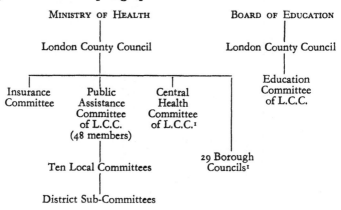

MINISTRY OF HEALTH   BOARD OF EDUCATION

London County Council   London County Council

Insurance Committee   Public Assistance Committee of L.C.C. (48 members)   Central Health Committee of L.C.C.[1]   Education Committee of L.C.C.

Ten Local Committees   29 Borough Councils[1]

District Sub-Committees

New Arrangements for London under the Local Government Act, 1931

(a) Public Assistance

The conditions of giving relief in the metropolis are greatly changed. It is intended, as soon as circumstances permit, that all assistance which can lawfully be provided otherwise than by poor relief shall be so provided; and that, furthermore, each form of assistance shall be in the hands of one, and not more than one, branch of the L.C.C. administration.

At once all domiciliary assistance to blind persons will be provided exclusively by virtue of the Blind Persons Act, 1920, and not by way of poor-law relief; and it is proposed that the same shall, as soon as practicable, apply to the mentally defective, and to assistance given under the tuberculosis and education powers of the L.C.C.

A *Public Assistance Committee* of the L.C.C. has been appointed having 48 members, of whom 32 are members of the L.C.C., and the remainder persons who are not

---

[1] For details of relation of these to each other, see text.

members of the Council, some of whom are women. This committee advises *inter alia*—

> on questions of public assistance policy, including the limitations of the duties of local committees and sub-committees appointed for public assistance;
>
> and undertakes the estimates of expenditure for London, controls the expenditure of the local committees and sub-committees;
>
> arranges for the care and maintenance of all persons requiring relief in institutions;
>
> advises as to the provision, classification, maintenance, and inspection of institutions;
>
> and arranges for the provision of domiciliary medical relief.

The county of London is now divided into ten *administrative areas*, instead of the 25 pre-existing poor-law areas, and each of them coinciding with the combined area of two to four metropolitan boroughs, or parts of boroughs. The population in these ten administrative areas varies from 247,590 (Greenwich and Woolwich) to 819,400 (Lambeth, Battersea, and Wandsworth). Each area has a *local committee*, consisting of from 32 to 50 persons, appointed by the L.C.C. from within or without its body. The local committee nominates and the public assistance committee appoints its chairman. The duties of the local committee, *inter alia*, are to

> supervise and co-ordinate the administration of relief by the district sub-committees;
>
> to keep under review the conditions of persons to whom relief has been granted; and
>
> to co-operate with voluntary agencies rendering analogous services in their area.

District or other Sub-Committees are required to be appointed by the local committee, consisting each of eight to ten members, who may be in part members of the local committee, in part others selected from a panel of names approved by the L.C.C.

The chief duty of these district committees is to investigate the case of each applicant for relief and to administer relief in accordance with general regulations.

It is believed that by these means it will be practicable to secure fairly equal conditions of poor relief throughout London. Evidently, however, there will continue to be the possibility of great divergence in the practice of these district committees, owing to varying interpretations of regulations as to the duration and character of relief to be given. This can only gradually be rectified.

(b) PUBLIC HEALTH ADMINISTRATION

Under the new conditions residential institutions hitherto provided by the Boards of Guardians and by the Metropolitan Asylums Board are taken over by the L.C.C., and its Public Health Committee, now to be known as the *Central Health Committee*, will be responsible for their maintenance and extension as needed.

The duties of the Central Health Committee are officially enumerated as follows :—

(i) The provision, classification, maintenance, and management of hospitals for the sick, and the making of arrangements for their visitation and inspection;

(ii) Consultation and co-operation with voluntary hospitals and other hospitals serving the county;

(iii) Dealing with cases requiring hospital treatment and their conveyance to and from hospital;

(iv) the periodical review of case receiving hospital treatment;

(v) The provision of local medical services;

(vi) The institutional care of children under the age of 3 years who are separated from their parents;

(vii) Laboratory services, medical instruction, and the training of nurses and midwives in connection with hospitals;

(viii) The direction of staff exclusively employed at hospitals, and of the district medical staff.

The provision and maintenance of mental hospitals is a gigantic problem in London, and is placed, as also for all county boroughs and other county areas, under a separate *Mental Hospitals Committee*, which undertakes the provision and care of mental hospitals, the care of harmless insane persons of the chronic or imbecile class, and of mentally defective and feeble-minded persons; also the provision of such laboratory and other services as are needed.

The functions of the *Education Committee* have not greatly changed.

From the preceding sketch of past and future administrative arrangements for London one can formulate some of the steps needed to secure increasing efficiency of medical administration. Some of these have already been indicated in part.

1. The medical officers of health and other special medical officers of each of the 29 boroughs need to be brought into closer liaison with the medical department of the County Council.

2. This, while providing for closer co-operation between all engaged in metropolitan public health work, and enabling each medical officer to come more completely in touch with the activities of others engaged in like work, is not inconsistent with autonomous work in each borough, local experimentation and advance being encouraged beyond the obligatory minimum standard in each borough throughout the metropolis.

3. The transference of poor-law work from the Boards of Guardians to committees of the County Council with local assistance committees functioning in each of ten metropolitan areas, if intelligently utilised, renders possible a larger mass of preventive work directed to the removal of the specific cause or conditions producing each case of destitution.

PRESENT MEDICAL ADMINISTRATION

ACUTE INFECTIOUS DISEASES

The same regulations as to notification of infectious disease as in England generally apply in London (p. 211). All such notifications are made to the borough M.O.H. He makes the needed investigation into each notified case personally, or through a skilled assistant. If the case is one of small-pox, he usually takes personal part in the needed field work. If hospital treatment is indicated, he arranges, with the consent of the doctor in attendance, for removal to one of the M.A.B., now L.C.C. hospitals. The practitioner himself may telephone direct to the offices of the L.C.C. to arrange immediate removal. We need not follow further the general line of inquiry pursued by the borough M.O.H. and his staff into the source of each infectious case and into the adequacy of the precautionary measures adopted. Some-times, however, these inquiries necessitate examination of other scholars in the school or classroom at which the patient had been taught. But the medical supervision of schools is the responsible care of the medical department of the County Council; and at this stage there may be needed active co-operative investigation by the borough and county health departments. This is rendered somewhat easier by the legal provision that the borough M.O.H. must within 12 hours send a copy of any notification certificate re-ceived by him to the L.C.C., and the latter is required to forward weekly to the County Council a return of the infectious diseases of which they have received note. The immediate intimations to the M.A.B. enable its officers to obtain prompt information as to the trend of an epidemic and the prospective need for providing beds in hospital.

The County Council plays a further important rôle in the prevention of epidemic diseases. Acute infectious diseases such as smallpox and typhoid or para-typhoid fever pay no respect to artificial boundaries between the constituent boroughs of the metropolis; and the medical officers of the larger authority can and do pursue investigations which facilitate and expedite the discovery of sources of infection, whether these are directly human or only indirectly so, as through specifically contaminated milk or other foods.

The M.A.B. (now the L.C.C.) is the chief public authority providing hospitals for infectious disease: its activities extend beyond acute infectious diseases. It also provides institutions for tuberculosis, for children suffering from ringworm and other specified contagious diseases, and for other children who require special treatment in hospitals or convalescent homes.

During 1927 there were admitted into its hospitals for acute infectious diseases 30,172 patients, the lowest number treated at any time during the year being 3,466, and the highest number 5,915. There are 14 fever hospitals, having an accommodation of 8,444 beds, and three smallpox hospitals, having a present accommodation of 1,740 beds. In 1927, 74·4 per cent. of the total notified cases of diphtheria and 86·3 per cent. of the total notified cases of scarlet fever in London were treated in M.A.B. hospitals.

Although measles is not at present a notifiable disease in most metropolitan boroughs, the M.A.B. hospitals are being used increasingly for treatment of cases of this disease.

Recently wards in the hospitals for infectious diseases have been utilised for the treatment of cases of puerperal fever and of poliomyelitis.

Fifty beds are allocated for the last-named disease at Queen Mary's Hospital, Carshalton, for the treatment of children entering into the second stage of this disease, or those who require correctional operations for deformities resulting from this disease.

In 1926–27 a unit of 100 beds was established at one hospital for the treatment of children suffering from the after-effects of encephalitis lethargica, and this is being continued. Arrangements have also been made for the admission of extra-metropolitan cases to this unit, the full cost of these cases being defrayed by the local authorities concerned.

At the request of the Ministry of Health, the M.A.B. have established at one hospital a clinic for the treatment by radium of cancer of the uterus. Similar treatment has also been given at one of the metropolitan poor-law hospitals. Patients to the above clinic so far have been received only from a metropolitan Board of Guardians.

The M.A.B. have also undertaken the treatment of ophthalmia neonatorum, and taken some part in the institutional treatment of cases of venereal disease in women.

The M.A.B. has had its own pathological and experimental laboratories, at which diphtheria antitoxin is manufactured, pathological specimens are examined for administrative purposes, and researches are undertaken. During 1927 some 437 medical students attended courses of instruction in fever; and 45 qualified doctors attended courses of instruction in hospital administration for the D.P.H. (diploma in public health) as required by the regulations of the General Medical Council.

Official Hospital Provision in London

Under the Local Government Act, 1929, the L.C.C. becomes the sole hospital provider for the metropolis. There only remain outside its jurisdiction the general and voluntary hospitals of London concerning which particulars are given on page 60 *et seq.* The Central Public Health Committee is entrusted with hospital provision, except in respect of mental hospitals.

The hospitals transferred from the M.A.B. are the following:—

	Aggregate Accommodation
11 Fever hospitals	6,771
3 Fever and smallpox hospitals	1,898
Hospital for oph. neon., marasmus, and enteritis	60
2 Institutions for venereal diseases	103
9 Institutions for tuberculosis	2,057
2 Institutions for sane epileptics	705
5 Hospitals and institutions for children	1,992
TOTAL	13,586

In addition, the following poor-law hospitals have been transferred from the 25 metropolitan Boards of Guardians:—

	Accommodation
North-western Area	3,786
Northern Area..	3,157
North-eastern Area	3,808
South-eastern Area	3,610
South-western Area	2,961
	17,322

In addition to the above 17,322 beds for the necessitous, much accommodation for the sick exists in institutions (workhouses) which provide also for the able-bodied poor. Among these are many maternity and mental patients. These institutions in the aggregate have 11,944 beds for sick persons and 10,067 beds for healthy persons.

The arrangements for some of the occupants of these beds will come under the Public Assistance and some under the Central Health Committee.

MATERNITY AND CHILD WELFARE

In London, as in the rest of England, the growth of hygiene and medical work directed to improve the safety of child-birth and the health of the infant and the toddler has been a special characteristic of the twentieth century.

In order of importance care of the mother before, during, and after parturition obviously should occupy the first place in time and in amount of attention; but care of the school child and of the infant has taken first place in official work. Metropolitan administration of the Midwives Act is under-taken by the L.C.C., there being no delegation to the Borough Councils. The duties of local authorities under the Midwives Act are set out on page 154.

Between 1913 and 1918 the number of midwives inti-mating each year—as required by law—their intention to practise in London was fairly constant, never more than 600. In the year 1927 the number was 870, and it was estimated that they attended 34,000 births. The number of qualified medical men residing in London in the same year was 8,248. What proportion—it must be large—of these doctors were not in practice, and what proportion of the remainder do not practise midwifery, can only be surmised.

As early as 1919 the proportion of the total births attended by midwives in London was estimated at 54 per cent. In 1927 the proportion was estimated as about 47 per cent. Medical aid was obtained in 21·8 per cent. of the total cases attended by midwives in 1928, as compared with 19·5 per cent. in

1927. In the year 1927–28 the Council's expenditure for medical aid called in was £4,060, of which about £966 was recovered. It is compulsory on the L.C.C. to compensate a midwife when she has been suspended from practice with the object of preventing the spread of infection. During 1927, £127 was paid to 19 midwives thus suspended from practice.

INSPECTION OF MIDWIVES

This is carried out for the L.C.C. by four women assistant medical officers, who pay special visits when puerperal pyrexia or ophthalmia has been notified in the practice of a midwife. During 1928, 2,115 visits were made by them, or an average of one visit for every 17 confinements attended by midwives.

During 1928, 787 notifications of puerperal pyrexia[1] were received, of which 42 cases proved fatal. The character of professional attendance in definite cases of puerperal fever, as given in the M.O.H.'s Report to the Council for 1928, gives a clue to the varying circumstances of parturition in London. (Fatal cases are given in brackets).

DISTRIBUTION OF NOTIFICATIONS OF PUERPERAL FEVER

Medical Practitioners	110 (19)
Certified Midwives	58 (10)
Doctor and Midwife	5 (2)
Hospitals and Poor-law Institutions.. ..	91 (17)
Medical Students	11 (1)

There were 19 other cases in which no qualified attendant had been engaged.

Each midwife is required to report any inflammation of the eyes of infants and to send for medical help if it occurs. In 1,421 instances medical aid was thus invoked in 1928, and in 59 further cases the responsible midwife failed to call in medical aid. Of the 1,480 cases, 444 proved to be ophthalmia neonatorum.

It is unnecessary to give further details of the supervision

[1] For definition of this, see page 168.

of midwives, except to mention that the L.C.C. has arranged courses of lectures and practical demonstrations in antenatal and postnatal work and in general midwifery during the autumn and winter months.

CARE OF THE INFANT AND TODDLER

In 1909 the Notification of Births Act came into force throughout London (p. 183). It provides that the parent, in addition to registering the birth of his child within six weeks of its birth, shall, within 36 hours after the birth, notify its occurrence to the M.O.H. of the metropolitan borough in which it occurred. This forms the basis of the system of home visiting of mothers and their infants, which has become general, and which forms the most important part of child welfare work in England.

These visits are made by health visitors appointed by the borough council of each of the 29 metropolitan boroughs. Similarly the infant welfare centres belong to the borough councils, or are supported and run by voluntary associations, aided by official funds, and working in collaboration with the official health visitors of the borough council. The L.C.C. give aid from the metropolitan rates to borough work. The L.C.C. is also interested in the early notifications of births received by each borough M.O.H., as nearly half of the births have been attended by midwives, and midwives are controlled solely by the L.C.C. Thus the officers of the L.C.C. make all the inquiries called for when midwives send for medical aid, when they are suspected of malpractice, when ophthalmia occurs in an infant born in their practice, and when puerperal pyrexia occurs among their patients. But the borough M.O.H. is also officially concerned in the same problems, if the morbid condition occurs in the practice of a medical practitioner, and the latter is required to notify such cases to the borough M.O.H. Evidently the position is unsatisfactory. Neither the officials of the L.C.C. nor the borough M.O.H. can completely investigate and take official action when needed respecting the complications of parturition and of the neonatal period, except after consultation with each other, and this may be difficult to arrange promptly. In every case residential institutional treatment has to be arranged through the L.C.C. unless this is provided by a voluntary agency. Thus an antenatal centre for expectant mothers is conducted by the Borough Council, while the provision of maternity beds rests with the L.C.C.

The Local Government Act, 1929, does not remove this unfortunate diarchy, but it should be practicable for the L.C.C. to decentralise arrangements in each of the 29 metropolitan boroughs, and thus secure closer supervision of midwives, greater personal contact between them and a sympathetic supervisor, and much closer co-operation between the midwives and the work of maternity and child welfare centres in each borough of the metropolis.

That such decentralisation of individual supervision will eventually be practised is certain.

The grants from the Government to borough councils and to voluntary agencies undertaking approved child welfare work on the basis of 50 per cent. of total approved local expenditure have ceased, and have been replaced by a block grant, the allotment of which rests with the L.C.C. This is intended, so far as work in non-residential institutions is concerned, to be allotted to the borough councils. Provision for patients in maternity hospitals, in children's wards, in babies' homes, etc., will be made by the L.C.C.

The matter is complicated by the large share taken by voluntary agencies in metropolitan maternity and child welfare work. Hitherto these have received grants directly from the Ministry of Health after local inspection; in future, contributions will be made at the will of the L.C.C. for voluntary residential institutions, and at the will of the borough council for local work in child welfare centres, etc.

A recent report of the L.C.C. enumerates six maternity hospitals, 35 mother and baby homes, 9 babies' homes, and several other voluntary institutions under voluntary management, and there are at least 68 associations in London concerned in voluntary child welfare work. It is estimated that the contributions of the L.C.C. to voluntary work will amount to £41,435, those of 26 metropolitan boroughs to £78,891.

The position is likely to be unsatisfactory to these voluntary organisations; and unless a broad-minded attitude is adopted by the borough councils, much valuable voluntary work will cease. Whether attached to official work or independently, this help from voluntary workers outside the governing bodies has a high social value.

The division of work between the borough councils and the L.C.C. remains unsatisfactory under the new conditions. Although not immediately practicable, the supervision of medical hygienic work, of which child welfare work is an important part, while remaining in the hands of the borough medical officials, should be so arranged that they act in this respect as officials also of the L.C.C. The detailed consideration of this problem is not needed for our present purpose.

In each borough the work of the sanitary inspectors impinges on that of the health visitors. They are both concerned in detecting sanitary domestic defects and in securing their correction; but health visitors confine themselves to judicious advice as to uncleanliness and overcrowding, and as to food storage, etc., which has immediate bearing on the health of the mother or her infant. The following statement, taken from the Annual Report of the M.O. to the L.C.C., in 1927, shows the number of these officers in London. Although the proportion to population varies considerably in the different boroughs, it is unnecessary to give these variations in full.

	Whole-time	Part-time
Sanitary Inspectors	{ Male 318	6
	{ Female 28	15
Health Visitors	Female 192	16

Three of the whole-time health visitors are also tuberculosis visitors.

The number of whole-time health visitors is equivalent to
1 per 381 births in London.

The borough work of maternity and child welfare work
in London may be best shown by taking a couple of
examples.

KENSINGTON had a population in 1927 of 176,700. Of the
total 2,148 births occurring in the borough in the same
year, 1,285 were notified by midwives. There are nine health
visitors, i.e. 1 per 239 births; but these, in addition to
advising mothers concerning their infants and helping in the
work of the seven infant welfare centres in the borough,
devote some time to visiting factories and workshops
where women are employed, and to visiting cases of ophthalmia, enteritis, measles, whooping-cough, and phthisis. Two
of them are employed on indoor work at the borough
tuberculosis dispensary. For a year an additional health
lecturer has been appointed to visit centres and give
health-talks.

The following statement by the borough's M.O.H., Dr.
Fenton, summarises the local activity's work on maternity
and child welfare:—

There were 2,549 births notified in 1927, of which 401
occurred in institutions outside the borough.

The number of visits made to infants under the age of 21 days	1,859
The number of visits made to infants under 1 year old	4,844
The number of visits made to children between 1 and 5 years old	7,404
Half-days at welfare centres	771
Special visits	2,415
Visits of inquiry *re* infection, etc...	502
Investigations *re* applications for a supply of milk	463

The borough has been mapped out in seven areas, in each
of which is a voluntary infant welfare centre. An official
woman health visitor has an office on the premises of each
welfare centre, where she keeps her records, and arranges
home visiting in consultation with the staff of the centre
and the voluntary committee.

The work done at these centres is for mothers and expectant mothers, and for infants and pre-school children. It is almost entirely consultative and educational in character.

SUMMARY OF TOTAL WORK AT SEVEN WELFARE CENTRES

Number of sessions which doctor attended for consultations 852
Number of sessions which doctor attended for special antenatal consultations 145
Total number of individual mothers who attended during the year 2,954
Number of individual mothers who attended antenatal sessions during the year 461
Total number of individual children who attended during the year—
 Old 1,923
 New 1,816
Total number of attendances of mothers for all purposes at centre (except for obtaining milk, etc.) 16,726
Total number of attendances of children for all purposes 40,721
Total weighings of children 36,108
Total attendances at doctors' consultations—
 1. Antenatal mothers.. 1,381
 2. Postnatal mothers 2,939
 3. Children 25,342

All the centres provide dental treatment, and each welfare centre endeavours, as far as possible, to make the scheme of dental treatment self-supporting. There is also a baby clinic in the borough, voluntary in organisation, in which some treatment is given: and by arrangement with the L.C.C. this clinic is used officially in the treatment of minor school defects and ailments.

There is in the borough a small in-patient hospital for infants with 20 beds, in which 120 infants were treated during the year. The Borough Council made a grant of £200 to the voluntary committee of this hospital, in order that two beds might be at the disposal of the infant welfare centres serving the borough.

A detached ward of 10 beds at the St. Mary Abbots Poor Law Infirmary (now Public Assistance Hospital) was opened as a maternity home for Kensington mothers. This is an example of anticipation of breaking down of poor-law restrictions and the extension of treatment in a poor-law institution to those who, though not technically paupers, require help. The Borough Council has hitherto paid 5s. per day to the local public assistance authority for each maternity case admitted, and the cost of any additional medical or nursing staff which this body has found it necessary to employ. In 1927, 126 women were confined in this home, i.e. about 5 per cent. of the total births in the borough. For 1927 the gross cost of the scheme to the council was £837; patients paid £346.

The official supply of milk continues to be in demand.

In Kensington the extent to which milk or meals are supplied can be seen from the following statement for 1927. The Borough Council's Sub-Committee made 531 grants of fresh milk at an estimated cost to them of £192. In addition, 140 packets of dried milk were supplied free at a cost to the council of £10 10s. Beyond this, £680 10s. worth of dried milk was sold to mothers at cost price; and 350 dinners were granted at a cost to the council of £8 15s. In checking the possibility of overlapping of charitable effort, the Council have found the "Mutual Registration of Assistance Society" of service, and they make an annual grant of £10 to this society.

The Kensington child welfare activities include two novel branches of work of much interest.

Epidemic Diarrhœa.—One of these is concerned with special measures for the control and treatment of zymotic enteritis. The scheme has been in operation for four years. A special physician has been appointed to render medical assistance during the summer months. This disease was made notifiable by the attending doctor to the M.O.H. when occurring in children under 5. The health visitors and voluntary workers at the infant welfare centres co-operate, and the services of the nurses of the voluntary Kensington District Nursing Association are requisitioned for home nursing of cases of this disease. Last year 41 cases were notified, and 20 of these were removed to hospital.

The district nurses attended 48 cases and paid 437 visits. There is evidence that fatality (case-mortality) has declined, and the scheme has had a valuable educational effect.

Acute Rheumatism.—The borough has been a pioneer in obtaining the Ministry of Health's consent to an order for a period of three years, making acute rheumatism (rheumatic fever) compulsorily notifiable to the M.O.H. by the practitioner in attendance. This has been done in order that a special physician attached to a local voluntary Children's Hospital may, with the help of voluntary workers, undertake the supervision and sometimes the treatment of patients with this disease. Meanwhile the borough officials investigate the possible environmental factors concerned in the causation of this disease. A rheumatism supervisory centre has been established, and a number of beds have been reserved in Kensington Infirmary for rheumatic patients. We cannot give space here for particulars of this interesting experimental scheme, but they are set out in Dr. Fenton's Annual Report for 1927.

BERMONDSEY illustrates public health administration on its medical side in one of the poorest of metropolitan boroughs. Only a few points concerning it need be detailed, as in most respects its child welfare work resembles that of other boroughs. It is a riverside borough, its inhabitants being occupied largely in the docks and warehouses on the riverbanks and in ancillary occupations, including the unskilled work associated with a vast number of warehouses. Its residential population is decreasing. It was 130,000 in 1901, and only 120,000 in 1921. Its dwelling-houses, apart from many huge blocks of tenement dwellings, consist of small houses, many worn out, often presenting a sordid appearance, and almost entirely destitute of the amenities of a well-assorted community in present circumstances.

The course of infant mortality is strikingly similar in Bermondsey and in Kensington.

Each of them began with a high infant mortality, that of Bermondsey being 160 and that of Kensington being 144 per 1,000 births in 1901–5. The reduction of this rate, comparing

1901–5 with 1927, has been 52 per cent. in Kensington and 58 per cent. in Bermondsey.

While the work for improving child health in Bermondsey is somewhat similar to that in Kensington and in other metropolitan boroughs, the question of intrusion on the sphere of the private practitioner comes in but little: for were it not for official and voluntary agencies, those who need the help now given would go largely unhelped.

Apart from child welfare work, a chief factor in securing improved social efficiency and comfort has been the change in the drinking habits of the people. For the whole country the improvement has been astounding.

The influence of this reduced consumption of alcoholic drinks in improving mother-care cannot well be exaggerated in securing a safer infancy and childhood. Although the argument cannot be developed here, an analysis of the factors which have reduced child sacrifice would be totally inadequate which left out of account our greater national sobriety. This is true, notwithstanding the still staggering facts concerning Bermondsey recently published by Dr. Albert Salter, M.P., for the borough. As a medical man, and otherwise, Dr. Albert Salter has for many years had intimate knowledge of its affairs; and, as a member of its rating assessment committee, he has been able to ascertain the total consumption of beer, spirits, and wine in the borough in a year. I give the final figures as he states them. In the year 1925 Bermondsey residents spent more on strong drinks than on bread, milk, rent, and taxes all put together. The exact figures are:—

	£
Alcoholic drink	1,350,000
Bread	230,000
Milk	182,000
House, rents, and taxes	742,000

This means that, in a year, 5,500,000 gallons of beer were consumed, and not quite 1,210,000 gallons of milk. For the 39,000 young children in the borough this meant a serious deprivation of what they need for satisfactory growth and development. The expenditure meant a *per capita* expenditure of over £11 a year, or for a family of man and wife and three children of £1 a week, which must be more than a fifth, and probably a fourth, of average weekly earnings. The hopeful features of this unnecessary expenditure are that it is less than formerly, and that something like half of it is due to the present higher taxation on alcoholic drinks.

In the light of these lurid social facts the decline of infant mortality in Bermondsey gives added importance and weight to the official and voluntary efforts to secure child welfare.

There is an excellent Tuberculosis Dispensary, with two whole-time medical officers and six tuberculosis nurses who carry out vigorously the functions attaching to this organisation. A new development has been the equipment of a solarium, where ultra-violet-therapy is largely utilised for tuberculous patients and for weakly infants and toddlers.

The M.O.H., Dr. King Brown, now retiring after many years of service, doubts whether the infant mortality rate can be brought below the figure 60, but in view of Swindon's present rate of 47 (p. 348), this statement is too pessimistic: certainly so, if the remaining incubus of alcoholic habits be removed or decreased.

Much good work is being done in providing dental treatment for poor mothers; two municipal dentists and several assistants are employed. This work has been carried on for seven years. The provision is in addition to that made by the L.C.C. for school children.

An assessment is made on patients, as also in the supply of milk. The scheme of assessment is based on the family net income. A large proportion of patients are treated at a merely nominal expense to them. Only a fraction of the toddlers needing dental treatment receive it, and the problem to be overcome is that of obtaining access to these, if the more advanced dental disease now found when school attendance begins is to be prevented.

There is much voluntary work in aid of the official hygienic agencies in Bermondsey. Among these is that of the District Nursing Association, which provides trained nurses for the sick poor in their own homes. In 1927 the Rotherhithe Association nursed 511 cases in this division of Bermondsey, paying 9,066 visits. Families in which the united family wages are under 40s. with children, or 35s. without children, are nursed gratuitously. For others a small charge is made, regulated by the amount of the weekly earnings of the united family.

SCHOOL MEDICAL WORK IN LONDON

The Education Act, 1902, transferred the control of elementary education from the *ad hoc* directly elected London School Board to the L.C.C., and made the County Council the education authority, thus adding greatly to its work as the chief metropolitan authority for sanitary and other purposes.

The present system of medical inspection and examination of school children in London as elsewhere in Britain has been built up and the treatment of defects discovered has been gradually increased, on the strength of the duties and powers conferred in the enactments quoted on page 197.

The magnitude of the work now being carried on may be inferred from the following statement of the professional staff engaged in it in 1928 :—

County Medical Officer and School Medical Officer,
Senior Medical Officer of School Division,
Chief Aurist (Principal Assistant M.O.),
Consulting Dental Surgeon (part-time),
Principal Assistant M.O. (part-time),
7 Divisional Medical Officers,
23 Assistant Medical Officers,
2 Assistant Aurists (half-time),
14 Assistant Medical Officers (6 sessions a week),
38 Assistant Medical Officers (3 sessions a week),
25 Temporary Medical Officers (part-time) for 11 sessions a week,
8 Medical Officers (part-time) at open-air and tuberculosis schools,
265 Surgeons and Anæsthetists at treatment Centres,
60 Inspecting Dentists (part-time).

In addition to the above, the school staff comprises also—

A second senior Medical Officer,
2 Consulting Surgeons (part-time)
1 Ophthalmic Consultant (part-time),
2 Divisional Medical Officers,

for examination of candidates, reference cases, Mental Deficiency Act cases, and cases under the Blind Persons Act.

In still another division several medical officers deal with laboratory work and with infectious disease administration.

The staff enumerated above would not be able to cope with the vast amount of medical work needed for three-quarters of a million school children did it not have the assistance of a very large body of voluntary workers, some of whose work is indicated on page 418. The amount of this voluntary help available in London is much greater than that which can be enlisted in most provincial areas.

Approximately one-half of the cost incurred in the work of the entire staff dealing with school hygiene is borne from national funds, and one-half from metropolitan rates imposed on the general public of London. Both, of course, are derived from the same source, but the expense of the two is differently distributed among the people. In London, in 1927, there were 970 elementary schools, and there were altogether 753,055 scholars in attendance at ages 3–14, of whom—

19·3 per cent. were aged 3–5 years,
20·4 per cent. were aged 5–7 years,
60·3 per cent. were aged 7–14 years.

The average attendance at these schools was about 88 per cent. of the number on the roll.

In addition, 1,280 children were on the roll of open-air schools, 115 on the roll of nursery schools, 273 in blind schools, and 836 in schools for the partially blind, 632 in schools for the deaf, 170 in schools for the partially deaf, and 10,326 in schools for physically defective and mentally defective children. The figures for higher education need not be given here.

During 1928, 207,254 routine inspections of children were made by the Council's medical officers, and, in addition, 37,650 children were inspected because of suspected illness or disability, and 2,036 were medically inspected at special schools. The total number of children medically inspected during the year was 357,424. In addition, every child in attendance is seen several times a year by the school nurse.

The Board of Education requires three medical inspections of each child during his school life. In London every scholar is medically inspected a fourth time when about to leave school. About one-third of the parents attend the examination of leaving boys, and nearly nine-tenths of parents attend the inspection of entrant infants. About 43 per cent. of the children examined in the three routine age periods of school life were found to need treatment. Many of these were referred for dental caries. Omitting these cases the proportion referred for the treatment of various ailments was 18·7 per cent.

Of the children examined in routine medical inspection the proportion found requiring treatment, omitting uncleanliness and dental disease, in the year 1927 was as follows:—

Age Group	Percentage Requiring Medical Treatment
Entrants	17·6
Age 8	21·6
Age 12..	21·5
Leavers (age 13¾)	18·3
In Total Elementary Schools	19·6
In Total Special Schools ..	19·0

The following is an incomplete list of defects found in the same year. Only a few of the largest items are given, and it will be borne in mind that one child may help to swell more than a single item on the list. Fuller particulars are given in the Annual Report of the M.O. to the L.C.C., page 172, year 1927, from which, and the report for 1928, most of the information in this chapter is derived.

ELEMENTARY SCHOOLS
Conditions Found to Require Treatment, 1927

	At Routine Inspections	At Special Inspections
Malnutrition	857	446
Cutaneous diseases	1,728	1,730
Defective vision (excluding squint) ..	20,873	3,520
Otitis media	1,939	908
Enlarged tonsils	10,057	2,630
Enlarged tonsils and adenoids ..	3,370	897
Dental disease	78,492	5,354
Tuberculosis	98	203
Deformities	916	272
All conditions requiring treatment ..	133,911	26,532

The extent to which treatment was secured for the defects found on inspection is shown on page 413.

The cleanliness work of the school nurses has outstanding value. During 1926 the school nurse made on an average six visits to each school, and examined at these visits 1,990,201 children, of whom 261,135 were uncleanly, and 105,570 were cleansed under the Council's arrangements.

In only 277 cases were legal proceedings required before cleansing could be secured.

Ringworm progressively diminishes in the schools as shown by the diagram on page 412, in which the 100 in 1919 implies 3,447 fresh cases, and the 20 in 1928 implies 684 fresh cases. In 1911 the number of fresh cases had been 6,214.

To attempt to particularise the different diseases and defects found in the course of inspection or otherwise among London school children would occupy more space than can be given. Full particulars are given in the Annual

Reports of the M.O. to the L.C.C. But as they have intimate
bearing on the relation between private and public medical

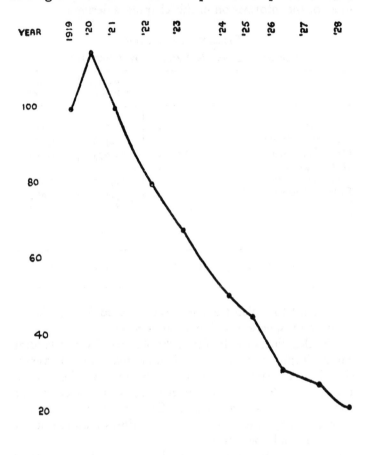

Decrease of Ringworm in London School Children

practice, we outline here the arrangements for giving treatment and set out in what circumstances payment for
treatment is expected.

TREATMENT BY THE SCHOOL AUTHORITY

In November 1909 the L.C.C. decided that in the treatment of school children presenting obvious defects when individually examined—that is, for every child in school three times during the nine years of school life—institutions already existing for the required purposes should be utilised, these institutions being given financial help when necessary in return for the treatment of school children. Agreements were entered into with a number of voluntary hospitals; and in districts where no hospitals were available it was

DEFECTS TREATED OR UNDER TREATMENT, 1927

	Under Council's Scheme	Otherwise
Ringworm of scalp	644	224
Other skin diseases	2,609	—
Eye diseases (excluding those mentioned below)		
Ear diseases (apart from operations and miscellaneous)	102,375	1,572
Errors of eye refraction, excluding operations for squint	38,000	1,593
Other eye defects	2,293	—
Defects of nose and throat	13,046	1,797[1]

generally found practicable to enter into agreements with voluntary local committees of medical practitioners, nursing associations, and dispensary and other committees for similar treatment. Arrangements of the second kind have been extended and amended.

In 1913 there were 28 centres at which treatment was provided for 73,000 cases,

In 1919 there were 53 centres at which treatment was provided for 160,000 cases.

At the end of 1921 the L.C.C.'s treatment scheme included 14 hospitals, 56 treatment centres, and a special dental centre; and in 1928 it included 17 hospitals and 68 centres.

[1] 1,692 at hospitals, 105 by private practitioners.

The bulk of treatment is carried out in the school treatment centres controlled by voluntary committees, the voluntary hospitals being unable, however willing, to cope with the mass of children's ailments calling for treatment. Furthermore, the treatment centres are more conveniently placed for children than the voluntary hospitals, these being situate chiefly in Central London.

The extent to which treatment by or on behalf of the Education Authority is effected is partially indicated in the table on page 413.

The special work done by the school dental service is shown below :—

Number of children inspected by the dentist, 226,146.
Found to require treatment, 158,992, or 70·1 per cent.
Actually treated, including re-treatment, 124,992, or 55·3 per cent.
Attendances by children for treatment, 206,663.
Fillings—Permanent teeth, 72,825.
         Temporary teeth, 354,152.
Administrations of general anæsthetics for extractions, 68,217.
Other operations, 24,994.

COMPARISONS OF RETURNS—DENTAL TREATMENT, 1912 AND 1927

Dental Treatment	1912 Six Centres	1927 Sixty-one Centres
New cases	9,799	124,992
Attendances	14,664	206,663
Teeth or Roots extracted	32,057	406,373
Extractions per child	3·26	3·24
Fillings	16,257	102,712
Fillings per child	1·65	0·82
Other operations	2,373	24,994
Other operations or treatments per child	0·23	0·18
General anæsthetics	2,533	63,635
Average operations per child ..	5·14	4·24
Operations per child compared with known incidence of caries	− 2·26	+ 0·85

In certain respects it is difficult to measure the increase in the medical care of school children, so much of it evades statistical analysis; but as regards dental care the table on page 414 is significant.

And that there has been improvement in the condition of the children's teeth is shown by the following diagram in which is shown, for the 12-year old group of boys, the proportion per cent. (lowest part of column) of children in whom no decayed teeth were seen, the number (dotted part) with not less than four carious teeth, and the shaded

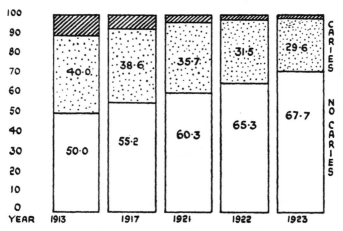

DENTAL CONDITION OF 12-YEAR OLD BOYS IN LONDON.
ELEMENTARY SCHOOLS

column showing the number with four or more carious teeth.

At present only half the school population is being dentally treated, and much educational work is needed still to overcome apathy or opposition on the part of many parents.

As yet there is no evidence of improvement of the dental condition of children on their entrance into school life, but that of school children is steadily improving, and this must be attributed chiefly to the official school dental service.

Many other branches of school medical work in London

would repay description. I must content myself with giving the following list of items, the work in connection with which is mentioned or described in the school section of the Annual Report of the M.O. of the L.C.C., 1927:—

Treatment of crippled children.
Arrangements for mentally defective children.
Care of rheumatic children and heart disease.
Classes for stammerers.
Convalescent homes and open-air schools.
Physical training of children and teaching of hygiene.
Cleansing arrangements.

THE LOCALISED SCHOOL TREATMENT CENTRES

The organisation of these localised treatment centres was undertaken by the local medical profession at the request of the London County Council. The doctors in a district formed themselves into a committee and manage each centre themselves. Initial grants were given to form these centres, and annual grants to maintain them, responsibility for the various kinds of work being adjusted among the doctors themselves, as well as the conditions of payment for it. In other instances when doctors could not make this provision, groups of charitable people organised committees to form and manage centres on similar terms. Dr. C. J. Thomas, of the L.C.C., gives the number of such centres at a recent date in London as 70, all voluntarily provided and managed, at which—

120,000 children annually receive dental treatment;
15,000 children attend in the throat, nose, and ear departments;
30,000 children have spectacles provided.

In addition, there are at these centres minor ailment departments where 90,000 children receive the daily attention of skilled nurses.

If parents cannot pay for spectacles, the cost is borne by voluntary spectacles associations working in connection with school care committees.

In 1921 the salaries of doctors and dentists attending at

treatment centres were modified in accordance with economic conditions, becoming as follows:—

Surgeons, £80 a year for one session of 2½ hours a week.
Anæsthetists, £75 a year for one session of 2½ hours a week.
Minor ailments doctors, £65 a year for one session of 2 hours a week.
Dentists, £60 a year for one session a week.

PAYMENTS OF PARENTS FOR MEDICAL TREATMENT

In 1926–27 parents contributed toward the treatment of their children the sum of £11,601, and this may be taken as approximately the amount contributed in other years.

Particulars of medical charges are embodied in the following extract from the regulations of the L.C.C. (Vol. II), E. 557.

CHARGES FOR MEDICAL AND DENTAL TREATMENT AND MINOR AILMENTS

(a) In accordance with the requirements of Section 81 of the Education Act, 1921, the following arrangements and charges shall be made in respect of the medical and dental treatment of children attending public elementary and day open-air schools:—

(i) Parents who, while not able to pay the fees of a private practitioner, are able and willing to pay the full cost of the medical or dental treatment of their children shall be enabled to do so.

(ii) The charges to be made to parents and guardians who do not pay the full cost to the council of the medical and dental treatment of children attending elementary schools, shall be:—

(1) Minor Ailments—no charge for the first period of a fortnight of treatment; thereafter 1s. for the first period of six months, and 1s. for each subsequent period of six months.

(2) All other cases, including dental cases, a charge of 2s., except that the charge shall be 1s. in those dental cases in which it is certified at the time of treatment that only slight treatment has been necessary.

(b) The charges specified in clause (a) of this regulation may be reduced from 2s. to 1s. in suitable cases, and may be remitted in full in respect of children whose parents have been ascertained to be necessitous by the children's care (school) committees or managing committees in the case of open-air schools; provided that, in those cases in which it is claimed that 2s. cannot be paid, the nurse at the centre may accept 1s. on account and inform the parents that inquiry will be made by the care committee into the family circumstances.

(c) In cases in which a certificate is produced to the effect that parents or guardians are regular subscribers to the Hospital Saturday Fund, the charges specified in clause (a) of this regulation may be reduced by 50 per cent. in the case of children attending public elementary schools and scholarship holders attending secondary schools and trade schools.

(d) In consideration of the payment by the Hospital Savings Association of a prescribed annual lump sum, the charges specified in clause (a) of this regulation shall be remitted in the case of children whose parents are subscribers to the association.

(e) The charges in respect of the medical or dental treatment of school children shall be collected, except in special cases, at the school treatment centres at the actual time of treatment. When this cannot be done, the charges shall be collected at the house of the parents or guardians by the school attendance officers.

VOLUNTARY AID TO SCHOOL MEDICAL WORK

A vast amount of assistance is given by an army of 5,000 to 6,000 voluntary workers, banded together as local care committees, without which the school medical service could scarcely accomplish much of its present work. The success of the work depends also largely on the co-operation of the teachers in each school and of the school attendance officers who visit absentees.

The opportunities for social contact with the children in school form perhaps the best means for giving the help which is needed to secure the integrity of healthy family life; and in bringing this about voluntary agencies have always been pioneers. The treatment of cripples in their hands proceeded far before it was undertaken also by public health and education authorities. The greatest advance is secured when voluntary and official agencies work hand in hand.

Success in school medical work depends on the extent to which children can be "followed up" and reinspected as needed. The vastness of the work may be gathered from some figures for 1924, when appointments were made for 146,394 children for dental treatment, 1,431,850 attendances were made at minor treatment centres, 12,980 appointments were kept at aural sessions, and 32,747 at refraction sessions. This was additional to the large numbers treated at general and special hospitals or during convalescence in the country through the aid of the Invalid Children's Aid Association and other voluntary organisations. A large part of this work of "following up" falls on the members of voluntary school care committees.

The success of "following up" is greatly helped by the invitation always given to parents to be present when their children are medically examined. Most parents are present, and the school nurse and representative of the school care committee, who are also there, at once get into touch with the mother.

This "following up" was admirably described as follows by Dr. C. J. Thomas, the M.O. of the L.C.C. in special charge of school medical work in London, in the Annual Report of the M.O. to the L.C.C. for 1920:—

The work of following up children suffering from minor defects is essentially one of education. It is tedious and prolonged, or never-ending. . . . There are those who would deal with the parents of children suffering from minor defects on a stern bureaucratic basis; they would have each child officially catalogued and enumerated, and would in a very short and prescribed time present a table in which should be shown each child accounted for either by the certificate of the school doctor that his edict has been complied with, or by the appearance of the parent as a unit in a statistically represented number of prosecution cases, some of which had undergone fines and some imprisonment. Such a system as this in London would inevitably defeat its aim; the London parent can be taught and, given time, can be persuaded—he cannot be driven. The fact that medical inspection in school is not compulsory of itself forbids such a system in dealing with those who voluntarily permit the examination of their children. Any manifestation of official overbearance would result in a wholesale withdrawal of children from the medical oversight in the schools which they are now enjoying. . . .

The duty of following-up has been delegated to the school

care committee, consisting of voluntary workers attached to every school. Each school care committee is given direct responsibility, and the whole of the school organisation, including teachers, attendance officers, organisers, and officials, is enjoined to give every aid to the voluntary workers in their devoted endeavours.

More recently Dr. Thomas, at a meeting of the International Conference of Social Work, Paris, August 1929, has elaborated his view of the right relation between voluntary and official workers in school medical work. He again stresses the point made above:—

In London alone is found an attempt to achieve the impossible and to weave an official system on a voluntary basis.

The London system, by its fundamental reliance upon voluntary effort, its eager acceptance of voluntary help and its subordination everywhere of the bureaucrat to the voluntary worker, has provided itself with a heart, as well as a brain, and presents the spectacle not of a machine, but of a living sentient organism.

This must, he rightly maintains, be associated with the condition that all social services in schools shall be carried out by the direction of the education authority, and in accordance with rules laid down by that authority.

A further condition ought to be fulfilled to ensure complete work. The family is one and indivisible: and the school social service must be closely interrelated to other social services in the same district. All social workers need to agree with the view that a disease or defect cannot be dealt with in isolation. This condition may be, and often is, a symptom a and consequence of an evil home environment: and medical treatment without an effort to combat parental ignorance or neglect, poverty, or insanitation, or alcoholic habits is doomed to partial failure.

In London the whole school medical service revolves around the care committee attached to each school, which is related to the Central Children's Care Sub-Committee of the Education Committee of the L.C.C. There are in London some 5,000 to 6,000 voluntary unpaid workers thus engaged.

Their utility is partially guaranteed, and indeed made possible, by the official workers associated with them, the voluntary workers being under the direction of a corps of trained organisers, who are salaried officials of the L.C.C. These are women who have taken diplomas in social science. They train new voluntary workers, and are always available to advise school care committees, and supplement their work. London is divided into twelve educational districts, in each of which there is an official district organiser, who directs the social services of the schools in her district and maintains relations on behalf of the children with the Poor-law Guardians, with the Tuberculosis Care Committees, and with the following, among other voluntary societies for helping children:—

The Invalid Children's Aid Association (I.C.A.A.),
The Society for the Prevention of Cruelty to Children (S.P.C.C.),
The Tuberculosis Care Committee,
The Children's Country Holidays Fund.

The success and continuity of this combination of voluntary and official workers depend in very large measure on the personality of the principal organiser, a lady who attends the Central Care Committee and is in direct touch with the education officer and the chief medical officer of the L.C.C.

SCHOOL NURSES

The work of the voluntary school committees is dependent, furthermore, on the work of the official nursing staff of the L.C.C. This includes one superintendent of school nurses, six divisional superintendents, and 350 nurses. A scholar may only come under medical supervision three times in his school life of nine or eleven years; but he is under the observation of the school nurse at least once every school term, or 27 to 33 times during his school life. The nurses discover many minor complaints which might otherwise be overlooked by teachers and not made the subject of special medical inspection. This is especially noteworthy in their discovery of otorrhœas, children found to have this being referred to the centre, where they are treated by ionisation or otherwise. The invaluable work of the nurses in securing body and head cleanliness, in the treatment of minor ailments, and in helping to "follow up" children needing treatment need not be further emphasised. A few words may be added as to

SCHOOL MEALS

These are commonly provided at schools for special children, at nursing schools, and open-air schools.

In 1925, 653,395 school dinners and 1,236,466 milk meals were provided, and the number of cod-liver oil "meals" was 179,363. These are always given on the recommendation of the school doctor, who keeps the child under observation. His weight is taken regularly by the school nurse.

Some payments are made by parents of non-necessitous children, and smaller amounts are obtained from parents of necessitous children in part payment for meals. In 1926–27 the total sum thus received was £39,892, of which about £32,000 was received from elementary and special schools (half of the total from each), and the rest from open-air schools. As to corresponding supply of milk and meals under maternity and child welfare schemes, see appropriate paragraphs.

TUBERCULOSIS

The administrative control of tuberculosis in London is somewhat involved. In the treatment and control of this disease the private practitioner must play an even more important part than in the control of acute infectious diseases of short duration which have natural limits to their course of a few days or weeks; and his relationship to the public health authority, and especially to its tuberculosis section, is delicate and liable to be associated with friction.

In London the practitioner is under a legal obligation to notify each case of tuberculosis to the borough M.O.H.

(one of 29 in London) as soon as he has determined its nature. In diagnosing his cases, he has available gratuitous assistance in at least two directions: (1) Any specimen of sputum will be examined and a reliable report sent to him from an official laboratory; and the specimen may be repeated from the same patient whenever required. (2) There is in each metropolitan borough a tuberculosis dispensary, to which is attached a whole-time tuberculosis medical officer, with whom gratuitous consultation can always be arranged, and, if needed, the aid of radiographic photographs can generally be invoked on the same terms. Furthermore, the practitioner is invited to allow family "contacts" with the notified patient to be examined by the tuberculosis officer, if he does not wish to undertake this task himself.

The Borough Councils and Tuberculosis Dispensaries

Only partial utilisation of the dispensaries as consultation centres has been made. The following gives a summary of specimen items extracted from an annual return made (for the year 1927) by the Ministry of Health, so far as it relates to London. Under each heading the figures given illustrate extreme cases in the 29 boroughs as compared with the average experience of London as a whole.

LONDON TUBERCULOSIS SCHEMES
Population, 1927: 4,541,000
A. Dispensaries

1. *Phthisis Death-rate:*
   (*a*) London 0·9, (*b*) Finsbury 1·6, (*c*) Hampstead 0·5 per 1,000 of population.

2. *Number of new cases of tuberculosis recorded in the year in the borough notification register per 100 deaths from tuberculosis:*
   (*a*) London 205, (*b*) Paddington 344, (*c*) Camberwell 169

3. *Number of cases of tuberculosis on the dispensary register on December 31st per 100 on the notification register:*
   (*a*) London 58, (*b*) Camberwell, 81 (*c*) Stepney 15.

4. *Number of contacts examined by the borough tuberculosis officer during the year per 100 deaths from tuberculosis:*
   (*a*) London 194, (*b*) Greenwich 385, (*c*) St. Pancras 92.

5. *Number of sputum examinations per 100 new cases and contacts examined:*
   (*a*) London 75, (*b*) Poplar 146, (*c*) Westminster 40.

6. *Number of X-ray examinations per 100 new cases and contacts examined:*
   (*a*) London 12, (*b*) Stepney 1, (*c*) Greenwich 43.

7. *Number of consultations at home, etc., per 100 deaths from tuberculosis:*
   (*a*) London 198, (*b*) Battersea 411, (*c*) Finsbury 50.

8. *Number of home visits by nurses or health visitors per 100 patients on dispensary register.*[1]
   (*a*) London 465, (*b*) Lewisham 243, (*c*) Chelsea 1,573.

9. *Number of insured patients on domiciliary treatment on December 31st per 100 insured persons on the dispensary register:*
   (*a*) London 57, (*b*) Stepney 78, (*c*) Chelsea 10.

B. INSTITUTIONAL TREATMENT

	London	England and Wales
Average number of beds available per 100 deaths from tuberculosis	61	58
Number of patients treated excluding observation cases per 100 deaths from tuberculosis ..	114	119
Percentage of pulmonary patients who were described on admission as T.B.	18·8	40·9
T.B. Group I	5·7	8·2
II	51·4	30·0
III	24·1	20·9

It will be useful to comment on this statement here. A similar statement for England is discussed on page 223. Under each heading the average experience of London as a whole is

[1] These figures are not strictly comparable owing to different classifications·

given first: then the two extremes in the experience of the 29 metropolitan boroughs are stated. Thus the phthisis death-rate which averaged 0·9 per 1,000 in the metropolis was 1·6 in Finsbury and only 0·5 in Hampstead. Taking the second heading, one wonders what differences of activity of administration, or of actual disease or discovery of disease, are represented by the contrast between Camberwell and Paddington. The differences between St. Pancras and Greenwich in respect of contacts examined should cause heartsearching in the former borough. Whether under the fifth heading the fewer sputa examined in Westminster imply slacker methods can only be surmised in the absence of local intensive inquiry. The vast variation in the utilisation of radiography in diagnosis is not surprising for so novel an auxiliary in diagnosis. But the varying number of consultations in different dispensaries speaks volumes as to the degree of friendliness established between the official medical staff and the doctors in the borough. Home visits to patients vary greatly, so likewise does the proportion between dispensary cases and total notified cases in the borough. It is remarkable that a poorest borough has the smallest proportion of dispensary cases. In the Ministry of Health's statement from which the above extracts have been made there is added the hope that the statement will be—

of use in considering whether their schemes for the treatment of tuberculosis need revision in any respects in order to secure the most efficient arrangements and full value for the money expended for that purpose.

The following statement abstracted from the Annual Report of the M.O. of the County of London for 1928 shows the total number of cases of tuberculosis dealt with in the 27 boroughs and the City of Westminster.

At the beginning of the year the number of patients on the dispensary registers of these municipalities was:—

Cases with diagnosis completed 23,466
Cases under observation 1,125

During the year the following new cases came under dispensary observation:—

Pulmonary tuberculosis	..	{ Adults	.. 3,681
		{ Children	.. 156
Non-pulmonary tuberculosis		{ Adults	.. 316
		{ Children	.. 457
Doubtfully tuberculous	..	{ Adults	.. 1,443
		{ Children	.. 598
Non-tuberculous	.. ..	{ Adults	.. 4,774
		{ Children	.. 4,313
			15,738

Total number (including contacts) under dispensary supervision during 1928 49,600

A large amount of good work is being done, but it remains inadequate. The work is still more inadequate for cases not seen at the dispensaries.

The following additional items are important. Home visits for dispensary purposes made by the—

Tuberculosis officers	..	..	6,706
Dispensary nurses ..	..	..	99,685

Thus home visits by the tuberculosis officer were equal nearly to two for each notified case of pulmonary tuberculosis: and the proportion for nurses was nearly twelve home visits during the year for every case dealt with at the dispensaries.

The number of specimens of sputum examined was 17,179, which is about one for every new case and contact examined during the year.

There are 41 medical tuberculosis officers in London, all except nine being whole-time doctors. They are clinically in control of the official tuberculosis organisation, while the M.O.H. of the borough is the administrative chief. The efficiency and completeness of the preventive measures against tuberculosis vary from borough to borough. In some boroughs there has been inadequate co-ordination between the dispensary and the health department of the borough, and the M.O.H. and tuberculosis officer act or possibly remain partially inactive separately from each other. There has also often been insufficient co-operation between the dispensary service and the school medical service. Nor can it be said that the tuberculosis officer in every instance has obtained and maintained personal touch with the medical practitioners in his area. But all these statements are relative, and there is steady improvement.

Co-operating with Private Practitioners

The main objects of the dispensary are diagnostic and consultative, and the success of the work depends largely on the degree in which the co-operation of private practitioners is secured.

One great difficulty is due to the vastness of London, and to the somewhat rigid separation of the dispensary organisation (borough) and the residential institutional organisation (county council). The general lack of observation beds to which tuberculosis officers can have access is especially felt. It will probably be remedied ere long.

In the "scheme for the treatment of tuberculosis in London" (revised 1922), prepared by the County Council and specifying the treatment to be carried out at the municipal dispensaries, it is stated that treatment at the dispensary as distinguished from diagnosis "shall as a rule be limited to patients whose continued treatment requires special knowledge or technical skill, and to those unable to obtain adequate medical attendance". Routine and continuous treatment is deprecated. It is added that—

patients who require treatment which can, consistently, be properly undertaken by a general practitioner of ordinary professional competence and skill, and who are either insured persons or can afford to pay for medical attendance, should not attend the dispensary for routine treatment.

The reference to insured persons who form one-third of the total population will be noted. As to these, see page 225.

The provision of dentures comes within the functions of

the dispensary medical service, when in the opinion of the tuberculosis officer their supply will materially conduce to the patient's recovery.

THE COUNTY COUNCIL AND INSTITUTIONAL TREATMENT OF TUBERCULOSIS

During 1928, deaths from pulmonary tuberculosis in London numbered 3,985. The number of adult applicants for residential treatment was 5,735, of whom 5,113 were accepted. These arrangements are organised by the medical staff of the London County Council.

Of the applicants

1,258 went to "observation" beds to determine the diagnosis, or to determine suitability for sanatorium treatment;
3,855 went direct to a sanatorium or hospital;
337 for various reasons failed to enter institutions; and
21 were awaiting vacancies at the end of the year.

The number of children recommended for sanatorium treatment under the Council's scheme has increased from 865 in 1923 to 1,081 in 1928. Of the last number 1,048 were accepted for treatment. The County Council's Education Committee have also six open-air schools for tuberculous children.

Besides official tuberculosis institutions, there are also several special non-official (voluntary) consumption hospitals (Brompton, Victoria Park, etc.), some of them with important sanatoria in the country which provide for many metropolitan cases of tuberculosis.

Furthermore—and in my view most important of all from the standpoint of preventive medicine—there is the accommodation for the hospital treatment of acute and especially of advanced and bedridden consumptives, who are the least able to dispose of their sputum satisfactorily, and who commonly live in crowded domestic rooms. This need in large measure has been met, for many years, in London and in the rest of the country, by poor-law infirmaries, and is being more satisfactorily met year by year. In

London more than half the deaths from pulmonary tuberculosis occur in hospitals (poor-law institutions, general and special hospitals, and asylums), the majority of these patients continuously or intermittently remaining in these institutions for long months before their death. Most of these patients spend a large proportion of their life-time of open tuberculosis in institutions. That this is a very large factor in the diminution of continuous massive infection of relatives and others, is too often overlooked. No recent return is available, but the following figures, taken from a report of the Public Health Committee of the County Council (July 1, 1920), may be taken as substantially correct for to-day.

In 1911, when a return was available, there were not less than 2,000 beds for tuberculous patients in the 29 London poor-law infirmaries. Accommodation was dislocated by war conditions; but in August 1919 there were beds in these infirmaries for 1,300 tuberculous cases, and at the end of 1919 it was estimated that the following number of beds were available in London, of which about 2,000 were in poor-law infirmaries.

Provided by	Beds Provided
Voluntary agencies in general and special hospitals and homes (not exclusively for London cases) ..	1,532
Poor-law infirmaries (now L.C.C.)	2,000
Metropolitan Asylums Board (now L.C.C.) ..	1,868
TOTAL	5,400

This is little more than one bed per 1,000 of population, an inadequate proportion for metropolitan needs.

The readjustment of official hospital provision in London following the transference of the work of the Boards of Guardians to the London County Council renders it practicable to utilise beds in the municipal hospitals (previously poor-law infirmaries) for the treatment of tuberculosis more fully and effectively than at present, including the provision of "observation" beds.

FINANCING OF TUBERCULOSIS ADMINISTRATION

The finance of all public medical work on tuberculosis rests with the County Council, which contributes to the 29 borough councils a share of their approved net expenditure on the dispensary organisation. This expenditure includes not only the cost of dispensary maintenance, including doctors and nurses, but also such expenditure as that on sputum flasks and paper handkerchiefs given to patients.

The County Council also organise post-graduate courses for tuberculosis officers, and "refresher" courses for tuberculosis visitors and nurses.

CONTRIBUTIONS BY PATIENTS

No charge is made for diagnosis and treatment at the tuberculosis dispensaries. For residential institutions the following scale is adopted. In the official regulations of the L.C.C. (London County Council) it is laid down that:—

ADULTS.—A contribution towards the cost of treatment shall be assessed, *if the circumstances of the case appear to justify the demand*, on—

1. The patient, or the person legally responsible for the patient, in receipt of an income not less than £160 a year.
2. The patient, having no dependents, and in receipt of an income less than £160 a year. Provided that no contribution shall be assessed on or in respect of (*a*) any insured person whose income is the main support of the family, and will be sensibly reduced while he is undergoing treatment, or (*b*) any ex-service man in respect of whom the Ministry of Pensions defrays the cost of treatment.

CHILDREN.—A small contribution, roughly equivalent to the *cost of maintenance of a child at home*, shall be assessed, if the circumstances of the case appear to justify the demand, on the parents or guardians of children dealt with under the Council's scheme.

The amounts received are small. For the maintenance of children in sanatoria, in each of the years 1926–27 and 1927–28, about £4,700 was collected for the whole of

London. Some further amounts are collected from the parents of children treated in special institutions.

The assessment for payment for both adult and child patients is fixed by a *local tuberculosis care committee* after considering the individual case. It is laid down in the scheme that any contributions made by patients or their relatives in respect of residential treatment shall be devoted to:—

1. Convalescent treatment of children;
2. Accessories to treatment and after-care of children; or
3. Any other purposes which may be determined by the Council in respect to the care of children suffering or suspected to be suffering from or predisposed to tuberculosis, or the after-care of child patients.

Under this heading help has been given in boarding out children living in contact with patients suffering from advanced pulmonary tuberculosis.

Payments are made by patients attending a tuberculosis dispensary, only when dentures are provided for a patient on recommendation of the tuberculosis officer. In such cases the help of the Voluntary Care Committee is again invoked, in determining a change appropriate to the patient's means.

Tuberculosis Care Committees

The County Council have made valuable use of the Invalid Children's Aid Association, which is concerned in securing treatment and convalescent care for sick children. In their scheme they also recommend that a care committee should be organised in connection with each borough dispensary to act as the organising centre of measures auxiliary to treatment. This committee is composed of official and voluntary workers, the voluntary workers predominating. The chief function of this committee is not the assessment of contributions by patients for residential treatment or for dentures, but—

to consider the economic position of the family of every patient suffering from tuberculosis as soon as he comes within the purview of the dispensary scheme, and to render such advice and assistance as the circumstances of the case dictate, with a view to enabling the family to adjust their circumstances to the new conditions, to maintain their economic independence, and to derive the fullest possible advantage from the medical treatment prescribed.

By the help of these committees children can be provided for during the stay of the mother in a sanatorium, help is given to families during the absence of the breadwinner, and in various other ways, as, for instance, in obtaining suitable occupation for the ex-patient.

Further comments on the treatment of tuberculosis are made in the general discussion for England as a whole. It is evident that in London a vast amount of valuable work is being done. Recent reforms in London local government will make much better work practicable. Closer co-operation between the borough councils and the County Council will be facilitated: the borough tuberculosis officers should be enabled to have observation beds; and the entire transfer of medical, including tuberculosis, work from poor-law authorities to the public health authority of London simplifies and greatly increases the possibilities of success. With such a large unit as London, however, there will still remain the possibility of ineffective working unless the borough medical officer of health and the borough tuberculosis officer are very intimately related to the central public health administration for London.

VENEREAL DISEASES

In November 1916 the London County Council initiated their scheme, based on the Government's regulations of the preceding February. This, with amendments and additions, is still functioning actively. This scheme had regard to the fact that London is the hospital centre for a large area outside the metropolis, and that a satisfactory scheme must provide treatment also for a large part of this external population. This was facilitated by two important provisos in the Government scheme for the whole country: (1) three-fourths of any expense incurred in the initiated treatment would fall on the imperial taxes, and only a fourth on the local taxes (rates); (2) the payment of the fourth part would be allocated on a *per capita* per patient arrangement between the local authorities whose inhabitants used a given treatment centre wherever situated. This second arrangement followed naturally from the condition laid down in the regulations that any person was at liberty to apply for treatment, whatever his financial position, and that this treatment must be given under conditions ensuring reasonable privacy and secrecy. It was found practicable for the L.C.C. to arrange for the councils of the counties of Buckingham, Essex, Hertford, Kent, Middlesex, and Surrey, and of the county boroughs of Croydon, East Ham, and West Ham, all bordering on London, to obtain the common facilities provided in a considerable number (at first 27) of voluntary metropolitan hospitals, both for in-patients and out-patients. The population thus served is approximately 8 millions. The same hospitals provided all laboratory facilities required in diagnosis and treatment (except for Kent) for the same wide areas. Mutually satisfactory financial arrangements were made by the L.C.C. with these hospitals. The hospitals also supplied salvarsan gratuitously to medical practitioners showing competence for its use in their private practice. The total expense of these arrangements and of educational work was paid by the State and the County of London in the proportions already stated, the outside authorities paying their share according to the number of patients from their areas treated in metropolitan hospitals.

Bearing in mind that the figures probably include a considerable proportion of extra-metropolitan patients, the following table shows the amount and increase in the amount of London's action between 1917 and 1927. The treatment, as already indicated, is given mainly at the various general and a few special voluntary hospitals, the staff of which (or the hospital) is being paid on an arranged scale for the services rendered to the London County Council.

	1917		1927
	Actual Number	Ratio (1917=100)	Actual Number
New cases treated in each year—			
Venereal	13,025	145	18,801
Non-venereal	2,360	431	10,164
In-patient days	63,932	176	112,413
Attendances	120,659	634	767,278
Pathological examinations—			
For treatment centres ..	13,988	767	107,512
For private practitioners ..	3,649	741	27,046
Medical practitioners receiving gratuitous supply of arseno-benzol preparations ..	108	—	446[1]

In the following diagram the course of events year by year since the national scheme came into operation in London is shown by relative figures. (The numbers represented by these figures can be ascertained by reference to the above table.)

It will be noted that there is some decline in the number of new venereal disease cases in recent years, though this appears to be having a check; the increase in number of in-patient days shows a more satisfactory treatment of severe cases.[2] The fact that the number of attendances has increased vastly, while the number of patients has not increased, is valid evidence of the increasing success in securing more protracted and thereby more efficient treatment. The great increase in patients who suspect they are—but are not—suffering from venereal disease gives further assurance that the treatment centres are more and more meeting with success.[3] A further satisfactory feature is the increasing resort

[1] There are 8,243 doctors entered as living in London. Many of these are retired, and many more would not undertake the treatment of syphilis.
[2] For special reasons the figures for 1929 are not quite comparable with those for earlier years.
[3] The reader should refer to the table on this page for the figures on which the diagram on page 435 is based. It must not be assumed erroneously that more non-venereal than venereal patients come to the clinics for treatment.

to gratuitous examination of pathological products (for spirochætes, Wassermann test, gonococci), eight times as

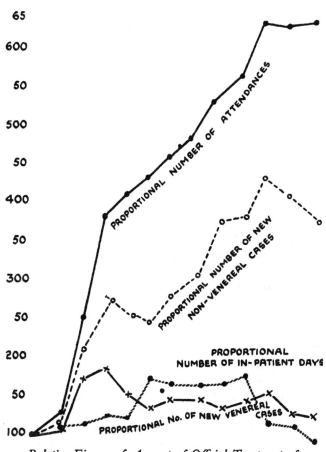

Relative Figures of Amount of Official Treatment of Venereal Diseases in London, 1917–29.

many specimens being examined in 1927 as in 1917 for treatment centres, and nine times as many for private practitioners.

Details cannot be given here of the linking up of maternity and child welfare work with that of the treatment centres. Although valuable work is being done in a few centres, there is great need for more general work for the discovery and treatment of syphilis in young children, in the pregnant mother, and especially for increased activity in the examination of mothers who have had still-born children. This will only be possible with the active co-operation of private doctors. A special phase of good work is the reception of patients for treatment in seven hostels, in addition to the treatment of venereal patients in the 24 metropolitan hospitals utilised in the general scheme. At these hostels female patients live who cannot arrange satisfactory routine treatment in their lodgings. Voluntary workers undertake the management of these hostels, the cost of which is paid out of official funds. In addition, at five of the above hospitals and at a separate clinic all-day clinics are now maintained, where patients can be treated gratuitously at any hour.

Subsidised by the L.C.C., lectures and addresses on various aspects of sex problems are given, and various publications are issued and films shown by the British Social Hygiene Council, acting as an indirect official agency. Notices are affixed in various public places warning as to venereal disease and stating where satisfactory confidential treatment can be had gratuitously.

The public-spirited action of the general medical profession, as voiced by the British Medical Association, in endorsing the facilities for the diagnosis and treatment of venereal disease of all applicants without distinction at the public expense has already been stated (p. 231). It should be added that, although the Government's regulations (under which the L.C.C. and other authorities arrange their venereal disease treatment schemes) prescribe that treatment must not be refused to any applicant, the medical officers of these treatment centres may properly suggest that patients, who are in good financial position and can obtain satisfactory treatment from their own doctors, should do so.

It may also be noted that the provision of free treatment under this official scheme does not apply to general paresis, to locomotor ataxy, or to other of the later non-communicable forms of disease.

In the London scheme it is specified that each hospital participating shall provide facilities for the instruction of medical practitioners and medical students free of charge. Too little advantage has been taken of these facilities: the medical practitioners are too busy, and the students' curriculum is too crowded. This tends increasingly to segregate the treatment of these diseases from ordinary practice.

In the original scheme of the Local Government Board, it was found necessary to limit the free distribution of salvarsan to private practitioners who were on the permanent staff of a hospital or who had a certificate of having attended a course of special instruction at a venereal disease centre, or who otherwise produced satisfactory evidence of experience in intravenous injections: and similar restrictions are still maintained.

The remuneration of medical officers in charge of venereal disease clinics varies according to the special views of each hospital staff from nil to four guineas a session. At St. Thomas's Hospital, where a clinic is in session each weekday from 8 a.m. to 10 p.m., the medical officer is paid on a whole-time basis. The British Medical Association have expressed the view that a payment of three guineas per session would be reasonable.

PART III
SCOTLAND

CHAPTER XXI

GENERAL ADMINISTRATION[1]

PRELIMINARY SUMMARY

The account of Scottish medical work, private and public, does not lend itself to satisfactory summary in a few lines; but some outstanding points may be mentioned in this incomplete précis.

Most of Scotland's special official medical activities are similar to those in England. The differences, and the recent changes, are indicated in the text.

Special attention may be drawn to the efforts for co-ordination of voluntary and official hospital work now in progress.

The medical side of sickness insurance work presents admirable as well as defective features, which are described on pages 454 to 470. There is too much "rush" work, and there exists the defective co-ordination with the out-patient work in voluntary hospitals which can be seen elsewhere. This should have been reduced by insurance medical work.

The medical service for the Highlands and Islands of Scotland is an important national contribution for providing medical care to remote districts in which, apart from the subsidies from national funds, this care would have been deficient or absent.

In Aberdeen there have been valuable advances towards unification of the public medical services of the city and county, both as regards hospital and consultative work. The hospital beds of municipal and public assistance hospitals, as well as of voluntary hospitals, have been made available for the training of medical students. Here and in other parts of Scotland there is a large measure of gratuitous provision of laboratory facilities for medical practitioners.

In Perthshire local bed-side nurses are employed also as public health nurses, and the combination works well and economically in its sparsely peopled districts.

[1] Date of investigation, September 1929.

In the royal burgh of St. Andrews there is an exceptional amount of co-operation between private practitioners and the child welfare centre, a complete record of each child's health status being thus secured.

Glasgow presents vast problems in its teeming population, densely housed and often extremely poor. Admirable work is being done in steadily improving its medical services. Owing to its large proportion of poor and of medically insured persons, there is relatively little friction as to the respective spheres of private and public medical work.

Details of the work of national insurance in Glasgow are given on pages 464 to 470.

In Glasgow, as in Aberdeen, there is already active co-operation between voluntary and official hospital services.

CENTRAL GOVERNMENT

In most respects the methods of central and local government in Scotland are substantially identical with those of England. Scotland has a large measure of Home Rule. The Scottish Department of Health in Edinburgh takes the place of the Ministry of Health in London; and this Department, like other Scottish Departments for various branches of administration, is under the Secretary for Scotland, who is a member of the British Government of cabinet rank. Scotland (Census, 1931) had a population of 4,842,544, of which 1,088,417 dwell in the city of Glasgow.

The Department of Health for Scotland is concerned with various branches of sanitation, such as control of food, supply, housing, river pollution, etc., and with the following medical services in which we are interested:—

> The Poor Law Medical Service.
> Public Health Medical Services, including—
>> Acute Infectious Diseases,
>> Tuberculosis,
>> Syphilis and Gonorrhœa,
>> Maternity Service and Child Welfare,
>> Special Medical Service for the Highlands and Islands.
> National Health Insurance.
> Medical Inspection of School Children.

A few points concerning each of these services may be noted. The insurance service will be described more fully.

Before giving some particulars of these various medical services, a paragraph is needed on—

SCOTTISH LOCAL AUTHORITIES

Relief of the destitute in Scotland has been administered by its 869 parish councils, the same number as the civil parishes into which the country is divided. There are 201 burghs in Scotland, all of which have had hitherto some measure of separate local government for public health work, etc.

In addition, there are 33 civil counties, which are responsible for the public health medical services outside the burghs. These counties are usually divided into districts, served by district committees, the latter administering public health and other services within their respective areas.

For education, including the medical inspection of school children, there have been 33 county education authorities, including all the burghs in the county areas, only the large cities of Glasgow, Edinburgh, Dundee, and Aberdeen having an education authority of their own.

A local insurance committee exists for each burgh with a population of 20,000 or over, of which there are 23, and for each county area (including all the small burghs therein), of which there are 31.

There are also 27 district boards of control, which have been formed for single large parishes or for combinations of parishes. These are responsible for the administration of the Lunacy and Mental Deficiency Acts. They are not, however, under the supervision of the Department of Health for Scotland, but of the General Board of Control for Scotland, which, in turn, is responsible to the Secretary of State for Scotland.

By the Local Government (Scotland) Act, 1929, parish councils, district committees of county councils, district boards of control, and education authorities have been abolished. Except in the four large cities, which have already education authorities, education is transferred to the county councils, while burghs under 20,000 of population retain only minor health functions, the major services being taken over by the counties. Burghs over 20,000 population continue to administer all the public health services at present vested in them.

A new body, the "District Council", is set up by the Act for the non-burghal (Landward) districts of counties, and they may exercise within their district, as agents for the county council, such duties in regard to poor-law, public health, lunacy, and mental deficiency as may be referred to them by the county council. Similar duties may also be devolved upon the town councils of small burghs which have not been abolished, but whose powers and duties have been restricted to minor administrative matters.

Local authorities are and will continue to be empowered to combine for the purposes of any scheme under the Health and other Acts.

From April 1930 the number of Local Government Authorities in Scotland is as follows :—

County councils (reconstituted) 31
Town councils of large burghs, containing population of over 20,000, and including the cities of Glasgow, Edinburgh, Dundee, and Aberdeen 23
Town councils of small burghs 173
District councils of non-burghal (Landward) districts of counties .. .. (*not yet fixed*)

Past and future administration may be illustrated by the conditions in the county of Perth :—

Past Administration

The population for the whole county area numbered at the 1921 census 125,503
    of which there were resident in burghs .. 57,698
    and in non-burghal areas 67,805

Number of civil parishes in county (total population, 125,5 3) 71

Number of burghs within county:—
1. With population over 20,000 (city of Perth, 33,208)   I
2. With population under 20,000 (total populations, 24,490)   II
                           — 12

County council   I
Number of district committees (total population, 67,805)   5
Number of education authorities (whole area)   I
Number of insurance committees   2
Number of district boards of control (whole area) ..   I

Administration after Reconstitution

County council—
  (*a*) For education (population, 125,503) .. .. ..⎱
  (*b*) For major health services, etc. (population, 92,295) ..⎰ I
Town councils of large burghs (city of Perth)   I
Small burghs   II
District councils   (*number not fixed*)
Insurance committees   2

The district committees in Perthshire, as in other counties, consisted of the county councillors for their own geographical part of the county, and of a member nominated from each parish in the district. This is an instance of partial indirect election of which examples are to be found in American experience.

While the district committees have now disappeared, small burghs obtain representation on the reconstituted county councils, but will only have a vote in connection with matters in which the county council are entitled to exercise their functions within the burgh.

In future, in Perthshire and throughout Scotland, the county councils will control all the sanitary and medical services, except a few minor services which will be left to the small burghs. Education (including medical inspection of school children) has hitherto been under a separate directly elected education authority for the entire county of Perth, including the city of Perth. It now becomes part of the work of the county council, under an education committee. A similar arrangement applies throughout Scotland. In the town of Perth, however, and also in all burghs in other counties with a population exceeding 20,000, the local public health authority retains control of medical services; though in school medical work there will be co-operation with the medical work of the county council.

The large cities, Glasgow, Edinburgh, Aberdeen, and Dundee, control all their sanitary and medical services through their town councils.

By the new Act of 1929 the final step has been taken to make each large local authority (county council and large city) the local parliament for all branches of local government. These will be:—

Poor-Law Administration.
Public Health Administration.
Education Administration.
Lunacy and Mental Deficiency Administration.

Each of these functions is now controlled by committees of the county or city council, subject only on matters of high policy and finance to the control of the entire council.

It will be noted that the local (county or city) control of the working of the National (Health) Insurance Act is not included in this unification of local government under a local parliament. It was recommended by a Royal Commission; but perhaps it is well—in view of the complex problems involved—that this final stage in unification should be deferred to a later period.

Insurance at present only extends to the employed population, and its cost is met out of contributions by employer and employee and the State. If insurance medical benefits are ever extended to the dependents of the insured, then it will become practicable to lift these benefits out of the insurance scheme altogether and to incorporate them with the medical services now administered by the reconstituted local authorities.

Poor-Law Medical Work

Domiciliary medical service is carried out by salaried medical officers, most of whom are engaged also in private and insurance medical practice. Indoor medical service is mainly given by whole-time medical officers. Poor-law infirmaries in many districts have greatly improved in quality, and their municipalisation will doubtless lead to further progress. The case of Aberdeen is given in some detail on page 490.

TUBERCULOSIS

Under this heading some details are given as to the areas visited by me. Institutional provision is made by both public health and poor-law authorities, a position which will now be rectified. The general position as regards notification of cases, tuberculosis dispensaries, hospitals, and sanatoria is not very dissimilar from that in England.

VENEREAL DISEASES

As in England, the most important feature has been "the provision of gratuitous, efficient, convenient, and secret treatment to all persons suffering or suspecting themselves to be suffering from venereal disease, who desire such advice and treatment". This has been associated with education of the people as to the prevalence and dangers and means of prevention of these diseases.

Centres for treatment have been provided in the large towns and some smaller towns, altogether more than 40. In Glasgow there are 16 approved centres, in Edinburgh 7, in Dundee 3, and in Aberdeen 2. Usually these centres are at voluntary general hospitals. In 1924, in all the centres officially recognised, 260 hospital beds were set apart for patients with these diseases. This is an incomplete statement, as many of the later manifestations of syphilis are treated in the ordinary wards. Free examination of pathological specimens is provided for all doctors. In 1927—

1,102 examinations were made for spirochætes,
23,202 examinations were made for gonococci, and
10,643 examinations were made for Wassermann tests.

That the centres are necessary and doing good work is becoming increasingly recognised. The treatment of venereal diseases in ordinary medical practice is unsatisfactory. The ninth Annual Report of the Scottish Board of Health for 1927 refers to the disquieting reports received from various centres regarding patients who had previously received private treatment that can only be described as inefficient; and particulars of such cases are given. In a report of this Board the following statement is made:—

Until the private doctor is able to treat with confidence and efficiency the ordinary forms of venereal disease, and to recognise as cases that should properly be transferred to a specialist, those that are unusually perplexing, aberrant, or obscure . . . it is eminently desirable that practitioners should refrain from dealing with cases that they have reason to think may be beyond their competence and skill, but should without hesitation pass them on to the clinics.

On the other hand, the medical officers of the clinics are urged and do, in fact, "keep in close touch with doctors sending cases to them". Thus in the Scottish Report for 1927 it is added:—

Nothing will more encourage the doctor in private practice to send cases to the clinic . . . than the knowledge that he will duly receive from the clinic information as to the conditions found and the treatment prescribed. At the same time, the patient should be encouraged to regard the treatment at the centre as having been done for him at the instance of his own doctor, to whose care he may return as improvement takes place. Of course, it is necessary to make sure that the suggested communication be made only to the patient's private practitioner and with the patient's consent.

One-third of the population, and probably an equal proportion of venereal cases, would be under the care of insurance doctors in the absence of venereal disease clinics. These doctors usually are more than willing to transfer their venereal patients, and a large number of doctors express their dislike for this class of cases. Some concern is being expressed as to the large proportion of "defaulters" at special V.D. clinics, namely patients who cease treatment before being medically certified as "cured"; and there is increasing demand for greater control over such defaulters.

ACUTE INFECTIOUS DISEASES

By the Scottish Public Health Act public health authorities are under an obligation to provide hospital accommodation for infectious diseases, and the position in England has recently been assimilated to this. Hospital provision for these diseases throughout Scotland is generally regarded as being adequate to the needs of the population.

MATERNITY AND CHILD WELFARE SERVICES

Of the births in Scotland nearly 40 per cent. are attended by midwives. Some details as to midwives are given in the local accounts, pages 482, 505, and 519. Under the terms of the Midwives and Maternity Homes (Scotland) Act, 1927, an obligation is imposed on any local supervising authority for midwives which has not in operation a maternity and child welfare work scheme to supply, after reasonable notice, a doctor or midwife to attend a woman in childbirth. Thus, as stated in the Scottish Board's Report for 1927, "every expectant mother in Scotland has now these services available to her during her confinement".

There are 4,525 practising midwives in Scotland, including those employed in institutions. These in 1926 attended 30,858 out of the total 92,581 total births in areas from which returns had been received by the Central Midwives Board for Scotland. The total births in Scotland were 96,669. In about one-fifth (6,366 cases) of the midwives' cases, a doctor was called in for help, mostly for delayed labour.

In 1927, in the whole of Scotland, there were 136 whole-time health visitors employed exclusively in maternity and child welfare work. In addition, 379 district nurses acted as part-time health visitors; while 62 whole-time health visitors had other duties in addition to those under this heading.

In 1926 health visitors made 786,341 home visits, 23,283 of which were made to expectant mothers, the balance being made to children. Nearly 75 per cent. of the children born during the year were visited soon after birth by health visitors, and on an average 5 revisits were made to each infant before it reached 1 year of age. In addition, there was some antenatal supervision of mothers representing 9 per cent. of the total births in Scotland.

One hundred and ninety-four maternity and child welfare centres have been provided by local authorities in Scotland, and the number of attendances at these centres in 1926 was 448,695.

Further particulars of these and allied services are given under local headings.

Further significant figures may be quoted as indicating the importance of pre-school supervision of children. According to the official report for 1927 of the Scottish Board, only 7·3 per cent. of the children aged 1–5 were visited at home. Of children suffering from middle-ear disease who attended Glasgow centres :—

In 48 per cent. the disease began in the 1st year of life;
In 27 per cent. the disease began in the 2nd year of life;
In 25 per cent. the disease began in the 3rd and 5th years of life.

School Medical Service

Prior to 1918 there were 79 separate school boards, but in that year, while their *ad hoc* character was maintained, 37 education authorities were constituted, one for each county. These were merged with county and city public health authorities in May 1930. In 1927 there were 3,411 State-aided schools, having 830,060 pupils in average attendance. At the end of 1927 these educational authorities employed :—

37 Chief school medical officers (S.M.O.), of whom 21 were also county M.O.H.
52 Whole-time and 12 part-time assistant S.M.O.
50 Part-time local practitioners.
43 Whole-time and 37 part-time dentists.
166 Whole-time school nurses, 29 school nurses doing other public work, and 471 district nurses doing part-time school work.

In addition, arrangements have been made for the following specialist services:—

30 Authorities employ 39 eye specialists.
11 Authorities employ 16 ear, nose, and throat specialists.
2 Authorities employ 3 skin specialists.
1 Authority employs 1 X-ray specialist.
1 Authority employs 1 orthopædic surgeon.
1 Authority employs 1 medico-psychologist.

A number of "minor ailment clinics" have been established. In these clinics in Lanarkshire 3,508 children were treated, and 29,290 attendances were made. There is a general consensus of opinion that, aside from their other benefits, these minor, ailment clinics "reduce very substantially the enormous burden of absenteeism".

Drug treatment of ringworm, etc., is provided by 22 out of 37 education authorities, and X-ray treatment by 18.

Twenty-six education authorities have made arrangements for the operative treatment of tonsils and adenoids.

Most education authorities have adopted schemes of dental treatment, and some treatment of eye refraction cases is effected. Some particulars are given under the local headings.

SCOTTISH HOSPITAL SERVICES

As already noted, hospital provision has been made both by the Poor-Law and the Public Health Authorities, the former for non-infectious diseases among the sick poor, and the latter for infectious diseases among all classes of the population. Along with these, much voluntary hospital accommodation is provided; and insurance patients, among others, avail themselves of these various hospital beds, the insurance medical service usually being limited to domiciliary attendance and treatment.

There are altogether some 25,000 beds for the hospital treatment of sick persons in Scotland. This figure does not include asylums and other institutions for mental disease. These are provided almost entirely by public authorities.

Of the above number, 9,000 beds in 100 general and 37 special hospitals are voluntary, 10,000 have been provided by public health authorities, 6,000 are contained in 230 poor-law hospitals and in beds for sick persons in poor-house buildings. The accommodation for tuberculosis alone amounts to 4,000 beds.

A recent official report ("On the Hospital Services of Scotland", 1926) gives further particulars, from which the following additional items are taken.

The main conclusion of the committee responsible for this report is that there are "many persons in Scotland who, mainly because there are not enough hospital beds, are unable to get at the proper time the hospital treatment which they need". This condition is not special to Scotland, but its social significance, and its importance in preventing private doctors from obtaining the best treatment for many of their patients, are evident. It signifies much prolongation of suffering owing to delay in securing the needed expert treatment; it sometimes means delay beyond the time when treatment is effective, and sometimes even death which might have been avoided.

The same report emphasises the fortuitous growth of the hospital system, and the fact that poor-law hospitals, hospitals of public health authorities, and voluntary hospitals do not work in entirely different fields, or supply separate needs.

There is needed a better integration of the hospital service, a process already partially effected for Aberdeenshire.

The committee concluded that 3,600 additional hospital beds were needed in Scotland.

The great teaching hospitals are associated with the medical schools at Aberdeen, Dundee (St. Andrews), Edinburgh, and Glasgow. These supply over one-third of the total voluntary hospital accommodation. The Scottish Hospital Committee, whose report has already been referred to, suggest the formation of regional hospital areas, centering upon the large teaching hospitals and supplemented by secondary and smaller hospitals throughout the area. It is anticipated that the poor-law hospitals, when transferred to the town and county councils, will also become available for teaching purposes, at any rate in the University centres.

RELATION OF THE PRIVATE PRACTITIONER TO PUBLIC MEDICAL SERVICES

This will be better understood after perusal of the chapters dealing with Sickness Insurance Work in Scotland and with the Medical Service of the Highlands and Islands, and the chapters illustrating local services in Scotland. The conditions are not very different from those in England, apart from the difficulties due to sparsity of population in a large part of Scotland. Dr. Kinloch, the recently appointed Chief Medical Officer of the Department of Health for Scotland, in his last Annual Report as M.O.H. of Aberdeen, discusses the subject of this paragraph. He regards the encroachment of public medicine on private practice as already practically complete; and the object of all parties in the State being to achieve an adequate health service for the whole community, he regards it as essential to incorporate the medical practitioner within the scheme. His conviction is that however complete may be the hospital and specialist services provided officially, they will "fail to provide an adequate medical service for the community until such time as the general medical practitioner becomes an executive officer within the service". This would imply the complete responsibility of the general practitioner for the health of the family, both its protection and the care for departures from health, with complete interlocking between the work of the private doctor and the statutory health authority, and also between the latter and voluntary agencies. The subject involved in this statement is deferred for discussion in a separate volume.

CHAPTER XXII

SICKNESS INSURANCE WORK IN SCOTLAND

THE system of national sickness insurance is practically identical in England and in Scotland, and it is unnecessary, therefore, to give full separate particulars for Scotland. A few sentences will suffice to introduce special items of experience in Scotland, derived in part from the admirable Annual Reports of the Scottish Board (now Department) of Health for 1924-27, and in part from my personal inquiries and from information supplied by Mr. W. Jones, of Glasgow.

Three parties are concerned in the finance of National Insurance for employed persons: the State (in Scotland the Department of Health), the employer, and the employed person. Its administration also is on a threefold basis: the State, the Local Insurance Committee (one for each county and large burgh), and the Approved Society.

The number of Approved Societies operating in Scotland at the end of 1927 was as follows:—

	Approved for Scotland only	Approved for Great Britain	Total
Friendly Societies	46	63	109
Industrial Insurance Companies and Collecting Societies	2	12	14
Trades Unions	12	54	66
Employers' Provident Funds	9	6	15
	69	135	204

Some of the friendly societies have branches. These number 402. The expenditure of these Approved Societies during 1924 was £1,253,000 for sickness benefit, and £767,000 for disablement benefit.

The Approved Societies carry on all the work needed for administering monetary benefits, and in this connection are intimately concerned to secure strictly accurate medical certification.

The insurance committees administer the medical benefits of insured persons in their area. This is a geographical unit, while unfortunately Approved Societies know no geographical boundaries. The control of the work of doctors by insurance committees is within the limited circle of the national conditions governing *per capita* payments; they are also concerned with disputes between insured persons and doctors, and between approved societies and doctors on matters affecting certification of sickness, as will be seen in what follows.

Each insurance committee is constituted as follows: three-fifths of the members represent insured persons, and are elected by the Approved Societies which have members resident in the county or large burgh; one-fifth are appointed by the council of the county or large burgh. The remaining one-fifth consists of two medical practitioners appointed by the local medical committee, one medical practitioner appointed by the council of the county or large burgh, and the balance are appointed by the Secretary for Scotland.

The insurance committee makes agreements with local doctors and druggists for the treatment of the local insured; and they are required to confer in certain circumstances with three other local committees: (*a*) the Local Medical Committee, (*b*) the Panel Committee, and (*c*) the Pharmaceutical Committee. Agreements in the main, however, are made on a national scale, and the functions of the local insurance committee are correspondingly restricted. Except in so far as they consult with the three last-named committees, their duties are little more than that of a cash-paying office for doctors and pharmacists.

The local medical committee is constituted by the doctors

in the area, not merely insurance practitioners. This committee must be consulted on general questions affecting the administration of medical benefit, particularly as to the range of services coming within the scope of the agreement with the doctors.

The panel committee represents solely the insurance practitioners of the area. It may be recognised as the local medical committee or be separate. These committees generally combine for the purposes of both.

The pharmaceutical committee is elected by the insurance pharmacists of the area.

The relation between the different bodies concerned in sickness insurance will be more clearly seen in the scheme on the opposite page.

The following table, compiled as at February 1929, is interesting as showing the distribution of medical practitioners who give a Scottish address for registration purposes :—

General Practitioners on the Panel	1,978
General Practitioners not on the Panel	209[1]
Consultants, Specialists, Teachers, etc.	388
Retired from practice	474
Dentists with medical qualification	76
Employed whole-time in Government service, Local Authority service, etc.	492
Not known to be doing any medical work in Scotland though their names remain on the Register at an address in Scotland	1,346
TOTAL	4,963

In the counties, and in the larger burghs, practically the whole of the doctors engaged in general medical practice are on the Insurance Panel. In the industrial districts of the large cities this is also true, but not in the better-class residential districts. In these latter districts only a small proportion of the population are insured, and doctors in these districts who join the Insurance Panel do so to enable

[1] Includes a number of persons who, though not on any panel list, are doing insurance work as assistants to doctors on the panel.

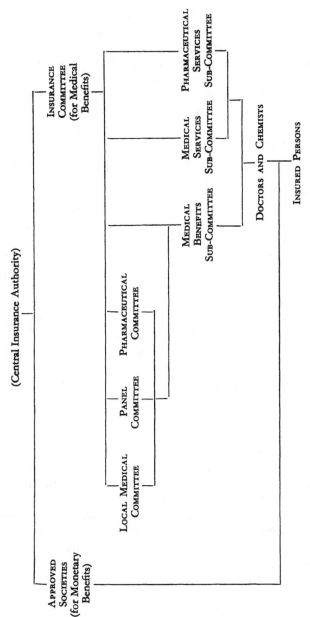

DEPARTMENT OF HEALTH FOR SCOTLAND

(Central Insurance Authority)

APPROVED SOCIETIES (for Monetary Benefits)

INSURANCE COMMITTEE (for Medical Benefits)

LOCAL MEDICAL COMMITTEE

PANEL COMMITTEE

PHARMACEUTICAL COMMITTEE

MEDICAL BENEFITS SUB-COMMITTEE

MEDICAL SERVICES SUB-COMMITTEE

PHARMACEUTICAL SERVICES SUB-COMMITTEE

DOCTORS AND CHEMISTS

INSURED PERSONS

NOTE.—The Local Medical Panel and Pharmaceutical Committees must be consulted on certain matters usually referred to them from the Medical Benefits Sub-Committee. The Services Sub-Committees deal wholly with complaints.

them to treat on a basis of certain payment domestic servants and younger members of well-to-do families who may be in insurable employment.

One million seven hundred and seventy-three thousand capitation fees of 9s. per head, together with a sum of £42,500 for ordinary mileage, were paid to insurance practitioners in Scotland during 1927, a total of £840,000. Payments to druggists amounted to £155,904, the number of prescription forms dispensed being 2,755,433. This expenditure was incurred for a little over one-third of Scotland's total population which, in 1927, was estimated at 4,894,700.

The limitations of statutory medical benefit are the same in Scotland as in England. Certain Approved Societies are, however, financially more prosperous than others and, on the strength of the second valuation of Approved Societies which has been made, are able to give additional benefits to their members, the most popular being dental and ophthalmic benefits. The dental benefit has been adopted in Scotland by societies having 1,200,735 members, or approximately 90 per cent. of all the Scottish insured.

The rate of grant to each claimant for dental benefit has varied in accordance with the amount at the disposal of the individual society for this purpose. It usually only represents a portion of the cost of dental work, including dentures.

Choice of Doctors

In England a doctor may not accept more than 2,500 insured persons on his "panel", and not more than 1,500 additional if he has a permanent medical assistant. In Scotland the same maximum figure applies in the case of the practitioner in practice, but the number allowed in respect of a permanent assistant is generally limited to one-half of this. Under the Medical Benefit Regulations, however, each insurance committee has the right, subject to approval by the Central Department, to fix a maximum lower than 2,500. In the city of Glasgow the maximum is 2,000, with 1,000 for a permanent assistant.

Patients had been allowed to change their doctor whenever they chose, but the phenomenal rise in payments for sickness benefits during the coal stoppage in 1926 led to restriction of this privilege. It is now necessary for an insured person who wishes to change his doctor to give two weeks' notice to the insurance committee, unless the first doctor has consented to an immediate transfer. This restriction does not apply when the patient has removed to a new district.

INCREASE IN INCIDENCE OF CERTIFIED SICKNESS

The great strike of transport workers in 1926 in sympathy with the coal strike put many industries out of action, and as unemployment insurance did not apply in these circumstances, there was greatly increased recourse to sickness benefits, obtained through medical certificates.

Since then claims on sickness benefits have remained high, as shown below. The attention of insurance practitioners has been specially directed by the Scottish Board (now Department) of Health "to the necessity for strict adherence to the statutory condition of incapacity for work on which correct certification of sickness claims depends". Professor A. Gray, Professor of Political Economy in the University of Aberdeen, who is also Chairman of the Consultative Council on National Health Insurance of the Scottish Board of Health, has also recently quoted figures given by the Secretary of State (*Hansard*, February 23, 1928) showing steady increase in expenditure on sickness benefits. Taking the index figure for 1925 as 100, it was 113·5 for 1926 and 117·75 for 1927. This increased expenditure was not associated with increased expenditure on drugs and medicines; which may be explicable on the supposition that there was no real increase of sickness, but only an increase in certification; or it may represent in part a change in the prescribing habits of the doctors. The figures as to cases referred to consulting doctors, some of which are given on page 461, are similarly open to a double interpretation.

In the debate in Parliament, in which the above figures were cited, a medical M.P. referred to "an inherent vice in the panel system", as responsible for the increased certification, this system in his view rewarding the easy-going, the not over-conscientious, and the flabby.

It is difficult to form a final judgment on the facts hitherto displayed. Various considerations arise. Thus there are years of greater and less incidence of disease, especially of catarrhs; again, the insurance system on a national basis might reasonably be expected to have a larger incidence of illness than was allowed for in the actuarial forecasts, which were based on the experience of the Manchester Unity Friendly Society during 1893–97, loaded by about 13 per cent. One has to remember that the members of the older friendly societies were the thrifty members of the community, while in the national scheme all wage-earners are included. It must be admitted that there is need for a higher standard of conduct on the part of many making claims on sickness benefit, and on the part of some certifying doctors. That there is need for accurate statement concerning each certified illness, and that the aggregate illness in every district should be made the subject of careful study to an extent which has hitherto not been attempted, is clear. This is extremely difficult in the absence of regional administration of sickness benefits, which at present is non-existent. Doctors need to be taken into the confidence of each insurance committee: discussion as to the basis of legitimate certification will always be valuable.

COMPLAINTS AGAINST DOCTORS

The Insurance Acts and regulations made under them provide the machinery for investigating allegations of neglect or improper certification on the part of an insurance doctor. For the investigation of these cases the local insurance committee is required to appoint a *Medical Service Sub-Committee*, constituted as follows:—

MEDICAL SERVICE SUB-COMMITTEE

Equal Numbers of:—
1. Doctors appointed by local medical committee.
2. Members appointed by and from members of the insurance committee who represent insured persons.
3. An independent chairman, usually one of the members of the committee appointed from the county or burgh council.

Such complaints are relatively few in number, and it is rare for punishment to be inflicted beyond some deduction from grants due to the accused practitioner. He has the right of appeal to the Central Authority. (See illustrations under Glasgow.)

A more serious difficulty arises in connection with alleged lax certification of unfitness for work; and still more, laxly continued certification of convalescent patients.

A number of district medical officers (medical referees) have been appointed to act as consultants to doctors in doubt as to certification, and to make inquiries into cases in which the officials of Approved Societies allege undue continuation of sick certification. Their duties are evidently delicate in character, though there is reason to think that the services of these officers are being increasingly welcomed by insurance doctors.

During six years these district medical officers have passed under scrutiny 165,266 cases (*Annual Report, Scottish Board of Health*, 1927). Of these 39 per cent. did not come forward for examination, and presumably returned to work. This may have been due in some instances to unwillingness to face impartial examination, in others to coincidence with previous intention to resume work. Of those examined, about two-thirds were found to be really unfit, and one-third were declared fit for work.

It is unlikely that difficulties in certifying unfitness for work will cease to be an embarrassing obstacle to the smooth working of national insurance until there is a completely linked-up service of general medical practice with consultant facilities and with hospital accommodation for more complete examination of dubious cases as well as for special forms of treatment. There is needed also local statistical investigation of the incidence of certification, in order that excessive sickness may be located for further investigation.

The extent to which, in special circumstances, medical certification may be excessive is evidenced by the fact that in 1926, a year of serious industrial stoppage, financial expenditure on sickness and disablement benefits in Scotland exceeded those of 1925 by 14 per cent., representing an increased cost of about a quarter of a million pounds sterling. Some of this increase doubtless represented increased sickness; much of it, however, must have meant resort to sickness benefit, when unemployment benefit (not obtainable in the circumstances of the strike) would have been the appropriate means of help.

INSURANCE MEDICAL WORK AND HOSPITALS

It might have been anticipated that the provision of domiciliary medical treatment for all wage-earners would have diminished the stress on the out-patient departments of general and special voluntary hospitals. No such relief has been experienced, so far as can be ascertained. The "rush" practice in private general work for the poorer people has continued, and many of these poorer people continue to crowd out-patient rooms for an independent, and especially for an expert, opinion. These out-patient departments have had their patients increased, furthermore, by school children referred to private doctors or hospitals, for it has become understood that neglect of treatment may carry with it legal consequences.

"Rush" practice continues in insurance work, and in view of the fact that the insurance doctor's payment is on a capitation basis, there is no strong inducement for him to prevent resort to hospitals. In cases when a consultation or special treatment is indicated, this is, of course, most valuable; but in the majority of instances more careful and less hurried work on the part of the insurance doctor would obviate the need for resort to hospitals.

But the existence of this continuous trend of insurance patients to hospitals, independently of reference there by their doctor, shows a chief weakness of insurance medical practice, namely, the lack of organised and regulated access to a consultant who has special skill in the department of medicine concerned in any case of difficulty.

"RUSH" MEDICINE

For doctors who wish to do good work and to avoid the necessity of sending out "bills", the national scheme offers admirable opportunity, and for them and their patients insurance works well, and for the societies to which the latter belong. But a "cheap doctor" is apt to do bad work whether for insured patients or for others.

The medical service sub-committee (see scheme on page 457) deals only with complaints submitted to it, and its members have no power of inspection, either as regards certification or treatment. As a means of defence, it has been suggested that Approved Societies should be authorised to submit for review the certificates of a doctor or doctors who might appear to them to be acting in a lax manner, but so far there is no power to do this.

Such complaints as come before the medical service sub-committee, if confirmed on investigation, are usually met by a monetary penalty. Exception to this is when a doctor has been so negligent of his practice that, under other powers vested in them, the medical service sub-committee represents to the central authority that a doctor's continuance on the panel may be prejudicial to the efficiency of the whole service. When such a representation is found proved, the central authority may either remove the doctor from the panel and authorise the persons on his list to make a fresh choice of doctor, or they may reduce the number on his list. Several doctors have been removed from panels throughout Scotland, and in at least one instance, a reduction in the number of persons on a doctor's list was imposed as a penalty.

THE SCOTTISH INSURANCE MEDICAL SERVICE AS SEEN IN GLASGOW

Mr. W. Jones, who was for some years the Clerk to the Insurance Committee for Glasgow, and was a member of the recent Royal Commission on National Insurance, which reported in 1926, has given me valuable particulars which are embodied in the following summary:—

Among the recent cases submitted to the medical services sub-committee, to whose reports I had access, the following may be cited in illustration of their work:—

1. A doctor was asked to attend this sub-committee because for several years he had failed to furnish summary cards in respect of persons on his list who were certified as incapable of work, contrary to the terms of his service as set out in the Medical Benefit Regulations.

The doctor attended the committee meeting, admitted the breach of duty, and no further action was then taken, but he was warned that any similar breach of the terms of service by him would be regarded very seriously.

2. An Approved Society complained that Dr. X had given a certificate in respect of A.B., an insured person on his list, which stated that he had examined the patient on September 25, 1928, when he had not so examined him, this man having been convicted two days previously and sent to prison for three months.

The doctor's defence was that A.B. was a "chronic", and had been ill for seven years with an injury to his back; that Mrs. A.B. called on the morning of the 25th stating that she wanted the certificate in order to obtain the money allowance from the Approved Society before its office closed on that day. He was told that A.B. could not come.

Dr. X admitted that, "in order to oblige patients, he had sometimes issued certificates before visiting the patients the same day, although he knew it was not strictly in order".

The sub-committee recommended that representations be made to the Scottish Board of Health, to the effect that £25 be deducted from sums owing to Dr. X for his insurance work.

3. An Approved Society complained that Dr. Y issued a voluntary certificate on Form Med. 40C on May 18, 1928, certifying that C.D. was incapable of work from May 13th, although he did not examine him until the 18th.

Dr. Y's reply was that when the patient saw him on the 18th with an incised wound of the neck, he said he received this on the 13th. The doctor found that the wound had been stitched, and this and other circumstances satisfied him that the wound had been received on the 13th. He told C.D. that he could not give an ordinary certificate, but he considered that the form mentioned above was appropriately used in this case. The sub-committee concluded that Dr. Y had inadvertently misinterpreted the use of this certificate, and a bulletin was issued to insurance practitioners generally advising them of its correct use.

The preceding illustrations are concerned with the relation of approved societies to medical practitioners, who are alleged by them to have granted improper certificates. Other cases arise from time to time where the insured person complains of neglect on the part of the practitioner; such cases are not altogether infrequent, but it is only occasionally that the questions raised are serious. Most often they occur when a medical practitioner fails to respond to a call for treatment, and complaint is made in order to recover fees which have been paid to another doctor.

A case may be cited which, although it was at first apparently trivial, gave rise to action raising it into a more important category. A doctor had failed to make a call on a patient when requested, and after having made a belated visit, failed to respond to calls for subsequent visits. Another doctor was called in, and fees amounting to less than £1 were incurred. A claim was made by the patient for recovery of this amount, but the doctor declined to admit liability. The case was heard by the medical services sub-committee, and in the course of the hearing it transpired that the doctor had used abusive and offensive language to the patient and members of his household. The medical services subcommittee found the complaint proved, and instructed that the amount of the fees be repaid to the insured person and deducted from the panel doctor's remuneration. He was also censured for his unprofessional conduct. Against this decision the doctor appealed to the Central Department, and the case was later heard by the then chairman of the Scottish Insurance Commissioners[1] and the medical member of the Commission, sitting together. They confirmed the findings of the insurance committee, and imposed a substantial additional monetary penalty. On the facts this decision was final, but on a legal question, that the definition of treatment in his agreement did not apply to his relationship to the patient in a general professional sense, the doctor appealed to the Court of Session (the Court of Appeal in Scotland). The Court of Session upheld the contention of the insurance committee, that treatment under the agreement between them and insurance practitioners covered the whole professional relationship between doctor and patient, as in the case of private practice. This decision is important, as it indicates that in certain circumstances disciplinary action in regard to a doctor's ethical relationship to his patient may be the subject of penal action under the National Insurance Act, just as in more serious cases this relationship may come within the disciplinary control of the General Medical Council.

The following are instances in which patients allege that Approved Societies have improperly refused to continue sickness benefit. As a rule, these arise because the approved society has referred the case for examination by the medical referee, who has declared the insured person to be fit for work, while the insurance doctor may still be continuing to grant certificates of incapacity. When the society discontinues payment, the insured person has a right of appeal under the society's rules to arbitration. These rules provide for reference to an arbitration committee, consisting of members of the committee of management of the society, or to an individual arbiter, jointly agreed upon between the society and the member. The cases summarised below are all instances dealt with by an individual arbiter; it will be seen that the duty may be delicate and difficult:—

[1] The Scottish Insurance Commission were formerly the central body responsible for the administration of National Health Insurance in Scotland.

1. E.F., aged 59, was last employed in the week ending February 7, 1925, and since then has been on more than one occasion on the sick list. From August 1, 1927, until May 16, 1929, he was continuously certified as "incapacitated for work in consequence of hæmorrhage due to tuberculosis".

On May 15th he was examined—apparently at the request of the Approved Society—by the medical referee, who reported that the patient had been examined by the municipal tuberculosis officer, and that following on this the referee stated "the insured person is not in my opinion incapable of work".

The man's insurance doctor on June 13th, however, certified that in his opinion the patient was "absolutely unfit for work involving any strain or exertion", owing to the liability to severe hæmorrhage.

On a re-examination by the T.O., including a new X-ray examination, some fibrosis was found, but no "evidence of any active disease".

The arbitrator's decision was that the man's "physical condition fits him only for employment of a light character. . . . Having regard to his age and the general difficulty of finding work, even for physically fit persons, at the present time, it may be difficult for him to get a job suitable for his physical capacity, but as he appears to be fit for work of some kind, he ceases to be entitled to receive either sickness or disablement benefit under the Health Insurance Acts."

2. G.H. had drawn sickness and disablement benefit from December 1923 until October 18, 1928, in consequence of impaired sight. It was certified that his right eye was apparently useless for vision, and that his left vision was very imperfect. Examined in July 1928 by Dr. O. on the instruction of the Scottish Board of Health, the verdict was that G.H. was not a blind person, and that he was fit for many kinds of work; but Dr. O. was unable to give many illustrations of this capacity. It had been suggested that G.H. should get training for some special work. Evidently medical opinion as to G.H.'s capacity for work differed greatly.

The arbitrator concluded that G.H. could not return to his former colliery work, though, apart from defective eyesight, he was in good health. G.H. was not wholly incapacitated for some forms of work, e.g. hawking, selling newspapers, and therefore, inasmuch as he "was not wholly incapacitated within the meaning of the Insurance Act, the society was justified in discontinuing payment of benefits".

3. I.J., aged 28, began to be ill June 6, 1927, when he was certified by his insurance doctor to be suffering from duodenal

ulcer. On October 14th he was examined by a medical referee, who reported that I.J. was making a good recovery. Payment of benefit continued until June 13, 1929, when I.J. was again examined by a medical referee, who stated that I.J. complained of pain after food, but in the referee's opinion he was capable of suitable work. On June 18th his insurance doctor gave I.J. a certificate declaring off sickness benefit.

I.J. says he is still attending Dr. C. at the Western Dispensary twice weekly, who is stated to have informed him that he might arrange for I.J.'s admission to the Infirmary if he did not improve.

The arbitrator, in his judgment, described the case as a difficult one. I.J. was probably not fit to return to his previous job as a builder's labourer, but that he could do lighter work.

Probably it would be difficult for him to obtain employment, and in that case I.J. would be eligible for unemployment benefit or its equivalent.

4. K.L., aged 44, a carter, was last employed in the week beginning December 18, 1927. He began to be ill April 30, 1929, with rheumatism, and was treated in a hospital until May 11th. His insurance doctor thereafter gave weekly certificates until June 10th, and on the 13th, at the request of the society, K.L. was examined by a medical referee, who said that, although the patient limped slightly, he was not incapable of work. The arbitrator confirmed this finding.

5. M.N., aged 32, from July 13, 1928, has been certified by his insurance doctor as incapacitated first for "nasal operation", and subsequently for "debility from phthisis".

On November 10th he was examined on behalf of the society by a medical referee, who said M.N. had chronic bronchitis and emphysema, with an old-standing healed tuberculosis lesion of the left apex, and that he was not incapable of work. Benefit was therefore discontinued as at November 9th, and M.N. appealed against this decision.

Full details of M.N.'s medical history need not be given. The arbitrator decided that he was in no worse condition of health than when he was last employed, and in his opinion the man should now seek to obtain some light occupation.

The preceding cases illustrate the difficulties of the doctor in certifying illness under the National Health Insurance Act. More is said on this subject in discussing the same problem in England (p. 125). It may be stated with confidence that gradually improvement is occurring. Most doctors are tending to be more careful and restrained in their certification. There is the constant temptation to oblige the patient. He may go to a more complacent doctor if his present medical attendant is rigidly honest; indeed, he often does, and so sickness claims based on medical certification mount up without, it is believed, a corresponding increase of sickness.

The employment of official medical referees has helped matters, but nothing short of a "change of heart", and an enhancement of conscientiousness, both on the part of insured persons and of certain insurance practitioners, can effect a complete remedy.

Mr. W. Jones, who has had considerable experience as an arbiter, gave it as his opinion that in Scotland the medical referees, who are officers of the central authority, do not "play for safety", but act with fair impartiality, although, naturally, their examinations are conducted with greater care than is usual by a panel (insurance) doctor. In cases of doubt they may also consult with, or seek the assistance of, a colleague in their examination of the patient.

There is a final appeal to the Department of Health for Scotland, both as regards complaints dealt with by the insurance committee in respect of certification and treatment, and from the decisions of arbitration committees of arbiters appointed under Approved Societies' rules, in cases concerned with the discontinuance of sickness benefit. The Department appoints a Final Arbiter to hear and decide appeals to them. Such appeals to the Department, however, are not numerous.

Financial Value of Insurance Practice

On the retirement or death of an insurance practitioner, his insurance practice finds a ready sale, along with such additional private practice as he may have, and commands the usual market value of from one to two years' purchase, according to circumstances and competition. The purchase of an insurance practice is regarded as a sound investment for the young doctor entering into practice on his own account, while the value of the practice is an important item in the inventory of a deceased doctor's estate. The Medical Benefit Regulations make suitable provision for the transfer of the insurance part of the practice to a successor, although each person on the list has a right, if he thinks fit, to exercise a fresh choice.

CHAPTER XXIII

THE MEDICAL SERVICE FOR THE HIGHLANDS AND ISLANDS

A LARGE part of the north of Scotland is mountainous, and its population sparsely distributed in hamlets and farms or small-holdings which are very difficult of access from towns and far from medical aid.

This is even more true of the islands off the mainland of Scotland. The sparsely distributed people are very poor. Many dwellings are primitive and unsatisfactory, primitive habits and customs survive, the dietary of the people is inferior, and the most stalwart of the people have migrated to other parts of Great Britain or have found homes in other countries. To add to these difficulties, it should be remembered that the benefits of the National Health Insurance Act have not hitherto accrued to a large proportion of the poorer people, "crofters", as they do not come within the definition of employed persons in the Act, except when they have a secondary employment.

In 1912 an official committee, called the Highlands and Islands Medical Service Committee, reported to the Government on the conditions found by them in these areas, and concluded that in view of their social, economic, and geographical difficulties, exceptional treatment was demanded. There was needed a medical, including a nursing, service aided by funds from the National Treasury. The inadequacy of the existing medical services was due to a number of factors, among which they enumerated inadequate remuneration, inability of the doctor to make provision for old age and infirmity, difficulties of locomotion and communication, insecurity of tenure of parochial appointments, difficulty experienced by doctors in obtaining suitable houses, and in obtaining deputies while away on holidays. These conditions meant that medical treatment and skilled nursing were beyond the reach of the average Highland family.

The recommendations of the committee were endorsed by the Government, and in 1913 Parliament voted an annual grant-in-aid of £42,000 to be administered by a newly formed body, the Highlands and Islands Medical Services Fund. This is not the only or the first instance in Britain of State aid in the treatment of disease or its prevention. Poor-law authorities in these areas, as elsewhere, already received help from governmental funds, and so likewise did local public health authorities in the treatment of acute infectious diseases and tuberculosis. Furthermore, for insured persons the State made some contribution to the sickness benefits financed chiefly from contributions by employers and employed. But the Highlands and Islands scheme is the only instance in which governmental assistance has been given, which "aims explicitly at the improvement of medical practice and services as a whole". Evidently arrangements to this end involved most difficult negotiations to fit them into existing services and to prevent the cessation of private practice which, aside from the scheme, would continue to exist.

The following general conditions were attached to the payment of grants to medical practitioners by the Scottish Local Government Board (now the Department of Health for Scotland).

(1) That within the area of his ordinary practice the doctor shall visit systematically, and when asked to do so, all persons in need of medical attention.

(2) That, in single-practice areas, he shall continue to give attendance to poor-law and insured patients in accordance with his agreements with the parish council and insurance committee respectively; and that he shall, when required by the Board, undertake on terms and conditions to be approved by the Board, such duties as the public health authorities of the district may desire him to perform.

(3) That wherever practicable he shall give, when required, personal attendance in midwifery cases.

(4) That he shall arrange for regular and systematic visits to certain localities on fixed days.

(5) That, in suitable cases, and according to circumstances, he shall provide himself with a motor car, motor-cycle, motor-boat, or other means of conveyance, and use it, so far as practicable, in his practice.

(6) That he shall give regular attendance at schools, or elsewhere, on such terms as may be agreed upon with the School Board or the Secondary Education Committee, with the approval of the Board for the treatment of diseases and defects disclosed by the medical inspection of school children.

(7) That he shall keep a classified register, to be supplied by the Board, and to be open to inspection by a duly accredited representative of the Board, of cases attended under arrangements with the Board, showing in each case the number of visits paid, the distance of the patient from his house, and the fees collected.

In accordance with the agreement as to conditions of service and fees obtainable from patients under it, the doctor himself runs the risk of the patient not paying the authorised fees, while the Highlands and Islands Medical Service Board, established under the scheme, makes itself responsible for the travelling expenses of the doctor in certain areas,[1] and in other special areas for a supplementary allowance to bring the doctor's income up to a "living wage". These two cases are explained as follows in a circular issued by the Board in August 1915:—

The claims of individual practitioners fall into two main categories: First, there is the case of single-practice areas in insular districts, or in wide and sparsely-populated districts on the mainland, where the services of separate doctors cannot be dispensed with, but where the total professional income is entirely inadequate either as a fair recompense for the work involved, or as an inducement to a suitable medical man to settle in the locality. Second, there is the case of multiple-practice areas or districts where there are several doctors whose practices overlap to some extent and who, in most cases, have patients of very limited means or insured persons living at a considerable distance.

In the first case it may be necessary to guarantee such a *supplement to the income* of the doctor as will bring his total

[1] In the instance given on page 476 the mileage based on some previous experience now fails to cover necessary travelling expenses.

emoluments up to a fixed sum after he has paid all rates and taxes (other than income-tax), and such approved charges under the heads of travelling expenses and house rent as, in the circumstances, may appear to the Board to be appropriate.

In the second case referred to above, the arrangement with the doctor will take the form of a payment in respect of additional work, and any increase in travelling expenses involved in giving medical attention at modified fees to patients living at a distance.

To secure payment of travelling allowances, the doctor is required to keep an exact account of his professional interviews. On his returns the periodical payments to the doctor are determined by officials in the Scottish Department of Health.

The objects of the scheme are two: (1) to secure medical attendance for the poorer section of the population at low uniform charges; and (2) to make it obligatory for every doctor entering into the contract to give medical services as they are required either by private patients or by local authorities within his normal area of practice. The fee allowed is 5s. for a first visit and 3s. 6d. for each subsequent visit, and the doctor may not charge more than this, though he can charge for travelling expenses.

The motor-car has rendered this scheme practicable, even though the fees are lower than they might be in unrestricted practice. In such practice it should be added patients also would be much fewer. Under the scheme there has been an enormous increase of professional visits.

According to an official statement on the fund, there are now 156 doctors under the scheme of modified fees, and in addition 24 doctors who receive mileage grants from the fund in respect only of the insured patients on their lists.

In 140 medical practices it was found that the giving of mileage allowances for the doctors' travelling expenses in all their private and public duties, when added to their poor-law salaries, and their capitation fees under the Insurance Act and fees from private practice, has sufficed to provide a living wage.

In 40 practices this would not have sufficed; and in these

instances additional grants were given to produce a net salary of £500 on the assumption that due diligence was exercised in expenditure on travelling and in the collection of fees from their paying patients.

The guaranteed income has had most beneficent effects, and this point must be emphasised. Parish councils can now obtain satisfactory doctors for the poor, and the standard of general medical work has been greatly raised. The sum paid to the 156 doctors works out at an average of rather less than £260 per doctor annually. The Board also spends £850–£1,000 a year in providing fully qualified deputy doctors for 30 doctors under the scheme, enabling the latter to secure a needed holiday each year. This expenditure has led to ready recruitment when vacancies arise.

For our purpose it is unnecessary to detail the subsidised nursing scheme which accompanies the medical provision. This service is partly supported also out of voluntary subscriptions.

Much has been done to aid in the provision of hospital beds; and in some instances grants have been given towards the provision of housing for doctors and nurses. Travelling surgeons and specialists have been also organised.

The following official statement shows the expenditure of the fund of 1927:—

SUMMARY OF EXPENDITURE FROM THE FUND IN 1927 £

		£
Medical Service	.. ..	.. 43,050
Nursing Service	.. ..	.. 13,300
Hospitals and Ambulances { Maintenance	..	.. 338
{ Capital	..	.. 6,000
Specialist Services (2 surgeons) ..	.. ..	.. 1,926
Houses for Doctors and Nurses—Capital	..	.. 1,890
Telegraphs and Telephones	.. .. ..	.. 153
Special Emergency Scheme	.. .. ..	.. 214
Special Tuberculosis Scheme	.. .. ..	.. 3,050

£69,921

Of that total £62,031 represents annual recurrent charges for maintenance of services. The remainder, amounting to £7,890 was paid in respect of capital works.

The scheme of special services for these special areas in Scotland was called for in view of their exceptional conditions, economic, geographical, and medical. Without it much suffering was untreated or unsatisfactorily treated. The service was urgently required in the interests of health in these areas; and its benefits are already visible. This experience shows the practicability—when through the Government the more prosperous is prepared to come to the help of the less prosperous part of a community—of supplying hygienic and medical services for people in relatively inaccessible places, for whom this could not be done in accordance with the usual rules of supply and demand. In the following note I give particulars of personal visits made in one of the more accessible districts under the Highlands and Islands Scheme. This area is much more accessible, and there is less poverty than in the more remote Highlands and Islands.

HIGHLAND MEDICAL SCHEME IN PERTHSHIRE

By kindness of Dr. D. J. McLeish, the County M.O.H. of Perthshire, I was introduced to Dr. Mackay, of Aberfeldy, who arranged for me to accompany him on his daily round on September 19, 1929. The day was gloriously sunny; and I had a marvellous view of parts of highland scenery, mountain and valley, river and loch, which are seldom visited by tourists. We went in Dr. Mackay's six-cylinder two-seater car, and travelled over 80 miles between 10 a.m. and 3.45 p.m. During this time six patients had been visited, and as only a few minutes were spent in resting, the difficulties of highland medical practice may be inferred. This particular area is much less difficult than some others under the Highlands and Islands Scheme.

A list of the cases in the order in which they were seen is not without interest.

1st Patient.—A young man completely deaf after influenza, the result of neuritis of the auditory nerve. Arrangements discussed as to future training of the patient.

2nd Patient.—A shepherd with quinsy. Dr. Mackay came

prepared for lancing the tonsil, but this was not needed. This patient had been seen last night after dark by Dr. Mackay's partner. He had been ill for three days with sore throat, and the telephone message for the doctor was only sent at dusk on the third day. (It may be stated here that local telephones are used largely for sending messages, and at each local post-office as we went on our round, Dr. Mackay looked out for a signal in the post-office window indicating that a "call" had been received.) This evening visit meant a 14-mile journey for the doctor there, and the same distance back. The man was known from past experience to be apt to call for help at unnecessarily late hours; but there is no machinery for making him—at least partially—responsible for this abuse of the contract conditions of work under the National Insurance Act.

3rd Patient.—A septuagenarian with chronic rheumatism. I am not certain whether this patient was seen by Dr. Mackay in his capacity as parish (poor-law) medical officer, or as an insured patient.

4th Patient.—A child who had previously been unsuccessfully vaccinated. Mother now declined to have vaccination repeated, as she had three older children in the house and no one to help her to attend to the vaccinée.

The case illustrated a further difficulty in vaccination in a district in which distances to be travelled are so great. The lymph obtained deteriorates with keeping after arrival from its centre for distribution; vaccination often necessarily is delayed for days, or even weeks, and the proportion of so-called "insusceptibles" is thus exaggerated.

5th Patient.—A man, aged 30, who had poliomyelitis four years ago and is still completely paraplegic. Apart from this he is well; but being unable to work, he requires a monthly medical certificate for his insurance society. Dr. Mackay had written to this society explaining that the patient's home was 24 miles distant from Aberfeldy in a direct line; and that medical certificates ought to be accepted at irregular intervals—sometimes in a week, sometimes with more than a month's interval—according as the doctor was making visits in the same district. This had at first been agreed to, but more recently objections had been raised. No medical treatment was needed for this patient, who was unwilling to accept the doctor's suggestion that he should go into town and learn some trade like basket-making.

6th Patient.—A gamekeeper's wife, expecting her second confinement next February. At that season the valley in which she lives may be almost or entirely impassable. The nearest telephone is 8 miles distant, and Dr. Mackay's house is 28 miles away. There is no nearer doctor. At to-day's visit, Dr. Mackay tried to persuade her to come into Aberfeldy to be confined. There are several houses in the burgh where women may be received for this purpose. She refused to come, although the possible contingent risks of the situation were clearly stated.

She is entitled to medical attendance under the Highlands and Islands Scheme at a maximum fee of two guineas, which includes any antenatal attendance or attendance for complications of parturition.

The only additional payment the doctor can claim is for mileage, and he incurs the risk of losing part or the whole of his fee, for the payment of which he must look solely to the patient herself or her husband.

A seventh visit was made during the day to the district nurse, who in attending to patients in this wide-scattered area has difficulties of travelling even greater than those of the doctor.

Medical attendance in the Highland District of Perth comes in part under the Highlands and Islands Scheme (p. 472) and is concerned chiefly with providing aid for the wives and dependents of men insured under the National Insurance Act.

The doctor's fee for a first visit, as we have seen, is 5s., and for subsequent visits 3s. 6d. each visit, irrespective of distance. This is in addition to what is received from the Government for expenditure in travelling. The scattered distribution of patients sometimes leads to shrewd calculation on the part of the patient as to whether it is cheaper to send for the doctor or to go to the doctor. A patient 18 miles distant recently sent to Dr. Mackay for a minor ailment, and explained to him naïvely that this was "cheaper" than would have been her difficult journey to his house.

In Dr. Mackay's practice there are about 60 confinements yearly, and his father states that this number has remained fairly stationary during his entire medical experience in this district.

The usual midwifery fee is two guineas. Scarcely any cases are attended by midwives, who cannot get a livelihood in this area. Puerperal eclampsia occurs occasionally; and it is difficult to suggest a workable scheme in such a widely scattered area which would allow of the examinations necessary to prevent or minimise this. It might, however, be possible to arrange medical antenatal visits paid for out of public funds for such cases as were notified by the district nurse to the doctor. In some cases attendance at a confinement has meant a three days' stay in the house, owing to nearly impassable roads.

In Scotland doctors do not as a rule dispense medicines. In this particular Highland practice the obtaining of prescribed remedies is beset with difficulty. The nearest druggist is at Aberfeldy, and there is no allowance for expenses of postage of bottles to distant patients who cannot come for their medicine. The second patient on the list previously given would have been the better for a narcotic, for he had not slept for two nights; but how to send for this?

The mileage allowance, which is common to the national insurance and the highland schemes, has been stabilised for a period of three years on the average experience of five years' medical practice, a certain estimated amount being deducted for mileage incurred in private practice. On the expiry of the three years' period, the grant for each practice will again be reviewed. In Dr. Mackay's practice the average number of miles thus estimated was exceeded last year by 2,000 miles. This excess is increasing as the possibilities of getting help are becoming better recognised by distant patients. Meanwhile every additional call increases expenditure by the doctor, and he is open to the temptation to reduce attendance really needed by distant patients. In a certain number of practices the annual grant from the Highlands and Islands Fund is not based on the amount of the actual travelling, but is a sum required to produce for the doctor a minimum net income, after payment of working expenses.

It is evident that there is much sending for the doctor under both schemes, for which attendance at the doctor's surgery might be substituted; and even when a doctor is required there is much disregard of his convenience and of the limitations of possibility of distant travelling. On the other hand, of course, there has been much gain in securing medical attention promptly to cases which otherwise would have been neglected. How to reconcile these conflicting considerations is a difficult problem. For complete success, a higher standard of education of the persons concerned is needed, and more particularly a greater realisation that the work is co-operative and can only attain its maximum success when each person concerned uses it with intelligence and sparing care.

In reviewing the Highland experience, there can be no doubt as to its beneficent working. But the doctors concerned in it still have many trials. They may have to travel several miles on foot through snowdrifts to reach their patients. They provide themselves with rubber boots for crossing flooded valleys and streams; they may be sent for 20 to 30 miles to see a case in which the only symptom is a blood-shot eye, as happened recently. Their work involves long and arduous days, travelling over by-roads never intended for motoring, in which the physical exertion of driving is no mean task. This I saw personally in a sunny, dry day; how much worse it can be with muddy roads, a biting north wind, and with snowdrifts can be imagined.

The Insurance Act with its capitation fees and the Highland Scheme with its subsidies have widely extended the possibilities of medical care. The average fee received by the doctors from the patients themselves has been lowered, but their practice has doubled. Formerly only farmers and hotel keepers and summer visitors could pay fees. Now a fee is obtainable in practically all cases; but there has been increased expenditure on the work, which must somewhat reduce the increase in the doctor's net income which has occurred.

From the point of view of patients, there has been great public benefit. Even if benefit is sometimes abused, much suffering is being assuaged, much illness is being curtailed, and lives are being saved which before the schemes of insurance and State aid were inaugurated were being sacrificed.

CHAPTER XXIV

ABERDEEN: COUNTY AND CITY[1]

THE city and county of Aberdeen are of special interest in this inquiry. In conjunction, they have in a degree anticipated some of the reforms of the Local Government (Scotland) Act, which came fully into operation throughout the whole of Scotland in May 1930. The relations existing between the private doctors and public health officials are cordial both in the city and in the county.

The entire county, including the city of Aberdeen, has an area of 1,261,521 acres. Most of its total population, 300,431 in 1931, is widely scattered in rural districts and in small burghs, with the exception of Aberdeen itself, which had a population of 167,259 at the census of 1931.

THE CITY OF ABERDEEN

It will be convenient first to outline the public medical arrangements for the city and then those for the county. Already there is a considerable amount of co-operation, especially in hospital services, between the city and the county, and shortly this co-operation will be more firmly established.

Dr. H. J. Rae has recently succeeded Dr. J. P. Kinloch (who is now chief medical officer of the Department of Health for Scotland) as medical officer of health of the city, and to him, to Dr. G. S. Banks, tuberculosis officer for the city and consulting tuberculosis officer for the county; and to Dr. J. A. Stephen, medical officer for mother and child welfare, I am indebted for much courtesy and for most of the information which follows.

Dr. Rae had been county medical officer of health for a number of years and, as already stated, had been closely

[1] Date of investigation, September 1929.

co-operating with the medical officer of health of the city, especially so far as institutional services were concerned, it being an accepted fact that rural areas cannot as a rule establish independent and efficient hospital units.

The city, prior to 1930, had three official authorities concerned with medicine: the Town Council, the Parish Council, and the Education Authority. To these may be added the local insurance committee, which is limited in its functions as elsewhere. All these have coterminous areas. Under the new Local Government Act, 1929, the three first-named become one in the Town Council, which in substance becomes the local parliament. The place of the education authority is taken by the Education Committee of the Town Council, but according to statute it must include eight members co-opted from without the Council, of whom three are specially interested in education.

The POOR-LAW MEDICAL SERVICE resembles that existing elsewhere. Its six parish doctors who give domiciliary treatment to the very poor are all also engaged in private practice. They each receive a salary of £70 to £80 per annum. The poor-law medical institutions are named later.

MIDWIFERY SERVICE

Of the 3,348 births in Aberdeen in 1927, midwives attended 670, and 1,975 were medically attended, a proportion of about 1 to 3. In addition, 528 were confined in the Maternity Hospital, and 173 were attended from this hospital at home.

Midwives in private practice sent for doctors in 158 cases, mostly for emergencies during and after confinement, but 11 during pregnancy, and 40 calls were in respect of the infant.

Midwives usually obtain a fee of 25s. for each case attended by them; doctors 42s.

At the Maternity Hospital the wives of insured persons pay 20s. for their ten days' stay and care in hospital; others pay what they can. This hospital is under voluntary management. Its non-resident medical staff are unpaid. The Town Council pay for a number of patients needing antenatal treatment and for confinement cases sent by them. The County Council also pay 30s. each for confinement cases sent by them into the hospital.

Puerperal mortality in Aberdeen is somewhat high. In a special publication issued by the Scottish Board of Health in 1928, Drs. Kinloch, J. Smith, and J. A. Stephen have discussed this problem as bearing on 34,653 legitimate births in Aberdeen, live and still, during 1918–27 and 3,331 illegitimate births, live and still, during the same period. For legitimate births the maternal puerperal mortality was 6 per 1,000, and it was 13·2 for the mothers of 1,000 illegitimate infants. It must be noted, however, that in these figures all deaths were included which occurred within four weeks of birth. It is noteworthy that in the practice of midwives the death-rate was 2·8, in the practice of doctors 6·9, and in in-patient institutional practice, 14·9 per 1,000 births. The institutional statistics exclude cases admitted from the practice of a midwife, doctor, or hospital district; but the midwives' statistics do include cases in which medical assistance had been obtained during birth.

The deaths from sepsis in doctors' cases were 1·45, in midwives' cases 0·75, and in in-patient institutional cases 4·5 per 1,000 births.

In commenting on these striking results Dr. Kinloch and his colleagues remark that there were no deaths among the 445 midwives' cases in which forceps were used. Nor do they think that the lessened instrumental delivery probably associated with the increased use of pituitrin in midwifery supports the view that traumatism is an important factor in the causation of puerperal sepsis. But they regard the institutional excess as probably due to contagion; and in view of their bacteriological findings they consider this to be due in considerable part to a streptococcal carrier condition in doctors. It is noteworthy, however, that excessive mortality in medical and institutional practice is not confined to the results of sepsis; and even when large allowance is made for trend of unfavourable cases away from midwives, the excessive mortality of doctors' and institutional patients is not explained altogether satisfactorily unless we assume that, because midwives are more truly obstetric, i.e. standing by, or for some other reason their practice is safer for their patients than that of doctors. Nor is it clear why midwives should, to such an extent, appear to be free from the carrier condition as regards hæmolytic streptococci. The conclusion arrived at in the report is that "the development of a new midwifery organisation in which midwives conduct all normal deliveries, and in which doctors provide the antenatal services and deal with obstetrical complications, will result in a significant reduction in puerperal mortality".

Maternity and Child Welfare Service

There are ten whole-time health visitors for the city. These in 1927 made the following visits. The live-births in that year numbered 3,348.

Infants under 1 year—	1st visits..	..	..	2,819
	Revisits ..	..	..	34,405
Children aged 1–5—	1st visits	..	..	555
	Revisits ..	..	..	4,112
Antenatal cases—	1st visits..	..	..	151
	Revisits ..	..	..	128

There are seven centres for child welfare work, two of these under voluntary management. A doctor attends each session, either Dr. Stephen or a lady doctor on his staff. Dr. Stephen gives fortnightly talks on mothercraft, a clinic being held afterwards. Very little treatment is given at the centres, what is given relating chiefly to nutrition. So far as is practicable, action is taken in consultation with private doctors. The relation between these and Dr. Stephen is so satisfactory that many of them send cases of marasmus, etc., to him for consultation or for hospital treatment. For such treatment 22 cots are reserved in a separate block of the City Fever Hospital, and 15 at the Woodend General Hospital. All of these are kept fully occupied. In addition, there are 42 cots for babies and 10 beds for mothers at Burnside Home.

There is very little friction between private doctors and the health visitors. When this arises, it is usually found that the mother has misinterpreted or mis-stated some official advice given to her; and frank intercommunication puts this right.

TUBERCULOSIS SERVICE

The relations between Dr. Banks, the tuberculosis officer, and the practitioners in Aberdeen are also excellent. This is illustrated by the fact that when a case is notified to the M.O.H. on a certificate which has appended to it the query, "Do you desire this patient to be examined by the T.O.", the answer usually is "Yes". A large number of patients are sent to Dr. Banks for preliminary examination and diagnosis. The standard of general medical work is good. Nearly all cases sent to the T.O. have records of several sputum examinations.

Aberdeen being a centre of the granite industry, special examinations of workers, including radiological, are in progress.

Dr. Banks visits patients at home with the doctor in attendance when they cannot attend the dispensary. He takes a radiological picture, 15 in. by 12 in., of the chest of a large proportion of all patients sent to him, and a reduced print of this is always sent, together with the T.O.'s report, to the private doctor, who is expected to return the print to him. A stamped envelope is sent for this purpose. About 150 of these are sent out yearly. There are three special health visitors for tuberculosis home visitation.

Institutional treatment for tuberculosis patients is provided at the Poor-Law Hospital and in 125 beds in separate blocks of the City Fever Hospital.

VENEREAL DISEASE SERVICE

During 1927 the free clinic at the Royal Infirmary treated 498 new cases. There is a second V.D. clinic at the Aberdeen City Fever Hospital, at which 166 new cases were treated in 1927.

An imperfect gauge of the proportion between private treatment of V.D. and treatment at the public expense is furnished by the number of specimens examined at the city laboratories. These relate to city cases only.

	Sent by Private Practitioners	Examined on Behalf of Clinics
Wassermann　..　..　..	200	4,983
Spirochæte..　..　..　..	4	600
Gonococcus　..　..　..	134	1,914
TOTAL　..　..　..	338	7,497

There is no social distinction in treatment. Dr. Bowie said he has had as many as five automobiles waiting outside for their owner-patients.

As in other parts of the country, private practitioners commonly are glad to be relieved of the treatment of these diseases. The clinic at the Royal Infirmary is conducted by a member of its staff who receives an honorarium for his services. His junior is Dr. Bowie, who also conducts the out-patient V.D. clinic at the City Fever Hospital.

The Fever Hospital clinic is conducted for patients who refuse to go to the Royal Infirmary, or who prefer to go to the City Hospital. Half of the patients received are sent by private practitioners; more than half of the male patients are medically insured and, as elsewhere, the method of payment of insurance doctors is not likely to impede the sending of patients to the clinics. It is said that 80 per cent. of female venereal patients are sent by private doctors.

In a current page of the register for both sexes I saw that

17 out of 20 of the patients entered on the page had been sent by private doctors.

Patients absenting themselves after partial treatment are written to, and if this is without result a sanitary inspector or health visitor calls on the patient. Dr. Bowie informs me that the number of patients who cease to attend before completion of treatment does not exceed 15 per cent., but that some of these "are probably quite cured, though they had not passed their final tests".

The V.D. scheme for the city of Aberdeen—of which only city figures are given above—is available for the entire county and for the north-eastern section of Scotland. Railway fares can be paid for distant patients, when a voucher to the effect that this is needed is received from the V.D. medical officer.

Laboratory Service of the City

No fee is charged for any work done for medical practitioners in this laboratory. In 1928 some 31,000 specimens were examined in it by Dr. J. Smith and his staff for the whole of North-East Scotland, including Orkney and Shetland, but omitting the county area of Aberdeen, the laboratory specimens from which are examined in the laboratory of Dr. Tocher, the county analyst.

The absence of fees has become practically universal, though in one annual report it was suggested that specimens from patients able to pay should be sent to a private pathologist.

The consultative services of the laboratory are valuable. Patients are sent to the laboratory for special examinations (see list at end of this section); and 8 to 10 private doctors visit the laboratory daily to consult as to specimens they wish to have examined, or as to the results of examination.

The appended extract from an official card sent to every doctor shows the completeness of the diagnostic service. Note also the extent to which sera and vaccines are supplied gratuitously to medical practitioners.

CITY OF ABERDEEN—HEALTH DEPARTMENT

CITY HOSPITAL LABORATORY

EXAMINATIONS

1. *Throat and Nose Swabs*
   (a) Microscopical and cultural examination for B. diphtheriæ.
   (b) Microscopical and cultural examination for other pathogenic organisms.

2. *Sputum*
   (a) Microscopical examination for tubercle bacilli.
   (b) Microscopical and cultural examination for other organisms.
   (c) Typing of the pneumococcus in cases of pneumonia where serum treatment is contemplated.

3. *Pus*
   (a) Microscopical examination for tubercle bacilli.
   (b) Microscopical and cultural examination for other organisms.
   (c) Microscopical examination of smears from urethral, vaginal, or eye discharges for gonococci.

4. *Blood*
   (a) Microscopical examination of blood film.
   Examination of red cells and differential leucocyte count.
   Examination for malaria and other parasites.
   (b) Enumeration of red cells and leucocytes.
   Estimation of hæmoglobin.
   (c) Examination by blood culture.
   (Blood which is allowed to clot in a tube is of little value for blood culture. For obtaining blood samples, the "Venuel" vacuum extractor containing nutrient bouillon will be issued on demand.)
   (d) Serum reactions.
   Widal reaction for Bac. typhosus, Bac. paratyphosus A., and Bac. paratyphosus B.
   Serum agglutination or food poisoning or other organisms.
   Serum agglutination for B. dysenteriæ.
   Wassermann and Kahn reactions.

(*e*) Chemical examinations.
   Estimation of blood urea.
   Estimation of blood sugar.
   Glucose tolerance test.
   For the glucose tolerance test, it is advisable, after making an appointment, to send the patient to the Laboratory.

5. *Urine*
   (*a*) Microscopical examinations.
      Microscopical examination of the centrifuged deposit.
      Microscopical examination for tubercle bacilli.
      Microscopical and cultural examination for organisms.
      Urines from female patients must be catheter specimens.
   (*b*) Chemical analysis.
      Qualitative analysis.
      Quantitative analysis.
      Urines for chemical examination should be preserved by the addition of a few drops of chloroform.

6. *Fæces*
   (*a*) Examination for intestinal worms.
   (*b*) Microscopical examination for the ova of intestinal parasites.
   (*c*) Microscopical examination for amœba histolytica or other protozoa.
   (*d*) Cultural examination for organisms of the typhoid, dysentery, and food poisoning groups.
   (*e*) General bacteriological examination.
   (*f*) Chemical examination.

7. *Cerebro-spinal fluid*
   A complete examination to include protein test, enumeration of cells, differential cell count, colloidal gold test, microscopical and cultural examination for organisms, and Wassermann reaction as required.

8. *Histological Specimens*
   Examination of tissues for pathological abnormalities.

9. *Examination of Gastric Contents*
   Chemical examinations are undertaken for the determination of the various constituents. Fractional test meals can be carried out on patients at the Laboratory.

10. *Water Samples*
   Full bacteriological examination.
   Full chemical examination.

11. *Milk Samples*
    Bacterial count.
    Cultural tests for B. coli.
    Chemical examination.

12. *Animal Inoculation for Diagnosis*
    Pus, sputum, and urine for tubercle bacilli.
    Milk for tubercle bacilli.
    Pathological material for B. anthracis.
    Investigation for presence of anthrax spores.

13. *Autogenous Vaccines*
    The cultivation and isolation of micro-organisms and the
    preparation of autogenous vaccines are undertaken
    from pathological material, collected from lesions of
    any specific infection.

Supply of Sera and Vaccines

The following biological products are issued by the Health
department free of charge to city practitioners, and are obtainable at the City Hospital Laboratory, or from the Chief Resident
Medical Officer.

1. Vaccine Lymph.
2. T.A.B. Vaccine.
3. Diphtheria Antitoxin.
4. Tetanus Antitoxin.
5. Sclavo's Serum—Anti-anthrax.
6. Anti-dysentery Serum—Polyvalent.
7. Anti-meningococcus Serum—Polyvalent.
8. Anti-pneumococcus Serum—Type 1.
9. Anti-streptococcus Serum—Puerperal.
10. Anti-streptococcus Serum—Scarlatina.
11. Anti-streptococcus Serum—Erysipelas.
12. Normal Horse Serum.
13. Botulinus Antitoxin.
14. Tuberculin.
15. Schick Test—Diphtheria toxin and heated toxin.
16. Diphtheria Prophylactic—Toxin-antitoxin.
17. Schick Test Toxin.
18. Scarlet Fever Prophylactic.

HOSPITAL SERVICE OF THE CITY

The position of Aberdeen in regard to hospital provision
is illuminating. Aberdeen is a University town with an
important medical school, requiring hospital beds and

out-patient departments for its medical faculty; and it has, in addition, voluntary provision in hospitals for special diseases. Further hospital provision is made for the destitute by the Parish Council; and for mental diseases and for infectious diseases by the Town Council.

During 1926 the Town Council and the Parish Council entered into a contract, in terms of which the former body has taken over the poor-law hospital buildings and in the future will treat all poor-law patients. This contract was made for a period of five years, but the Local Government Act of 1929 will make the combination permanent. These hospitals have been reconditioned, and now function as modern municipal hospitals. The City Fever Hospital is being extended at an estimated cost of £57,000; and the Royal Infirmary, the Maternity Hospital, and the Royal Hospital for Sick Children, all voluntary institutions, are in process of extension, an appeal for £400,000 for this purpose having been initiated. The Scottish Board (now Department) of Health made it a condition of their approval of the scheme of fusion that the Town Council should seek co-operation with the University and the voluntary hospitals in making their plans, that the teaching school should have full access to the appropriate local authority's institutions, and that the Town Council should offer to engage the services of the recognised teachers of the Medical School of Aberdeen. After much negotiation all this is in process of being accomplished, and the following beneficent results will accrue:—

1. The hospital provision for the destitute is merged into that for the general public.

2. The voluntary principle is maintained for the existing voluntary hospitals; and

3. The material in all municipal hospitals is made available for teaching purposes, to members of the staff of the voluntary hospitals, who are also teachers in the medical school.

4. The combined hospital arrangements have been made available under special arrangements for a large part of

North-Eastern Scotland. Thus a large step has been taken towards the organisation of regional hospital provision.

Some incidental items in the co-operative arrangements may be cited. Dr. Bowie is a V.D. officer at the Municipal Fever Hospital and at the Royal Infirmary. His salary is paid by the Town Council.

Dr. Banks, the T.O. of the city, lectures to University students on tuberculosis. They are required to attend his clinics during 18 hours for special practical instruction. Dr. Stephen is also a part-time lecturer at the medical school, and medical students attend at the municipal Burnside Home for Children or at the City Hospital at least six times to receive clinical instruction in children's complaints and in preventive methods.

The city M.O.H., Dr. Rae, has been appointed head of the public health department of the University and lecturer on public health. There is a course of 120 lectures on public health and infectious diseases for medical students, chiefly given by a whole-time lecturer, Dr. Berry, who is also an assistant M.O.H. of the city. Lectures on fevers are given at the City Hospital by Dr. Rae, Dr. Berry, Dr. Smith, the bacteriologist, and by the hospital visiting physician.

At the Woodend (late Poor-Law) Hospital there are 180 beds for general cases, and 160 for tuberculosis. Five honorary surgeons of the Royal Infirmary attend patients here in addition to the three resident medical officers. Each receives an annual honorarium of £200. A physician attending medical patients from without receives £300, and a further doctor (at £100 per annum) is retained for cases of pneumothorax.

The T.O., Dr. Banks, attends the tuberculous patients without any additional salary beyond that of T.O.

At the City Fever Hospital there are 300 beds, for whom 70 nurses are provided, including probationers. These are trained at the hospital, including an adequate course of theoretical instruction. The course of three years is followed by an examination and a certificate of competency from the General Nursing Corporation for Scotland. Unfortunately this training hitherto has not counted for a general nurses' certificate, for which two additional years' training is demanded—an instance of uneconomic redundance. Here, as elsewhere, it is clear that the period of nursing training might be curtailed were it not that probationers are required to do work which ought to be done by the domestic staff.

At the Fever Hospital is a special ward containing 22 cots for wasting children. Every child admitted is kept isolated until a negative rectal swab (for dysenteric organisms) is obtained. An additional precaution taken in this block is the rigid division of staff into "feeders" and "cleaners", which minimises contact enteric infections.

Cases of puerperal fever are treated in this hospital. Blood cultures and cervical cultures are taken in each case, and meanwhile Hobbs' glycerin local treatment is carried out.

School Medical Service

This, as already indicated, is being merged into the municipal service. Hitherto it has been a completely separate service in the city, Dr. George Rose—who has kindly given the information below—being its whole-time medical officer. There is also a whole-time assistant M.O., and there are two whole-time dentists, a part-time oculist, a part-time aural surgeon, and 4 school nurses. There are 27 schools in Aberdeen, including 4 secondary and 3 special, having 26,184 children in average attendance.

At a minor ailment clinic a number of minor maladies are treated. Apart from this but little treatment of children is attempted except for defective teeth.

The Administrative County of Aberdeen

Much of what has been written on the city applies also to the county. The tuberculosis medical officer is consulting officer in the same capacity in the county, and it is hoped that the medical officer for mother and child welfare in the city will soon act in a consulting capacity for similar service in the county. Joint arrangements for hospital beds exist. The V.D. scheme is common to the two, as also to the whole of the north-east of Scotland.

In the county itself, under the stimulating influence of Dr. Murison, the clerk of the County Council, amalgamated activities have been secured. A joint committee for public health services has been organised for some years, containing representatives of:—

> The County Council,
> The Education Authority, and
> The Town Councils of Burghs within the county,

ensuring a common service for public health, for medical inspection and treatment of school children, for venereal diseases, and bacteriological work. The whole county, except two burghs, has a single organisation for maternity and child welfare work.

Poor-law medical work will now be joined with the services named above under one organisation.

The conditions of medical and nursing service in the county are determined by its sparsely scattered population. This may be illustrated by its *Nursing Service*. There are 38 district nursing associations affiliated to a county nursing association, and employing 41 nurses. The network of nurses is as yet incomplete, only about three-fourths of the county being covered. Ten further nurses are needed. These district nurses not only nurse the sick in their districts, but also carry out all nursing and health visiting required under the three statutory schemes of:—

> Maternity and Child Welfare Service,
> Medical Inspection and Treatment of School Children,
> Tuberculosis Scheme.

It is claimed by Dr. Rae, in his last Annual Report for the county, that in its circumstances this system presents the following advantages:—

1. By one nurse doing the manifold duties required the work is centralised, there is economy both in time and in money,

and, what is more important, overlapping and friction are avoided.

2. The district nurse already knows the mothers and can obtain their sympathy more readily than can a full-time health visitor.

3. If the district nurse is the only nurse visiting the home, then there is no undue encroachment on the privacy of the home.

4. The visitation of the home by the district nurse, health visitor, tuberculosis nurse, and school nurse in different persons must lead to confusion of advice, with the result that the advice given will probably be ignored.

Each district nursing association receives £80 per annum from the County Council for the statutory services of its district nurse, voluntary subscriptions, etc., making up her total salary, including the salary for her work in home nursing. The total salary is £180–£200. All the nurses are fully trained, and none of them are registered as or act as midwives. They are forbidden to act in confinement cases except as maternity nurses, for which a payment of 5s. to 10s. is obtained.

There are only three registered midwives in the county.

The *Infant Welfare Work* is not yet fully developed, but such work as is done depends on the help given by the district nurses, and on the co-operation of voluntary workers and medical practitioners. A certain number of children needing hospital care are admitted to the institutions of the Aberdeen Town Council, and some patients also to the City Maternity Hospital.

Tuberculosis Services.—As in other rural counties, the dispensary or anti-tuberculosis centre does not play the important part as a sorting-house which it does in cities. The city T.O. undertakes radiographic work for the county.

The *Venereal Disease* scheme is identical with that of Aberdeen.

School Medical Service.—There are about 26,000 school children in the county, and about one-fourth of these require medical attention when they first enter school. Dr. Rae looks for the remedy of this serious position in the possibility of an extension of the National Insurance Act to dependents and the inclusion of the general practitioner in a comprehensive scheme for the prevention of disease.

The methods by which school medical work is secured in many cases may be gathered from the following official notices :—

COUNTY OF ABERDEEN—PUBLIC HEALTH SERVICES

I

To the Parent or Guardian of

This pupil's teeth require treatment. If you desire to obtain treatment for the pupil please sign the Form on the back of this Card, and return immediately to the Head Teacher of ....School.

The charge for treatment will be 1s.

School Dental Surgeon

I hereby consent to treatment of

(*Name of Pupil*)...

by the School Dental Surgeon.

I am prepared to pay...........................

(If you cannot afford to pay the whole charge, as stated on the other side, please say what you are prepared to pay.)

Signature...

Date...........................

To be filled up and returned to the Head Teacher *immediately*.

II

To the Parent or Guardian of...

This child has been found to have Defective Sight. As this defect will interfere with the child's progress in school work, and may cause headaches and general ill-health, you are advised to consult a Doctor immediately, or send the child to the School Oculist—the place, date, and time of his visit will be intimated later.

If glasses are found to be necessary, you should not obtain them without a Doctor's prescription.

Medical Officer

Date------------------------------

III

To the Parent or Guardian of--

The Medical Officer finds that this child suffers from *Adenoids and Enlarged Tonsils*. Not only may defective speech and defective hearing result from such a cause, but permanent disfigurement to the appearance of the face, mouth, and nose as well. You are advised to consult a Doctor without delay.

Medical Officer

When help in obtaining spectacles is required, the following form is used:—

(To Parent or Guardian.)

MEDICAL TREATMENT—DEFECTIVE EYESIGHT

I beg to enclose prescription received from the oculist employed by the above committee for school spectacles for
named thereon in order that the same may be provided for as soon as possible.

I have to state that if you are in a position to do so at your own expense it is open to you to get the spectacles from any source that you may select, but if you prefer to take advantage of a contract which this committee has made for the supply of spectacles for the children for whom they will require to make provision, they can be ordered through this office on your returning here the prescription along with a remittance for the sum of 4s. 6d. to cover the cost and postage. The committee will not be responsible for damage to spectacles in course of post. Spectacles will be despatched from this office as soon as they have been supplied by the contractors and examined and passed by the oculist. The committee cannot guarantee when they may be delivered, but there will be no avoidable delay, and therefore it is not necessary that any inquiries should be made on the subject.

Any parent or guardian who is unable to procure the spectacles without assistance should send an application for such assistance, along with the prescription, to the Clerk of the School Management Committee for the Area in which his or her place of residence is situated (in your case Mr.   ), stating the applicant's circumstances and the grounds on which such assistance is required, and the S.M. Committee will thereafter report to this office whether, in their opinion, the Committee should contribute the whole or any part of the cost.

Yours faithfully,

(*Signed*) _____

Chief Medical Officer

CHAPTER XXV

I

THE COUNTY OF PERTH[1]

PERTHSHIRE contains some of the most romantic scenery in Scotland: a marvellous kaleidoscope of mountain and forest, of river and lochs; and in this county the problems of medical attendance on the sick and of preventive medicine present many special difficulties, shared to an even greater extent by the still more remote parts of the highlands and islands of Scotland, which are included in the scope of the State subsidised scheme described on pages 471 to 480.

Perthshire has a total area outside its burghs of 1,589,254 acres, its estimated population in 1928 being 67,498.[2] The burghs in the county have an estimated population of about 60,000.

The major public health work of the burghs, each of which at present has a part-time M.O.H., has now come into the hands of the County Council (see also p. 445), the entire executive work being carried out by the county M.O.H. and his staff.

Perthshire—as also Aberdeenshire—anticipated by local initiative the new advance in co-ordination and unification of local administration for all purposes (see p. 444), so far as its officers were concerned. The separate authorities have continued, but the educational and public health medical staff were amalgamated and placed under the executive control in Perthshire of its county M.O.H., Dr. D. J. McLeish, who formerly had been the school medical officer. The amalgamation was made without serious opposition; public opinion was in favour of it; and there can be no doubt that it ensures greater efficiency, with more economical use of the medical and nursing staff. As separatist

[1] Date of investigation, September 1929.
[2] The census (1931) population of the entire county was 120,777, of its burghs 58,012.

views as to the need for keeping educational medical work distinct from other medical branches of public health medical work still persist, the pioneer action of the two county councils named above, confirmed now by like legislation for the entire country, is noteworthy.

MEDICAL STAFF OF THE COUNTY

Public Health	*Education*	
County M.O.H.	The same	
Deputy M.O.H.	The same	} Whole-time.
2 Asst. Medical Officers.	The same	
	Dental surgeon	

2 Dental surgeons (part-time).
Oculist (part-time).
2 Clinical Assistants (for medical and dental work).
2 Nurses (whole-time) for the burgh of Perth.

It is convenient to describe the arrangements for PUBLIC HEALTH NURSES at this point before giving details of individual public medical services. Except in Perth itself, the entire public health nursing work is carried out by district nurses, under the County Superintendent of Nurses, helped by three full-time public health nurses.

The Perthshire Nursing Federation was formed in December 1919. It is a voluntary organisation to promote co-operation between existing district nursing associations in the county, and to help in the formation of further needed local nursing associations. Its organisation is like that of the county nursing associations in England.

It arranges to carry on the public health nursing needed throughout the county, and for this purpose secures annual grants from the County Council. These amount at least to £35 per nurse in districts where all the public health work and school and nursing work, capable of being done by them, is undertaken by the district nurse. Tuberculosis visits are paid for separately at the rate of 1s. per visit.

In the year 1925–26 there were 55 district nurses in the county. Of these 48 were in affiliated districts; and 37 of them were fully trained, and 28 were Queen's Nurses, which means that they had special training in district nursing in addition to their three years' hospital course.

Of the 44 district nursing associations at the same date, 39 were affiliated to the federation. Of the 39 affiliated associations, the nurses in 27 were doing all public health and school work, and in two others were undertaking school work alone or child welfare and tuberculosis work alone.

In a few outlying districts the headquarter staff of the federation, consisting of superintendent, assistant superintendent, and two emergency nurses, undertake local public health and school nursing; and in 1925–26 this central staff did the following work:—

106 Visits to district nurses.
351 Meetings and interviews on nursing subjects.
147 Meetings and interviews on varied matters.
24 Antenatal visits.
3,399 Visits for child welfare work.
1,594 Visits to school children (327 of these were for infectious cases).
180 Inspections of schools.
416 Visits to tuberculous patients.

The following is a summary of work done by the nurses of the district nursing associations in the same year:—

68,490 Nursing visits.
1,849 Ante- and postnatal visits.
13,750 Child welfare visits.
1,198 Tuberculosis visits.
4,461 School inspections and visits.

The difficulties as to transport of nurses are only gradually being overcome. Exact accounts are kept of visits made by the nurses and of the time occupied in:—

1. *Public Health Work.*
   Expectant and nursing mothers.
   Child welfare.
   Tuberculosis.
   School children.
2. *General Nursing Work for Insured Patients.*

The County Council pays at least one-fifth of the total cost of each district nurse. This is about £200 for salary, housing, and travelling. The grant made to the federation for this purpose is given conditionally on the whole-time nurses at the central offices of the federation making all the first visits to notified cases of tuberculosis, thus ensuring uniformity of investigation of these cases. These central nurses also fill up emergency gaps in local staffs, and take holiday and sickness duties.

The chief funds of the local nursing associations are derived from local subscriptions. The County Council arranges that all local nurses shall have the opportunity of attending special courses of instruction for health visitors in Edinburgh or Glasgow.

It will be noted that the district nurse is a "sick nurse" as well as a public health nurse. Many medical officers of health in England strongly object to this combination, urging that sick nursing—especially during an epidemic of influenza, or even with a single home-treated case of pneumonia—prevents the nurse from steadily performing her daily duties as a public health nurse. There is force in this contention in towns and other populated districts which are not too sparse; but in scattered rural districts, and still more in the highland districts of Scotland, the combination is justified and is in fact economical of effort and more efficient than a dual system of service. Without the combination it would be almost impracticable—as well as terribly extravagant of time and effort—to serve the scattered population of rural Perthshire.

MATERNITY WORK

In the entire administrative landward county 892 births occurred in 1928 (population, 67,498), and of this number only 32 were attended by midwives.

Of the 15 midwives in practice, eight were district nurses. A few additional births were attended by district nurses in the unavoidable absence of the doctor. Four deaths occurred in the year from conditions associated with child-birth, but only one from sepsis, this being a patient who was confined in Dundee.

Of the births in the county 3·4 per cent. were still-births. The extent to which home visiting of expectant mothers and infants is carried on is shown below. The figures should be related to the 1,177 births in the year in the landward county and the eight small burghs included in the maternity and child welfare combination.

Expectant Mothers.—No. of 1st visits	.. .. ..	655
No. of revisits	.. .. ..	1,011
No. who consulted a doctor	..	325
Infants.— No. of 1st visits	.. .. ..	1,164
No. of revisits	.. .. ..	8,572
Children 1–5.— No. of 1st visits	.. .. ..	797
No. of revisits	.. .. ..	8,001

There are no antenatal or infant consultations or tuberculosis clinics in the county. With its scattered population their establishment would be futile. The practical alternative is that the functional essence of these agencies should be carried throughout the county under the doctor's hat and the nurse's cap, and that these two should be in effective collaboration.

A few patients are sent to lying-in institutions.

The infant mortality rate in the county is low. In 1928 it was 49 in the landward county, and 57 in the burghs, as compared with 86 for Scotland as a whole.

TUBERCULOSIS WORK

In 1928 the number of deaths from tuberculosis in the landward county was 43, of which 34 were pulmonary, equivalent to a total death-rate of 0·63 per 1,000 of population. In the same year in the entire county, excepting the burgh of Perth, 110 cases of tuberculosis were notified to the M.O.H. Of these cases 17 per cent. were only reported within a month of death; and in 28 per cent. of the total deaths from tuberculosis no notification had been received.

It will be seen that while the incidence of tuberculosis is low, the supervision of cases of this disease is difficult, owing in part to failures in notification and in part to the scattered distribution of the population. Most of the newly notified cases are seen personally by the county M.O.H., who decides in consultation with the medical attendant when institutional treatment is indicated. Owing to difficulties in making appointments, the M.O.H. has arranged to examine such patients alone. The doctors trust him, and the arrangement works well.

First visits by nurses are made by the central nursing staff, subsequent visits by nurses of the district associations. In 1928, 2,474 such visits were made, many of these not only for supervision and advice, but also for nursing. In addition to the monetary grant by the County Council to each nursing association, an additional *per capita* payment of 1s. per visit is made for each visit by a nurse. Friction between the visiting nurses and the private doctor is rare.

It may be noted that prior to 1922 five special tuberculosis nurses were employed exclusively for these cases; but the work was scanty and its distribution scattered, and on the advice of the county M.O.H. district nurses are now utilised for this work.

Venereal Disease Work

There are two free treatment centres for all comers, one in Stirling, and one in Perth, the latter at the Royal Infirmary (a voluntary hospital). In 1928 only 24 patients were treated at these centres. They made 591 attendances.

There appears to be little venereal disease in the county; but it is likely that some patients, whose home address is untraced, are treated at other centres outside the county.

School Medical Work

There are 15,258 children in average attendance at 169 elementary schools in the county; and to undertake the medical work for these, the staff, in addition to Dr. McLeish, acting as principal school medical officer, consists of three assistant school doctors (whole-time), an oculist (part-time), two dentists (whole-time); also two separate school nurses for the burgh of Perth.

The details of medical and dental inspection need not detain us. There is a school clinic in Perth, and much treatment of minor skin and other such ailments is carried on by nurses in different parts of the county.

Sometimes it is difficult to persuade private doctors that they are being "fed with work" by the school doctors, though this is so. Very rarely is there friction, and quite recently the Perth Branch of the British Medical Association passed a resolution approving of the school medical arrangements, and stating that they had no desire to undertake school medical work.

In rural parts of Perthshire very often poorer patients with minor ailments are sent by the private practitioner to the district nurse, to receive her continued care.

The *Poor Law Medical Work* in the county is not very extensive since national insurance was introduced.

National Medical Insurance is regarded in the county as having been the salvation of the country doctor, whose income previously was very small. This is so, although the position of the rural doctor under national medical insurance is not nearly so favourable as that of his urban confrère.

To Dr. McLeish I am indebted for giving me every facility for making inquiries in Perthshire and explaining its public health arrangements; as well as for arranging my visit to Dr. Mackay (page 476).

II

THE ROYAL BURGH OF ST. ANDREWS

St. Andrews is a small town on the east coast of Scotland, occupying a somewhat isolated position, separated from Edinburgh and Dundee by broad estuaries. It has a population of about 10,000[1]; but nevertheless, apart from its

[1] The census (1931) population was 8,269.

celebrity as the Mecca of golfers, it is also well known as the centre of an ancient University, and the home of the James Mackenzie Institute for Clinical Research.

It finds a place here, because in St. Andrews has been developed, probably more completely than elsewhere, a complete medical supervision of a large portion of its population through every period of life. It has, in nucleus at least, a State medical service, in which the private medical practitioners of the burgh play a predominant part.

The child welfare scheme is the organisation around which this service has been built up, with the continuous co-operation of the well-known Institute for Clinical Research, founded by Sir James Mackenzie.

The M.O.H., Dr. Matthew Fyfe, is also bacteriologist to the institute, and thus there is a constant linking up of the activities of the child welfare institute. There were only 119 births during 1928, and every case can, therefore, be given a "personal touch".

Clinics are held twice weekly in the child welfare centre, and there were during the year 1,229 attendances of children under 5 years of age. Of the total babies born 88 per cent. received the benefits of this service.

In addition, 73 special clinics were held at the James Mackenzie Institute. These were for children over 2 years of age; 331 children attended.

The general practitioners in the burgh are in contact with these clinics, and supply information as to any acute illness attended by them. As stated in the Annual Report for 1928 of Dr. Matthew Fyfe, M.O.H., the system of regular observation from birth affords the opportunity of calling the attention of the mothers to conditions which require medical attention and nursing in the home, and it is found that in almost all cases they put the children under the care of the family doctor when asked to do so.

No treatment is given at the clinics.

There is also an antenatal clinic conducted by the general practitioners of the town, expectant mothers consulting the doctors of their choice.

The spirit actuating the Institute for Clinical Research, that of endeavouring to detect the earliest departures from normal health, is carried into the whole of the work of personal hygiene in St. Andrews, and fortunately the general practitioners of the burgh have actively co-operated in this effort. From this point of view it is regarded as highly inadvisable to deprive private doctors of their facilities for all-round treatment, thus avoiding the risk of diminishing their clinical acumen. The ideal in Dr. Fyfe's words is that "it is not the specialist, not the public health official, but the general practitioner who is the true custodian of health".

The records kept in this burgh are exceptionally complete and continuous. Most of the children of the burgh are followed up from infancy to school age; they are then kept under observation during school life, the school medical officers adding to the previous record of each child, which is stored in the clinical institute; and, lastly, this continuous record becomes available for the insurance doctor or private practitioner, who in St. Andrews continues to add to the record. Thus for over 80 per cent. of the younger inhabitants of the burgh there is available a dossier of health and disease, ready for research and for the guidance of the physician when seeing a patient at any period of life.

Dr. Fyfe remarks that "one of the more pleasing effects which have been produced by the local policy has been the removal of that barrier of suspicion which too commonly exists between general practitioners and public officials".

This note is inserted here as a striking example of what can be done in a small town where there is good leadership and the attitude of constant co-operation is encouraged. If a similar spirit could be evoked in rural communities, and still more in densely populated cities, public health work would become more successful than it has hitherto been.

CHAPTER XXVI

THE CITY OF GLASGOW

GLASGOW, in 1931 (census), had a population of 1,088,417 persons. Thus in Great Britain it stands next to London, Birmingham coming third. To attempt in these pages an adequate description of its medico-hygienic arrangements is impracticable; and I propose to restrict myself to points at which public administration comes into touch with private medical practitioners, and in which there are, therefore, possibilities of friction. The social circumstances of the population determine in large measure the possibilities of friction between private and public medical work. For the very poor these possibilities do not arise. Medical practitioners are willing to be relieved of the large mass of gratuitous medical work which in the past they have done. Now that a third of the total population are insured for medical attendance, on a *per capita* basis, sick or well, there is little opportunity for friction when practitioners are relieved of some of their work by tuberculosis and V.D. clinics provided at the ratepayers' and taxpayers' expense, or when the out-patient departments of voluntary hospitals—as is the general experience—continue to receive patients, among others of the insured class, in numbers which show no diminution.

Glasgow is one of the largest ports, as well as a centre of vast miscellaneous industries, many of which employ large numbers of unskilled workers. It is somewhat cosmopolitan in its population, and receives large numbers of immigrants from Ireland, whose standard of life has been below that of the average Scottish worker.

It is densely populated; the proportion of dwellings consisting of only one or two rooms to a family being very high. Its birth-rate was 20·6 per 1,000 in 1928, and its death-rate from all causes was 13·7, from tuberculosis (all forms) 1·13 per 1,000, on the basis of the M.O.H.'s estimate of Glasgow's population. Its infant mortality in the same year was 107 per 1,000 births.

At the end of 1928, about 3 per cent. of the total population were resident in institutions, and of the total deaths 45 per cent. occurred in hospitals.

These hospitals are:—

I. *Voluntary*—

Royal Infirmary	782 beds
Western Infirmary	600 beds
David Elder Infirmary	43 beds
Victoria Infirmary	400 beds
Elder Cottage Hospital	29 beds and 5 cots
Royal Hospital for Sick Children ..	288 cots
Royal Maternity and Women's Hospital	145 beds
Royal Maternity Cottage Hospital ..	23 beds
Royal Samaritan Hospital for Women	154 beds
Glasgow Hospital for Women ..	32 beds
The Eye Infirmary	108 beds
Ophthalmic Institution	30 beds and 6 cots
Ear, Throat, and Nose Hospital ..	52 beds
Royal Cancer Hospital	62 beds
Lock Hospital	60 beds and 30 cots

II. *Official*—

(a) *Public Health Department*

The infectious diseases, excluding tuberculosis	1,406 beds
For tuberculosis—	
In hospitals	973 beds
In sanatoria and homes	188 beds
In poor-law institutions	218 beds
(b) *Parish Council* (Poor-Law), in various institutions (excluding lunacy)	2,327 beds
(c) *Education Committee*	12 beds

Most of the voluntary hospitals have out-patient departments or dispensaries, often crowded with general medical and surgical cases and patients with special diseases.

The venereal disease clinics at each of these hospitals or infirmaries are in fact official organisations in voluntary hands, and do the same work as is done in the special Corporation clinics for V.D. In addition, there are five special tuberculosis clinics under official management, and 14 clinics for maternity and child welfare in different sections of the city; these also are official. These are in addition to the school clinics and small school hospital mentioned on page 520.

In actual fact any difficulty experienced by private practitioners has been chiefly with the voluntary and not with the official dispensaries and hospitals. These even more than official dispensaries deprive the private doctors of patients who otherwise would come to their private surgeries, and there is the further objection that touch is lost with patients whom the practitioner has sent to a hospital. The position in this regard is somewhat complicated. Very often the practitioner himself is in fault when he receives no report concerning a patient sent by him to a hospital, inasmuch as he has sent no report of the patient's history with him to the hospital, and has not specifically asked for a report. In view of the multitude of cases coming to each out-patient department the physician seeing new patients cannot be expected to send personal letters about these "into the blue". Not infrequently, when this appears desirable, patients will say they have no doctor, or do not know his name, or do not intend to go back to the same doctor. On the other hand, a personal letter from a doctor to a particular physician at the hospital will bring an answer.

To a good family doctor it is galling to lose touch with patients when special treatment which is impracticable at home necessitates his sending them to a hospital. In view of this and similar difficulties the local medical committee for Glasgow (under the National Insurance Act) have formed a *Hospitals Sub-Committee*. This comprises eight members of the local medical committee, the superintendents of the four chief voluntary infirmaries of the city, and the M.O.H. The aim of this committee is to investigate methods for establishing a closer relationship between private and hospital doctors in the interest of their patients, and they have published a brochure (*Notes on Hospital and Infirmary Arrangements, Glasgow*, A. MacDougall, 1927) which gives information as to methods of procedure. The salient direction when sending a patient to a dispensary or special department for opinion or treatment is "send note containing name and address and a brief summary of salient points in condition. . . . A professional card is not a substitute for a letter." The following note is also important: "National health insurance patients, except in cases of urgency, are not attended to unless referred by the practitioner responsible for their treatment".

The following extracts from the same brochure illustrate special relations with official hospitals and clinics :—

When a patient is sent in with diphtheria, reference should be made to any previous antitoxin treatment....

When a case of tuberculosis is notified, the patient is visited by a nurse to obtain certain information, and to arrange for examination of the patient by the T.O. at a dispensary or, if too ill, at home. . . . Should the practitioner desire to continue the treatment of the patient, the T.O. does not visit.

If the practitioner does not wish the nurse to call, he is asked to supply certain medical and sociological particulars. . . .

A practitioner wishing it will be supplied with a copy of the records of institutional treatment. . . .

When sending a V.D. patient to a clinic for treatment it will greatly help if the doctor sends a short history of the patient and his previous treatment.

Further comments on some of these points are made in later paragraphs.

The due co-ordination of the work of voluntary hospitals with that of private practitioners is a task of colossal magnitude in a city as large as Glasgow. It implies mutual helpfulness and a readiness to devote time to interchange of experience and opinion. On both sides this is difficult, owing to the overwork both in hospital and private practice, particularly the worst form of overwork, which is work against time—"rush work".

The relation of insurance practitioners to hospital and other agencies is considered in a separate chapter.

Official medical agencies for the sick poor in Glasgow, as elsewhere, have hitherto been under the control of the

Parish Council; under that of the Corporation for acute and chronic infectious diseases, including tuberculosis and V.D., and maternity and child welfare; and under the Education Authority for school children. These agencies are now brought under a single local parliament, the City Council of Glasgow.

An interesting example of what has already been accomplished in collaboration between public medicine and voluntary medical charity is that of provision for maternity cases. The demands on the Glasgow Maternity Hospital (voluntary) were in excess of available accommodation, while at the Stobhill Hospital[1] (poor-law) there was suitable vacant accommodation, and with the approval of the Scottish Local Government Board (now the Department of Health), the accommodation of the two hospitals in 1925 was arranged to supplement each other in meeting the public need. In this wise development there has been some departure from the legal position of poor-law administration, under which, strictly interpreted, the dependents of an able-bodied man, even though he is destitute, are not entitled to assistance at the expense of the poor rates. But Glasgow has determined to look at the matter broadly and provide hospital accommodation urgently needed, until there is some statutory provision charged with the duty of ensuring that hospital provision is available to all persons requiring it and unable to pay for it (see *Seventh Annual Report, Scottish Board of Health*, 1925, p. 265).

In Scotland public health authorities already have the statutory duty to provide hospital accommodation for all infectious patients needing it.

The above illustration of valuable co-operation between voluntary and official hospitals has been followed in recent years by increasing co-operation between the Parish Council and the Town Council in providing hospital beds and treatment for tuberculosis and pneumonia.

[1] Stobhill Hospital has some 1,700 beds, and is the largest hospital in Scotland. So far as legal restrictions permit, it is already a first-class general hospital.

The City Council, which is the chief local governing body in Glasgow, and since April 1930 is the sole one, consists of 113 members selected by direct vote of ratepayers, divided into councillors and a smaller number of bailies, who are also magistrates. Its Public Health Committee consists of the Lord Provost and 37 members elected from the Council. They control the public health activities of the city, subject to financial control by the Council as a whole. The Committee has the following sub-committees for detailed consideration of different branches of work:—

> Hospitals and Sanatoria.
> Maternity and Child Welfare.
> Venereal Disease.
> Meat and Fish Inspections.
> Smoke Abatement.
> Accounts.
> Works.

There are no co-opted members on the Maternity and Child Welfare Committee. This is legally required under the English Law. The above committees will soon be entirely remodelled. The chief secretary of the Department is Mr. William Jones, without whose collaboration and guidance the medical staff would be submerged in executive secretarial detail.

The able chief of the public health staff of Glasgow is Dr. A. S. Macgregor, M.O.H., to whom I am indebted not only for most of the information in this report, but also for his courtesy in sparing me much time and in giving me access to files in his department.

He has the following whole-time medical staff:—

> 1 Assistant M.O.H.
> 4 Divisional Medical Officers,
> 1 Port Boarding M.O.
> 5 Tuberculosis Clinical Officers.
> 10 Child Welfare Medical Officers.
> 1 Child Welfare Medical Officer for Venereal Diseases

All the maternity and child welfare doctors are women, including one who is concerned wholly with administrative work.

At one welfare centre, in addition, two medical women, who are also in general practice, are employed, as well as a part-time woman dentist.

There is also a consulting oculist.

The above staff does not include the staff of the four large infectious diseases hospitals, which have a resident medical staff of 19.

In addition, these hospitals have visiting surgeons, aural surgeons, and oculists.

MATERNITY SERVICE

In 1928 the deaths classified as due to maternal causes occurred at the rate of 8·8 per 1,000 births. In 1926 the rate was 6·7, the excess in 1928 being due to excessive mortality from sepsis in one of the lying-in hospitals of the city.

In 1928 there were 289 midwives in practice in Glasgow, 108 of these being in practice prior to December 1914, and without recognised certification of competence. Of the total 23,649 births registered in 1928, about 41 per cent. were attended by midwives. Among these cases 120 cases of puerperal fever occurred; and in 2,496 instances, or about 24 per cent. of their cases, requests were made for medical aid in emergencies. Of these cases the emergency arose :—

> During pregnancy in 107 instances.
> In labour in 1,682 instances.
> In lying-in period in 288 instances.
> In respect of the child in 404 instances.
> Unclassified in 15 instances.

The fees paid to practitioners in 1928 amounted to £1,632 5s., of which amount £366 8s. 6d. was subsequently recovered by the Corporation from the patients. The calling-in of medical practitioners for emergencies does not show the marked increase manifested in some other areas.

CHILD WELFARE SERVICE

The infant mortality rate in 1928 was 107 per 1,000 births, which, although it represents a decline of 35 per cent. as compared with Glasgow's average experience in 1901–10 is not satisfactory in comparison with other great towns. Comparing its statistics for 1927 with those of Birmingham, the next largest city in Great Britain, the infant death-rate from respiratory disease was double, and that from diseases of the digestive system nearly 26 per cent. in excess in Glasgow.

There are 14 centres for mothers and infants in the city, at which are held 71 weekly consultations, of which 13 are antenatal clinics and 6 ultra-violet light treatment centres. At the infant consultations the total attendances in the year were 127,879, an average of 50 at each consultation.

Supplies of milk were given to expectant and nursing mothers and to children under 5 when (1) the medical officer of the centre certified this was necessary; (2) the case was necessitous; and (3) there was regular attendance at the child welfare centre. Grants of fresh milk in 1928 were made free in 36,421 cases, at a reduced price in 1,216 cases, and 219 applications were refused. Grants of dried milk were made free in 159 instances, and at a reduced price in 4 instances.

At the Royal Maternity Hospital 4,431 mothers attended its antenatal consultations, and 1,172 patients were admitted to its antenatal wards. At the antenatal clinics held in the official child welfare centres 503 consultations were held during the year, and 2,651 primary attendances were recorded.

Home visiting is done by health visitors, all infants born at which a doctor has not been in attendance being visited. In 1928, 15,392 infants under 1 year were visited for a first time, those classified "well" at this visit not being revisited. Evidently home supervision and counsel by skilled nurses are not very complete in Glasgow. The health visitors for infants do not undertake tuberculosis visiting. Dr. Macgregor attaches importance to this separation of duties. The city population is compact, and the separation of duties involves but little extra travelling. Furthermore, the division of duties makes it possible for the health visitor to be present at each consultation, which is very valuable when making her subsequent home visits.

At the centres infants and toddlers found to need treatment are referred to their own doctor, or to the various voluntary hospitals of the city—Children's, Ear and Throat, Eye and Dental. It is hoped shortly to combine activities in these directions for scholars with similar care for the school child.

Many minor conditions are treated at the centres. For the majority of patients the average practitioner in Glasgow cannot undertake some classes of cases. He has not the time for it; and if he had, the heads of families concerned could not remunerate him on a scale which would give a "living wage". This applies particularly—

(*a*) To the regulation of the diet of infants and young children; and

(*b*) To minor surgical, and especially septic or contagious conditions, e.g. impetigo, sores, eczema, pediculosis, etc.

The same remarks apply—

(*c*) To the dental needs of the majority of school children.

Not only in Glasgow, but very generally, dentists are very willing to be relieved of the majority of these patients. In regard to all the above groups of cases it is broadly true that if the public health and school authorities did not treat, using their nursing staff—which is usually lacking in the private doctor's surgery—very largely to assist in this work, the cases would continue to be neglected.

Speaking generally, the doctors in Glasgow do not object to the child welfare work of the Corporation. It has been stated above that parents would not pay doctors for most of the conditions now being treated at infant clinics. This results from economic conditions, in part also from the unwillingness of parents to spend money on "minor" complaints. Whenever the benefits of medical insurance are extended to dependents, the position can be revised, and each family doctor may possibly be made responsible for keeping the family well, and for detail in the treatment of minor complaints. Even then much of the work thus devolving on him could be done by a nurse.

TUBERCULOSIS SERVICE

During 1928 there were 954 deaths from pulmonary tuberculosis, and 1,724 new cases were notified.

During the year the number of cases of pulmonary and non-pulmonary tuberculosis admitted to institutions was as follows :—

Local Authority's Hospitals	1,429
Sanatoria	418
Poor Law Institutions	819
	2,666

altogether several times the number of deaths.

There are six special dispensaries for tuberculosis, in which 1,236 sessions have been held. Two hundred and forty-four new patients attended, and made 51,406 subsequent attendances during 1928. Health visitors made 46,182 home visits to tuberculosis patients.

There is said to be practically no complaint by general practitioners of the official tuberculosis work, except that institutional beds for their patients sometimes cannot be had. Many doubtful cases are sent to the dispensary for diagnosis, and X-ray photographs taken in these cases. Dr. Macgregor states that the practice is now growing up of cases not being notified by the private practitioner until after a dispensary consultation has taken place. The tuberculosis staff still encounter patients—this is not surprising, though regrettable, in a large city—who have been attended at a doctor's private surgery for a long period with a cough without any sputum or chest examination, and without reference to the pathological and consultative facilities always available.

A report is sent by the tuberculosis officer to every practitioner who has sent a patient with a letter giving particulars and asking for it.

VENEREAL DISEASE SERVICE

This disease is treated gratuitously for all comers at all the chief voluntary hospitals in the city, as well as at two *ad hoc* centres. These are all staffed by salaried part-time medical officers. Altogether there are 19 of these, including two pathologists. In 1928, 801 patients were admitted into hospital, and 5,343 patients were treated as out-patients for these diseases. There is not much private practice in these diseases. Attempts have been recently made unsuccessfully to obtain legislative powers to secure the continued attendance at the clinics of persons who cease coming when active symptoms have disappeared; and it is likely that these attempts will be renewed. If compulsion is to be attempted it should not be limited to patients attending clinics. The problem presents very serious difficulties. Three years ago a special nurse visitor was appointed to visit women and children who ceased attendance before their treatment was completed, to endeavour to bring them back to the clinic. This has been successful in about 50 per cent. of the cases visited.

During the year the following pathological examinations were made at the municipal laboratory for the physicians at various clinics:—

Wassermann tests	8,378
Spirochætes	761
Gonococci	13,823

Similar specimens are examined gratuitously for all medical practitioners.

BLIND PERSONS

Throughout Great Britain these are entitled to a pension at the age of 50. The working of the Blind Persons Act is in the hands of a joint committee composed of the local public health authorities of Glasgow and the south-west of Scotland. A central clinic has been established in Glasgow, conducted by four consulting ophthalmologists, at which is decided the treatment and future of blind persons, and the giving of pensions at the age of 50. This is the first clinic of the kind in Scotland.

SCHOOL MEDICAL SERVICE

This has hitherto been in charge of the independent Glasgow Education Authority; but it is now being transferred to the new Education Committee of the Corporation. I am indebted to Dr. E. T. Roberts, who has been the whole-time school medical officer for Glasgow for the last 20 years, for the following information.

There are nearly 162,000 children in the elementary schools; and, including intermediate schools and residential institutions, the total number of pupils for whom the Education Authority was responsible in 1927–28 numbered 190,880.

During the year 142,847 breakfasts, 458,734 dinners, and 122,536 teas were supplied to necessitous children at various centres, and boots or clothing, or both, were supplied to 23,508 children.

The medical school staff consists of Dr. Roberts and a deputy M.O., of 12 assistant medical officers, and of 4 dentists, all of whom are whole-time officers. In addition there are the following part-time officers: 2 aurists, 4 oculists, 3 dentists, and 1 inspecting M.O. The methods and intervals of medical inspection do not differ from those in other towns.

Medical treatment is based on the rule that only necessitous children will be treated whose parents are unable to pay a private practitioner, or to obtain from a voluntary agency the help they need.

The standard of ability to pay for treatment which has been adopted is 12s. income for every member of the family. Thus a man with a wage of £3 a week, with a wife and three children, would have his school children treated gratuitously.

This scale means that a very high proportion of school children can be treated gratuitously. If an operation is needed, as for tonsils and adenoids, the upper limit of wage eligible for free treatment is increased by 20s.

In practice the Education Authority has been compelled by circumstances to take on considerable non-medical charitable work as well as treatment of disease. Neither the Parish Council nor the Society for Social Service (a voluntary body) has been equal to the prompt and adequate supply of food, clothing, etc., in many instances, and the Education Authority has supplemented their work.

On the medical side parochial medical facilities for children were inadequate and the voluntary hospitals were overcrowded with patients. Furthermore, attendance and prolonged waiting of children at these centres were most undesirable. For adenoids sometimes an interval of several months occurred before operation was possible.

School clinics were therefore initiated with the broad limitations indicated above; and in view of the difficulty of securing prompt operations in voluntary hospitals a school hospital having 12 beds was started for operation cases. At this hospital there are operations thrice weekly; each child with adenoids is kept in for two nights, one before and one after the operation, longer if necessary. Other operations are for abnormal turbinates, but mastoids are not undertaken.

For eye cases, refraction and other work is done by part-time specialists in the school service.

Any treatment needed can be enforced under Section 12 of the Children Act, 1908, neglect to provide this on the part of the parent being construed as cruelty. The following warning notice is sent in such cases to parents:—

EDUCATION AUTHORITY OF GLASGOW

MEDICAL INSPECTION AND TREATMENT OF CHILDREN

Warning to Parents and Guardians regarding Medical or Dental Treatment

Parents and Guardians are warned that any person over the age of 16 years who has the custody, charge, or care of any child, and wilfully neglects such child in a manner likely to cause unnecessary suffering or injury to health, is guilty of a misdemeanour, and is liable on conviction to various penalties.

At Glasgow Sheriff Court some time ago, a parent was charged with neglecting his child by failing to have certain decayed teeth extracted. This parent had received warning from the Education Authority that in the opinion of the School Medical Officer the condition of the child's teeth was causing suffering and injury to his health. The parent had refused to provide the dental treatment, and had also declined to allow the Education Authority to give the necessary treatment. The Sheriff imposed a fine of £5, with the alternative of 10 days' imprisonment.

Director of Education

For children whose parents are receiving parish relief there is no difficulty as to free treatment.

Dental treatment is given by school dentists for a large number of school children, especially in the schools in poorer districts, where as many as 90 per cent. of the children may be necessitous.

PART IV

IRELAND

CHAPTER XXVII

IRELAND[1]

PRELIMINARY SURVEY

From the point of view of public health and of medical care for its population Ireland in its entirety presents a number of interesting features.

In the past it has been a chief home and centre of typhus fever, from which this bane was carried from time to time to England and Scotland, and even to America. The epidemiological history of typhus in Ireland, and of the more chronic infection of tuberculosis, is most instructive; but for this I must refer readers to official reports and to my study on "Poverty and Disease, as illustrated by the Course of Typhus Fever and Phthisis in Ireland," which I contributed to the *Proceedings of the Royal Society of Medicine* (Presidential Address, Epidemiological Section, October 1907). Typhus fever now prevails in Ireland to a limited and declining extent. In 1880 it caused a death-rate of 179 per million of population; while in the year 1927-28 only 13 cases were recorded in the Free State and six in Northern Ireland.

The medical points of special interest displayed in Ireland are three:—

1. Ireland as a whole has a dispensary (including domiciliary) system of medical treatment for all "poor persons"; and from one-third to one-half of the population —in rural districts, and perhaps also in towns—are treated under this system.

The dispensary doctor is empowered to call in a consultant physician or surgeon if need arises; and institutional treatment is also given when patients cannot be safely treated in their homes.

2. The provision comprises also a salaried midwife in most dispensary areas, with provision in critical cases for

[1] Date of investigation, April 1930.

assistance by a skilled obstetrician, when the dispensary doctor as the first consultant thinks this necessary.

In its dispensary service Ireland possesses a national medical and midwifery service for a large part of its total population, supported out of rates and taxes.

Notwithstanding the deficiencies of this dispensary service, it has been of inestimable social service to Ireland; and were it abandoned some similar provision would need to be recreated.

3. The British Sickness Insurance Act, 1911, provided in Ireland a monetary sickness benefit, but not medical attendance, as in Great Britain. Medical certification was provided for, as set out on page 536.

These three circumstances give special interest to Ireland, in studying national provision for medical aid in relation to the private practice of medicine. Before giving further details, the governmental system of Ireland must be outlined, and a short statement given of other aspects of medical governmental work than those enumerated above.

GOVERNMENT AND SOCIAL CONDITIONS

Prior to 1922, Ireland's affairs were controlled much as in England and Scotland, with differences arising out of its poverty and the political and religious disputes between North and South, and between Ireland and the British Parliament. Ireland's poverty has been extreme, and prior to the Potato Famine of 1845–47 its population of about 8 millions were most of them dependent on a single tuber for subsistence. In 1928 the population of the Free State (Saorstat Eirann) was estimated at 2,949,000, and that of Northern Ireland at 1,250,000. A continuous stream of emigration had transferred a large part of Ireland's population to America and other countries.

This is not the place to describe the efforts of the British Parliament to secure land reform, improved housing, and other reforms, for which British funds were very largely used.

Except in some remote sparsely peopled western districts,

where the people live a precarious life in boggy and stony areas, there has been steady improvement in the standard of living. As the result of liberal housing subsidies in the past the standard of housing has been greatly improved, and the single-room hovel, except in a few areas, has disappeared. But in towns conditions are unsatisfactory, and perhaps especially so in the poorer part of Dublin.

Ireland for wage-earners and the small peasant proprietors remains a land of relative poverty; and even for those above this level it is a much poorer country than Scotland (in the main) and than England. This fact has governed public health and medical developments in Ireland. It must always be remembered that Ireland, outside a few towns, remains a chiefly agricultural country; and that it has not yet, as a whole, found the prosperity in intensive and co-operative agriculture which Denmark has created.

Prolonged political dissatisfaction of a section of the Irish population became rebellion; and in 1920 there followed the giving of a measure of self-government to the greater part of Ireland, going far beyond the Home Rule which the Irish through their representatives had been willing to accept, and which would have been given at a much earlier date but for the rigid and bellicose opposition of the Protestant North of Ireland. The new constitution of Northern Ireland was based on the Government of Ireland Act, 1920; and the Free State was created separately in 1922.

Ireland was thus divided into the Irish Free State (Saorstat Eirann) and Northern Ireland.

Each of these has a representative Parliament, and separate central official departments for the supervision and partial control of local government, but Northern Ireland is still part of the United Kingdom, and continues to send representatives to Westminster. The Irish Free State has the same degree of independence as other countries outside Great Britain within the British Empire; and Northern Ireland has been given similar separate status as regards local government, but certain services, e.g. Customs, Post Offices, are reserved by the British Government.

The Free State is divided into 27 administrative counties and 4 county boroughs; while Northern Ireland has 6 counties and 2 county boroughs.

Until recently the unit of administration outside the larger towns, both in the north and south of Ireland, was the rural district, and it still remains so in Northern Ireland. The rural district is a subdivision of the county, and is controlled by members of the district council, who are *ex officio* Guardians of the Poor. This is like English Government of the recent past; and, as in England, county councils were entrusted with certain special work, detailed for Ireland in the Tuberculosis Prevention Acts of 1908 and 1913, in the Midwives (Ireland) Act of 1918, and in the Medical Treatment of Children Act of 1919. In Northern Ireland the last-named Act was repealed by the Education Act (Northern Ireland) Act, 1923, which gives somewhat wider powers to local authorities. In 1925 rural district councils were abolished in the Free State, and their powers, duties, and debts transferred to county councils.

Local boards were set up under the new regime for the relief of the poor. County health districts were created with local boards of health, omitting urban areas. These local boards are formed of 10 members of the county council, elected by an ingenious system of proportional representation. In the more highly organised counties three committees are formed, a Public Health Committee, a Hospital and Dispensary Committee, and a Home Assistance Committee.

A full-time county M.O.H. under the 1925 Act was required to be appointed for each county; and this officer is already at work in more than half the counties.

Centrally local affairs are supervised, and through grants and in other ways controlled by the Department of Local Government and Public Health for the Free State; and a steady improvement in local sanitation and general health is occurring.

There is a Parliamentary Minister and a Permanent Secretary of the Department; and the Principal Medical Adviser is Dr. Edward F. Stephenson, to whom I am indebted for valuable assistance and guidance. The Central Health Department is divided into three branches, with Dr. Stephenson at their head. The branches are:—

1. *Preventive and Public Health Branch.*
   Executive office staff.
   A consultant pathologist.
   Three medical inspectors (general).
   One medical inspector (tuberculosis and venereal disease).

2. *Curative Medical Charities Branch.*
   Executive office staff.
   A pharmacist.
   Three medical inspectors (also engaged in public health work).

3. *Institutional Poor-Law Hospital.*
   Executive office staff.
   Two medical inspectors.

In Northern Ireland, outside its two county boroughs, Belfast and Londonderry, and 32 additional urban district councils, its six counties are divided into 32 rural districts, each with a rural district council, responsible for sanitary administration, and with the boards of guardians for relief of the poor. County administration is not so advanced as in the Free State.

We may next briefly outline the public medical services, apart from those of sickness insurance and for the sick poor. In the large towns there is a varied provision of voluntary hospitals supported by subscriptions and endowments; and attached to these hospitals in Dublin, Belfast, and Cork are medical schools with a distinguished record in medical education.

The provision for infectious diseases and for pathological examinations, which are made somewhat incompletely by public health authorities, need not be specially detailed.

MATERNITY AND CHILD WELFARE WORK

The crude birth-rate in the Free State in 1928 was 20·1 per 1,000 of population. The number of legitimate births per 1,000 married women aged 15-45 was 271 in 1927-28, as compared with 229 in Northern Ireland, 183 in Scotland, and 138 in England and Wales. The infantile mortality was 68 per 1,000 births, that of Northern Ireland being 78, of Scotland 86, and of England and Wales 65. It was somewhat high in towns—in Dublin 96, in Limerick, Wexford, and Tralee 117 per 1,000 births. In Belfast it was 101 per 1,000 births.

As in England, local authorities since 1915 have been encouraged to make arrangements for attending to the health of expectant and nursing mothers and children under 5 years of age; and grants for this purpose of 50 per cent. of approved expenditure have been given by the Central Government.

In the year 1927-28 £17,303 was disbursed by the Government of the Free State for this purpose, and £4,882 similarly by the Government of Northern Ireland. Most of the work has been done by voluntary agencies, and in the Free State especially by the 105 district nursing associations which work outside Dublin. The work is not yet completely developed, and great arrears need to be overtaken. In Dublin a model child welfare centre has been opened, given by the Carnegie Trust, which is intended as a model for the rest of Ireland, and a whole-time pediatrician and gynæcologist has been appointed for maternity and child welfare work. He will work in close unison with the Rotunda and other maternity hospitals in Dublin. In Belfast, as in Dublin, there has been, until recently, no medical officer in the public health department devoting her or his whole time to this special work. There are three part-time medical officers who attend the six infant welfare centres in Belfast. These meet weekly.

These and allied facts for Belfast are contrasted with corresponding facts for other towns in the following table, the details of which are taken from an unprinted return supplied by Dr. Chas. Thomson, the newly appointed medical superintendent of health of Belfast, to whom and to Dr. Barron, his second in command, I am indebted for showing me the municipal work of Belfast and the important prospective developments which are contemplated by the municipality, guided by Dr. Thomson:—

	Belfast	Birmingham	Bradford
Population	415,151	976,500	288,500
Infant Welfare Centres ..	6	27	12
Weekly Sessions	6	88	17
Medical Officers for Maternity and Child Welfare—			
Whole-time..	0	9	4
Part-time	3	19	2
Health Visitors for Maternity and Child Welfare Work	10	81	20
Antenatal Centres	0	0	5
Sessions	0	40[1]	7
1d. rate produces	£7,000	£25,805	£9,976

1d. rate produces in Dublin (population, 319,700) £10,546.

I was informed that the local branch of the British Medical Association recently addressed a letter to the Corporation of Belfast. In this, referring to a recent report by the Medical Superintendent of Health advocating greatly needed increase of child welfare work, they strongly objected to the fact that they had not been consulted in regard to these proposals, and deprecated the projected encroachment on their work which they assume is about to occur. Their efforts presumably will be directed towards securing a rota of part-time doctors for the child welfare centres. Dr. Thomson is opposed to this, as in recent experience he has found that private practitioners may fail to keep their appointments at the centres. There is little doubt that progress in Belfast will follow a course similar to that through which English communities have already passed.

[1] These are held in infant welfare clinics.

Medical practitioners in the city and county of Cork had somewhat earlier made representations to the central department in Dublin, alleging that the appointment of whole-time medical officers of health for the city and the county was leading to encroachment on the work of private medical practitioners, and especially of specialists for eye, ear, and throat cases, and in orthopædics. They urged the limitation of the work of officials "as much as possible to the prevention of disease", and urged that health visitors should be definitely "responsible to a local practitioner for patients dealt with by them".

The discussion of maternity work in Ireland may be better understood after its dispensary system has been described.

School Medical Work in Ireland has only recently been begun. It was not until 1919 that the Public Health (Medical Treatment of Children, Ireland) Act placed this duty on county and county borough councils in what is now the Free State. Since then there has been much activity in some centres. In Dublin the general and special hospitals are utilised for the treatment of eyes, ears, and throat.

In Dublin two school medical officers and two school nurses were appointed in 1928. Voluntary hospitals are paid 30s. for each operation on tonsils and adenoids. In Cork a scheme has been working for four years, a school medical officer supervising the pupils at 39 schools, and in this borough (population, 78,500) considerable treatment has been effected.

In Northern Ireland there are schemes for the medical inspection and treatment of school children in all except two counties.

In Belfast much more has been done, for information concerning which I am indebted to Dr. T. F. S. Fulton, the school medical officer, who for seven years has carried on admirable work with an inadequate staff. As in other parts of Ireland, the educational, and to some extent public health, work is hampered by religious jealousies. In Belfast, in 1924–25, of the total 64,407 pupils, 45·1 per cent. were

Presbyterians, etc., 31·1 per cent. were Church of Ireland (Protestant Episcopal), and 23·8 per cent. Roman Catholic. Large sums are being spent on new schools, which are badly needed; and meanwhile medical activities remain somewhat cramped. There is a large amount of unemployment in Belfast.

Owing to the inadequate school accommodation, children under 6 are at present not admitted, and defective children under this age fail to be discovered. Dr. Fulton has three assistant school medical officers, with four other part-time doctors doing special work. He finds this staff inadequate for full development of the work. There are 14 school nurses, three of them employed on clinic work.

At first, Dr. Fulton informed me, there was much antagonism to the school medical work, but this was due largely to ignorance of the procedure. As elsewhere, it has been found that very little treatment is carried out by the school medical service which would otherwise fall to private medical practitioners. This is true especially of the minor ailment clinics which meet three times weekly. Formerly a small charge was made, but this has ceased, as it was found that such cases were not treated elsewhere.

One specialist is appointed who does both the eye work and the cases needing operations on tonsils and adenoids among school children. The parents are first invited to secure private treatment, but this is seldom obtained. Some cases go to voluntary hospitals, but the officials of the local hospital, the Royal Victoria Hospital—like the officials of the corresponding Royal Infirmary in Edinburgh—have requested the school medical service to undertake their tonsil and adenoid cases.

When the school medical work began, a deputation from the teaching hospitals waited on the Education Committee, proposing to do this work on a *per capita* basis. Experience proved that it was difficult to obtain from the junior staff of a voluntary hospital records useful for public work; and now the entire transfer of this work to official clinics has been urged by the voluntary hospitals themselves.

A charge of 5s. is made to parents by the Education Committee for each operation on adenoids and tonsils, and of 3s. 6d. for adenoids alone. This includes two nights in a bed at the clinic. Often the charge is remitted. No charge is made for testing refractions, but 7s., the cost of spectacles, is charged, smaller sums being accepted in many cases.

Although there is little or no friction with private practitioners, friction sometimes arises with dispensary doctors. In Belfast these doctors have too many patients to attend, and they sometimes resent the sending of patients to them by the school doctors, thus giving them additional work without added salary. The cases thus referred are those in which the school examination has shown that continuous medical care is needed. The Guardians of the Poor have also asked the Education Committee to pay for the expense of operating on adenoids in school children, who have been referred to the former for treatment as "poor persons". This has been refused.

Evidently there is need for co-ordination, and some measure of unification of all medical services carried out at the public expense.

Dr. Fulton's experience is that school medical work has materially increased the practice of private medical practitioners. It has doubtless also increased the work of dispensaries and hospitals. These results of experience, I believe, hold generally true in different countries.

TUBERCULOSIS WORK

The death-rate from tuberculosis is somewhat high in Ireland, and although much valuable anti-tuberculosis work has been done, it is only partial in its distribution and extent. Unfortunately tuberculosis is only notifiable when tubercle bacilli have been discovered. Only a few counties are without specially trained tuberculosis medical officers. In the Free State there are 21 central tuberculosis dispensaries, with 142 branch dispensaries; and 126 institutions are approved for the treatment of tuberculosis. Altogether 2,190 beds are specially reserved for tuberculosis, and 5,757 beds are stated to be available as required. In 1927–28 the total central disbursement in aid of anti-tuberculosis work was £41,276.

In Northern Ireland the death-rate from tuberculosis in 1928 was 1·37, as compared with 1·41 in the Free State. Much anti-tuberculosis work is being carried on, there being special schemes for this purpose in all areas except the county borough of Londonderry. The Central Government contributed about £27,000 last year towards the cost of these schemes in Northern Ireland. The work carried on by Dr. A. Trimble, the chief tuberculosis officer, and by the five assistant medical officers in this department of the municipal service of Belfast, appeared to me of high quality. In 1928, at the tuberculosis institutions, 1,816 new patients were examined, and 585 contacts, while 32,869 reattendances were made by old patients. Patients are only treated when sent by a private practitioner or dispensary doctor. Unfortunately some doctors only send patients when they can no longer pay fees, and in other instances patients are sent who have been under treatment for months, but no physical examination or examination of sputum has been made. As there has been hitherto no medical benefit in the Sickness Insurance Act as applied to Ireland, arrangements are made with private practitioners for the notification and the domiciliary treatment of cases of tuberculosis, and the municipality pays practitioners for this work.

In 1928 the number of tuberculous patients being treated for tuberculosis under the official scheme in Belfast were:—

At the Institutes..	1,875
Under domiciliary treatment	2,702
In sanatorium and hospital	281
In open-air schools	114
	4,972

A table is given in Dr. Trimble's Report showing that of 936 patients with tuberculosis living at home only 160 occupied a separate bedroom, while of the same total only

243 occupied a separate bed. Evidently greatly extended work is needed.

Venereal Diseases

In Northern Ireland, in 1928, £6,463 were disbursed by the Central Government for the expense of approved expenditure (75 per cent. of the total expenditure) by local authorities on the treatment of venereal diseases. Five thousand eight hundred and ten patients presented themselves for treatment, of whom 2,318 were not suffering from venereal disease.

In Belfast there is a fully organised scheme, similar to English schemes. In the Free State similar conditions hold good. There are four treatment centres in the Free State, two of which are in Dublin. Central disbursements of £6,414 were made in 1928.

Evidently these schemes are only partially developed.

Sickness Insurance in Ireland

The National Insurance Act, 1911, for unemployment and sickness applied to Ireland as well as to Great Britain; but in view of its existent system of dispensary, including domiciliary medical care for "poor persons", medical benefit was excluded, and the weekly payments for employers and employed were made lower than those in Great Britain in view of this omission. From January 1930 local insurance committees were abolished, the administration of medical benefit then becoming centralised.

Medical certification being an indispensable safeguard for receipt of monetary sickness benefits, arrangements had to be made for this. Evidently a system of direct payment for each medical certificate of (*a*) inability to work, (*b*) resumption of ability to work, with (*c*) intermediate weekly certificates of continued inability would tend to excessive claims, and a system of payment for certification was devised in virtue of which a lump sum was allotted for medical certification, and the payments for each doctor were paid on a basis proportional to his work. In the Free State the

insured population is about 400,000, out of its total population of 3 millions; and the sum available for certification
is £23,000, which is found to work out at about 4½d.
(9 cents) for each certificate given by the 1,941 doctors who
have agreed with the Insurance Commissioners for the
Free State to issue certificates.

In Northern Ireland certification prior to 1930 has been
paid for on a similar scale.

Up to the end of 1923 the cost of medical certification was
defrayed out of State Funds, but from that date it was
decided that a part of the cost should come out of the
insurance funds, and in the Free State some reduction in
the pool out of which doctors were paid was negotiated
with representatives of the Irish medical profession.

In Northern Ireland conditions are similar; but legislation passed by its Government in 1930 provides for a
supplementary medical benefit from July 1930 onwards,
separate payment for certification then ceasing. This has not
been approved for the Free State; and although a majority
of the Committee on Health Insurance and Medical Services,
which reported in February 1927 to the Minister of Finance
of the Free State, favour similar supplementary medical
benefit, reasons to the contrary are given by minority
members of the committee, and no action has yet been
taken. This difficult point is discussed on a later page.

Separate certification of sickness by doctors who are
not—otherwise than through certification—related to the
Insurance Commissioners of the Free State or of Northern
Ireland is stated to have been associated with a considerably
heavier experience of sickness among the insured than in
Great Britain.

In both Ireland and Great Britain there has been much
increase of certified sickness. In the Free State the costs
of benefits and of administration for the insured were
£479,949 in 1923 and £712,968 in 1927. A part of the
increase is explicable by the giving of some additional
benefits in recent years; but other reasons exist. It has been
urged that emigration of the more healthy; that the lowered

health following war and civil war; and that lax certification explain the result. It is difficult to form a valid conclusion as to the relative weight of these and other possible factors. Undoubtedly lax medical certification occurs on a large scale both in Great Britain and Ireland; but if, as is stated, recent increases are heavier in Ireland than in Great Britain, it would appear likely that this laxness is more common in Ireland than in Scotland and England.

As in Great Britain, medical referees have been appointed to consult with and to check the certificates of the certifying doctors, but too recently to be able to say with what benefit.

Dr. Wm. J. Maguire, Medical Commissioner of the National (Health) Insurance Commission for the Free State, gave me valuable information, much of which is incorporated in these pages; though all expressions of opinion are my own. The same remark applies to Dr. Stephenson, to whom I am very specially indebted.

THE DISPENSARY SYSTEM OF IRELAND

This is part of the Irish organisation for poor-law relief, though more elastic in its distribution than the material relief given by boards of guardians. When the Royal Commission on the Poor-Law reported on Ireland in 1909 (Cd. 4630) there were 159 unions in Ireland divided into 740 dispensary districts, containing 1,208 dispensaries or dispensary stations. The number of officers engaged in the dispensary service in 1907 were:—

> 807 Medical officers,
> 48 Compounders of medicines,
> 640 Midwives;

and in that year 654,877 new cases were attended, of whom 169,376 were visited in their own homes. The salaries of dispensary officers amounted to £96,529 (averaging about £118 for each medical officer), with £15,320 for payment of substitutes, and £18,109 for medicines and appliances. In that year the estimated population of Ireland was 4,388,451.

In the year 1927-28, in the Free State, 648,856 new cases were attended by the dispensary service, 126,289 of these at patients' homes; and the dispensary service in the Free State comprised 634 medical officers, 41 compounders of medicine, and 656 midwives. The total amount expended was £298,650, of which £219,597 was paid in salaries to the three classes of officers.

In Northern Ireland, in the year 1928-29, the dispensary officers attended 182,917 new cases, 56,869 of these at the patients' own homes. The amount disbursed in medical officers' salaries in Northern Ireland was £41,861, on an average £248 for each officer per annum.

Some of the conditions of medical aid under the dispensary system may be gathered from the following notes of interviews with two dispensary medical officers in the Free State and two in Northern Ireland. To the four medical officers interviewed I am much indebted; and my conferences with them gave me a vivid impression of the valuable work they are doing for "poor persons", in circumstances in which it is difficult to think that any other machinery would be more or equally effective.

1. Dr. O'Connor is the dispensary medical officer for the dispensary district of Colbridge, about 11 miles distant from Dublin. It is rural in character, its population of 4-5,000 being scattered over a wide area. More than half this population receive free medical attendance, for which Dr. O'Connor receives a salary of from £200 to £280 a year. In addition, he receives small payments for giving insurance certificates, and, like other dispensary officers, he acts as local M.O.H. under the county M.O.H. for a salary of £10-£20. His duties as M.O.H. are almost nominal, but it is evident that under improved conditions his services may become valuable in preventive medicine. All the labourers in the district are insured, and all when sick are dispensary patients outside the national insurance scheme. Sometimes small farmers are also dispensary patients. The doctor does his own dispensing, drugs, etc., being supplied by the county council.

Permits to obtain dispensary attendance are given by the

local relieving officer (called the "home assistance officer", who receives a salary of £85–£100 a year), or by the local elected member of the county council, or by one of a number of "wardens" who are unpaid, and who have been chosen by the county council for this local service. The doctor seldom finds it needful to protest against the nominations for medical aid, dispensary or domiciliary, made from these several quarters. Dr. O'Connor has no evidence that he loses private practice through the elasticity of dispensary recommendations. The fact is that the scope for private practice is very limited. Nor has Dr. O'Connor found cause for friction in the examination of school children by the very progressive Kildare County M.O.H., Dr. Harbison, followed in many cases by treatment in hospital or elsewhere. The county tuberculosis officers' activities are welcomed.

Dr. O'Connor has been a dispensary doctor in two districts altogether for fifty years, and is still active and competent; and were his work typical of that for the whole of Ireland, one would find it difficult to suggest improvement, except as regards institutional treatment. The former Poor House has been renamed "District Hospital". There is also a county hospital, and a county home for the aged and defective.

There is need here and elsewhere for ensuring surgical competence in the staff of these hospitals. Colbridge being near Dublin, urgent cases can be sent to its hospitals.

The dispensary doctor has power to send for a consultant in special cases, including operative midwifery, and to pay a fee of two guineas. The dispensary midwife receives a salary of about £60, and may have 30–35 gratuitous confinements in a year, and perhaps eight private cases. Both she and the doctor are allowed to engage in private practice.

There is a district nurse supported by a voluntary organisation, with the aid of grants for work done under child welfare and tuberculosis schemes. Some patients contribute to the cost of the nurse.

2. Dr. Paul Blake is the dispensary doctor of the district

of Clane and Kinahoe, in the county of Kildare. The district has a population of about 2,000, and half of them are dispensary patients. Dr. Blake receives a salary of £300 (including payment for dispensing), and of £15 as local M.O.H. He receives £52 for travelling expenses. He has been a dispensary doctor for 13 years. The nearest doctor to him is six miles distant; there is no competition for the scanty private practice which is obtained. There is a midwife in the district, who has 20 to 30 dispensary confinements and 4 or 5 private confinements in the year. Many patients travel to Dublin for special consultations. There is no friction with the doctors engaged in public health medical work.

Dr. Blake's work as M.O.H. appears to be limited to reporting to the county M.O.H. an occasional nuisance or overcrowding.

I conferred with Dr. Harbison, the whole-time county M.O.H. of Kildare, in which the above dispensary districts are situate. He is a whole-time public health official, and is rapidly improving the health administration of this county. His work has been greatly helped by a five-year graduated grant from the Rockefeller Foundation. Largely through the impetus of this it appears likely that a complete county administration will be established. There are 19 district dispensary medical officers in the county of Kildare. Altogether these serve a population of 58,000 scattered over an area of 418,000 acres. There is one well-organised county hospital.

Dr. Harbison has three whole-time medical officers in his department. One acts as assistant M.O.H., one is school medical inspector, and one is engaged in tuberculosis work. In addition, there are two whole-time public health school nurses; and six district nurses of the Local Nursing Association follow up school children and tuberculous patients for after-care. There is one whole-time sanitary inspector, and a number of part-time sanitary inspectors, who will be replaced by a whole-time officer.

3. Dr. Burns is dispensary doctor for one of the 16 dispensary districts of Belfast. Some dispensary doctors acts also

for neighbouring rural areas. There are about 450 medical practitioners in Belfast, including consultants. There are 170 dispensary doctors for Northern Ireland, and 550 doctors who certify for sickness insurance under the Insurance Act. The number insured in Northern Ireland is 335,000 (total population, 1¼ million).

Dr. Burns receives a salary of £225. He attends at his dispensary each week-day at 10–12, whether few or many patients. On some mornings he may see 150 patients; probably the average is 75. His dispensary visiting list averages 15–20. The recommendations for treatment are made as in the Free State. Sometimes it has been found necessary to ask the relieving officer to cancel a recommendation for free treatment.

In an industrial area such as Belfast there is some evidence of the feeling of poor-law "taint," and even very poor patients will sometimes somehow pay for an additional private doctor. Many of them also pay to a contributory scheme for hospital treatment in a general hospital.

4. Dr. J. Carson Longbridge is dispensary doctor for Belfast R.4, an entirely rural area, of some eight by four miles. The arrangements are somewhat similar to those elsewhere. He has not experienced much aversion to medical attendance from the dispensary, and this appears to be generally true for rural areas. Hospital treatment is given in the Belfast Infirmary (poor-law) and can be obtained also at general hospitals.

HISTORY OF THE DISPENSARY SYSTEM

Although contained within the poor-law, the dispensary from its beginning pursued a partially independent existence.

In 1838 Ireland was divided into 130 poor-law unions, this number being increased to 163 in 1850. The present area of the Saorstat comprises 131 unions. The feature distinguishing Irish from English poor-law administration has been the fact that out-door, i.e. home relief, financial, and medical, in Ireland has been given rather than institutional relief in a much higher proportion of the total cases of destitution. This has been so, although relief of the able-bodied is provided only in the workhouse.

The Poor Relief (Ireland) Act, 1851, better known as the Medical Charities Act, laid the foundation of the poor-law medical service. Under this Act each union was sub-divided into dispensary districts, a medical officer being appointed for each, who was required to give gratuitous medical advice, treatment, and medicines to "poor persons" resident in the dispensary district. The Act, while conferring this right on the poor, did not define the term "the poor", but evidently it was intended to be and was accepted as being of wider interpretation than "the destitute," for whose condition material relief can be given. Furthermore, medical relief, unlike material, did not disfranchise the recipient. Since 1918 disfranchisement for any form of relief has been removed.

In an official report on "Poor Law, etc., Relief in Ireland," 1909, by the Medical Commissioner of the then Irish Local Government Board (Dr., now Sir T. J. Stafford), appear the following remarks which throw light on the need for a very liberal view of the need for medical aid:—

It will hardly be disputed that we may include among the grades of persons who properly come within the Medical Charities system all the agricultural labourers, inasmuch as their wages, which average about 10s. a week, are not sufficient to enable them to buy the necessary food, clothing, and fuel for themselves and their families, pay house rent, and at the same time make provision for medical attendance. The unskilled labourers in the towns and cities are also unable to maintain themselves and their families and pay the doctor out of their wages. Most artisans and their families, domestic and indoor servants, small farmers, and petty tradesmen may also possibly be included.

So impressed was Sir Thomas Stafford with the difficulties of the situation that he concluded:—

The only method I can see for meeting the extreme circumstances of the poorer unions, and at the same time bringing the dispensary Medical Service in general up to a high standard of efficiency, and keeping it in that state, is to convert it into a National Service.

This conclusion has been endorsed by other commissioners who have made inquiries into the circumstances of Ireland. Thus, although the economic condition of Ireland has improved since the last two quotations were written, the trend of the "Final Report of the Committee on Health Insurance and Medical Services", presented to the Free State Government in 1927, is in the same direction. The committee's report refers to a previous sub-committee's report, in which was adumbrated a scheme for "a State Medical Service following on the lines of the recommendations of the Irish Public Health Council of 1920". The report then states that the committee regard this as "the ideal solution of the problems" as to the medical services of the State; and continues that it was only because of being "disappointed in the expectations of a medical service of national scope" embracing both the insured and "poor persons," that the committee had turned to an alternative proposal for providing medical treatment for insured persons, viz., on the lines of a "panel" system, as in Great Britain. It should be added that the committee thus reporting was one of national distinction; including among its members Dr. Maguire, the Medical Commissioner on Insurance, and Dr. Stephenson, the Medical Adviser of the Board of Local Government and Health. The last-named, however, adhered to the "ideal" scheme, regarding the institution of "medical benefit (under the Insurance Act) as unnecessary and superfluous".[1] This view, with which, in the circumstances of Ireland, I agree, is rendered the more feasible by:—

REFORMS IN THE DISPENSARY SYSTEM IN THE FREE STATE

These may now be indicated.

1. The chief reform is the reformed method of appointment rendered statutory by the Local Authorities (Officers and Employees) Act, 1926. Under this Act the former power of boards of guardians to appoint their own medical

[1] At the annual meeting of the Approved Societies' Association of the Free State, held in December 1929, a resolution was passed expressing the view that "a National Medical Service should be instituted in the Free State".

officers is removed, and the same rule applies to boards of health, which have now replaced these boards. Boards of health may promote officers already in their employment, but new officers can only be appointed on the recommendation of the Local Appointment Commissioners, who set up selection boards for the purpose. Each candidate must have satisfied the Commissioners either by examination or otherwise that he possesses the necessary qualifications for his office. Thus medical officers and surgeons of county hospitals are required to have had experience which includes the performance of major operations, and a medical officer of health must possess a diploma in public health.

This removal from small local and county authorities of the power to give local medical appointments has rendered impossible the jobbery and incompetence in choice of the past. If the system is maintained in its integrity, the future of the dispensary service is bright.

2. The salaries of dispensary officers have been fixed in accordance with a scale adopted by the Department of Local Government and Health, and accepted by the associations of the medical profession.

3. Arrangements have been made for independent payment of deputies, to allow of holidays and when sick leave is required.

4. Facilities have been arranged for providing postgraduate instruction to dispensary medical officers.

5. The dispensary medical officer is relieved from attendance at the now non-existent local committee. He is supervised by the medical inspectors of the central authority and by the board of health. Local authorities can promote and may suspend a medical officer but cannot dismiss him.

6. The dispensary medical officer has become pensionable on the civil service scale, *plus* added years for good service.

The objections to the dispensary system are based chiefly on its association with the poor-law, which for the Irish has had many sinister associations. These objections, now chiefly sentimental, are most felt in towns. In rural areas gratuitous medical attendance has become an accepted practice; and it has undoubtedly been the means of greatly reducing the amount of human suffering in Ireland.

It doubtless is sometimes perfunctorily carried out by individual medical officers who have little impetus in the hope of paying practice to improve their standards of work. The same danger exists wherever there is a population of poor persons without a large admixture of paying patients. It exists under the insurance panel medical system in England in some areas. Such conditions call for improvements in the conditions of service, as well as for a higher conscience in medical work; they do not show the need to abolish an established service, which is doing beneficent work in circumstances of great difficulty.

It should be added that there is great need in many areas for improved dispensary buildings, and that many of the poor-law infirmaries or hospitals are radically unsatisfactory structurally, and their staffing sometimes even more so. Reform, retarded by financial stringency, is occurring, and especially action is being taken to improve county hospitals, and to link these up with the large general hospitals attached to the medical schools of the Free State. In Northern Ireland a considerable number of poor-law infirmaries are being reconstructed.

RELATION BETWEEN DISPENSARY AND INSURANCE WORK

At this point we reach the burning question as to whether a medical as well as the present sickness benefit should be included in national sickness insurance. Northern Ireland has already taken this step. I interviewed Major Connoch, the Permanent Secretary of the Ministry of Labour; also Major Harris, the Permanent Secretary of the Ministry of Home Affairs (including Health), and Dr. Patrick, the Chief Medical Officer of this Department, from whom I received much courtesy. In conversation with these and many others It was clear that this action is not unanimously approved. it is perceived that the "panel" doctors to be appointed by free choice of patients will be doing much work which has hitherto been done at the expense of the State by the dispensary doctors, while the wives and families of the insured will need still to be treated gratuitously by the dispensary doctor. It is likely that 75 per cent. of the insured persons in Ireland are dispensary patients. There is the further point that in urban centres dispensary doctors who admit insured persons on their "panels" are likely to receive an excessive number of the more sickly section of the insured, and thus will be handicapped as compared with panel doctors who are not also dispensary doctors.

In the negotiations that have occurred it has been pointed out that dispensary doctors will be relieved of insured patients, while their salaries cannot be reduced, and it has been suggested that this being so, dispensary doctors should have a smaller capitation allowance for each insured person on their panel than other doctors receive, and this has been arranged, a reduced annual capitation of 7s. 6d. (about $1.80) being paid to dispensary doctors for each insured person on their list. There will be no reduction in the existing salaries of dispensary doctors.

These points illustrate the difficulties of the situation. My own view is that the institution of a medical benefit in the circumstances of Northern Ireland is a mistake, and would be so if extended to the Free State.

For (1) 75 per cent. of the insured are already being treated under a system which potentially and probably actually is as satisfactory for the patients as "panel"practice. It is better in some important particulars, because the patient when this is needed has the right—

> (a) to institutional treatment, and
> (b) to the services of a consultant.

(2) The panel system will give, as in England, an unfortunate separation between the medical care of the insured person and of his dependents, at least so far as conditions of medical service are concerned.

The ideal method would doubtless be to take the dispensary service entirely out of the poor-law, and the hospitals associated with it likewise. With the help of such improvements in this service as are within practicable reach, there could then be furnished a medical service for all who were eligible for sickness insurance, or are below this status. It need not be a free service, but might be made, except for the destitute, a contributory service on the lines which have been successful by voluntary arrangement in providing general and special hospital treatment in so many towns in the British Isles.

Such a dispensary service with improved dispensary buildings would have in each area a dispensary or health centre, at which poor persons and the insured would consult with their respective doctors; and at which could be assembled the municipal and county work of maternity and child welfare centres, of tuberculosis clinics or institutes, and school clinics. The bringing of these varied activities under one roof and under one county or municipal management would give the further important advantage that the dispensary and panel doctor could forthwith have the advantage of consultations with doctors specially skilled in ophthalmic, dental, ear and throat, and other diseases.

MATERNITY WORK IN IRELAND

As already stated, there is an official midwife in most dispensary areas throughout Ireland, and midwives are now required to possess the same qualifications as midwives in England. The midwife can call for the services of the dispensary doctor when required, and the latter is authorised to send for a further consultant when needed.

DEATH-RATES PER 1,000 BIRTHS

Year	From Puerperal Sepsis	From Accidents ot Pregnancy and Childbirth
1918–27	1·70	3·17
1928	1·74	3·19

The above figures for the Free State are given, and although in view of possible ambiguities of classification their significance is not quite certain, it would appear that mortality in childbirth is high in Ireland.

There does not appear to be competition between midwives and doctors in most areas. Midwives as a rule have smaller areas than doctors; their salaries are from £52–£72 per annum.

The whole country is covered by this official midwifery service, though in some areas unregistered midwives, so-called "handy women", are still employed, occasionally private doctors "covering", i.e., abetting this illegal work. In the inaccessible parts of Western Ireland, where the official midwife is not within reach, the Lady Dudley Nurses (affiliated to the Queen's Nurses) undertake midwifery work, by arrangement with the central authority.

During the last three years post-graduate courses have been arranged at the Rotunda Hospital for midwives, and midwives are given leave of absence, with allowances for travelling and maintenance, and a substitute is provided.

I visited this hospital, and its working was explained by Dr. Bethel Solomons, the Master. It is perhaps the most famous lying-in hospital in the world, and admirable training is given in it to midwives, medical students, and doctors (post-graduate). It has also a gynæcological department, and special beds for sick children. Although I cannot spare space to describe its work, I was deeply impressed with the value of this charity.

From this institution in 1928–29, 1,805 births were attended in the mothers' homes, and 2,034 in the institution, while the births registered in the city of Dublin were less than 4,000. As there are two other maternity hospitals in Dublin, it would appear, even after allowing for rural patients, that but few women can be attended by doctors in the ordinary course of family practice.

Patients admitted to the hospital are expected to pay two guineas weekly, but no patients are refused. Country patients are admitted free on production of an official order from the dispensary doctor, or the clerk of the rural district council. A charge of 5s. is made for the signing of each maternity certificate required to obtain the maternity benefit under the National Insurance Act. From this source last year £578 was obtained, and £3,505 was obtained from in-patients. Some money is earned from pupils' fees, and the Dublin Corporation and Government contribute together £100. The remaining total ordinary expenditure of £10,805 in 1928–29 was derived mainly from invested funds and from voluntary contributions.

Throughout rural Ireland it is evident that little mid-wifery practice is in the hands of general medical practitioners, though they are called for in difficult cases.

Nursing Arrangements

These call for only a short notice. The British organisation of the Queen's Nurses continues and flourishes under separate Irish management. All these nurses, numbering 207 for the whole of Ireland, are fully trained. There are two training-halls for nurses in Dublin—one Catholic, one Protestant. Each nurse, after three years' training as a nurse and after having obtained the qualifying certificate of the Midwives Board, receives six additional months' training in district visiting, including a month's attendance at an Infants' Clinic in Dublin. In the greater part of Ireland the Queen's Nurses do no midwifery (see also p. 549). The nurse in rare instances acts for two or three dispensary districts. She does bedside nursing, and, in addition, acts as health visitor, school nurse, and visitor for tuberculous cases.

Miss Kavanagh, who, in the absence of the Superintendent of the Queen's Nurses, gave me valuable information, described the special difficulties in Western Ireland, and particularly in Connemara, where the difficulties resemble those of the Highlands and Islands of Scotland, but without the special governmental aid which has been given in the latter instance.

Miss Kavanagh stressed the importance of the public

health nurse doing actual nursing. Parents are suspicious, but welcome aid in sickness; and this forms the best introduction for subsequent advice and guidance on health.

The extent to which the nursing needs of Ireland still need to be met may be gathered from the following figures quoted by Miss Kavanagh:—

	Number of Queen's Nurses
Free State (Population,[1] 2,949,000)	207
Scotland (Population,[1] 4,893,000)	800
England and Wales (Population,[1] 39,482,000) ..	8,000

[1] In 1928.

SUBJECT INDEX

INDEX OF PROPER NAMES